Fundamental Statistical Methods for Analysis of Alzheimer's and Other Neurodegenerative Diseases

T0122843

Fundamental Statistical Methods for Analysis of Alzheimer's and Other Neurodegenerative Diseases

Katherine E. Irimata
Brittany N. Dugger
Jeffrey R. Wilson

Foreword by Marwan Sabbagh

Johns Hopkins University Press
Baltimore

Katherine E. Irimata is serving in her personal capacity. The work for this book was initiated and conducted when she was a student at Arizona State University. The views expressed are those of the authors and do not necessarily represent the views of the National Center for Health Statistics, the Centers for Disease Control and Prevention, or the US government.

Datasets referenced in this book and available through https://www.public.asu .edu/~jeffreyw/ are for educational use only. These are a limited excerpt from the National Alzheimer's Coordinating Center (NACC) database. Further distribution or reproduction of these data, research analysis for publication, or any other purpose beyond the specific examples provided in *Fundamental Statistical Methods for Analysis of Alzheimer's and Other Neurodegenerative Diseases* are strictly prohibited. Persons wishing to access the NACC database for scientific research must visit the NACC website, www.alz.washington.edu, to apply for access.

© 2020 Johns Hopkins University Press
All rights reserved. Published 2020
Printed in the United States of America on acid-free paper
9 8 7 6 5 4 3 2 1

Johns Hopkins University Press
2715 North Charles Street
Baltimore, Maryland 21218-4363
www.press.jhu.edu

Library of Congress Cataloging-in-Publication Data
Names: Irimata, Katherine E., 1990–author. | Dugger, Brittany N. (Brittany Nicole),
    1982– author. | Wilson, Jeffrey (Jeffrey R.), 1953– author.
Title: Fundamental statistical methods for analysis of Alzheimer's and other neuro-
    degenerative diseases / Katherine E. Irimata, PhD, Brittany N. Dugger, PhD,
    Jeffrey R. Wilson, PhD. Foreword by Marwan Sabbagh, MD.
Description: Baltimore, Maryland : Johns Hopkins University Press, 2020. | Includes
    bibliographical references and index.
Identifiers: LCCN 2019020304 | ISBN 9781421436715 (paperback : alk. paper) |
    ISBN 9781421436722 (electronic) | ISBN 142143671X (paperback : alk. paper) |
    ISBN 1421436728 (electronic)
Subjects: MESH: Statistics as Topic | Biometry | Alzheimer Disease | Neuro-
    degenerative Diseases
Classification: LCC RC523 | NLM WA 950 | DDC 616.8/31100727—dc23
LC record available at https://lccn.loc.gov/2019020304

A catalog record for this book is available from the British Library.

Special discounts are available for bulk purchases of this book. For more information, please contact Special Sales at specialsales@press.jhu.edu.

Johns Hopkins University Press uses environmentally friendly book materials, including recycled text paper that is composed of at least 30 percent post-consumer waste, whenever possible.

To Kyle.   KEI

To my biostatistics students, present and past.   JRW

To the numerous persons who are working to alleviate the burdens of these devastating diseases, to the patients, and especially to the caregivers who face the overwhelming challenges of everyday life. We hope this book will allow more persons to aid in analyzing data and have constructive dialogues with statisticians to unlock the secrets of these diseases.   BND

Contents

Foreword

This book is a timely and important contribution to the field of statistics and Alzheimer's disease (AD) research. Drs. Irimata, Dugger, and Wilson do a deep dive into the statistical methodology behind clinical trial design for Alzheimer's disease studies.

The reader will spend time learning complex statistical principles, but I caution the reader to step back for a moment. While we are mired in p-values, these concepts have far-reaching consequences. We in clinical research live and die by statistics. Our decisions of outcomes, efficacy, treatment decisions, go / no go decisions, and drug development strategies are based on statistical plans. We value a priori data and eschew post hoc or secondary data. Our statistical analysis plans remain fluid, and we pain over sample sizes and power calculations.

The consequences are real. There has been no new drug approved to treat AD in the past 15 years. Many drugs have shown promise in phase II trials, only to fail in phase III because the phase II results cannot be recapitulated. Why might that be? There are many reasons, but fundamentally, we rely on the slope and trajectory of the placebo group. In many cases, the placebo group does not decline or change in the predicted or modeled manner. When that occurs, the delta between treatment and placebo becomes more difficult to demonstrate.

We use statistical plans to predict outcomes. The challenge is that we often have incomplete data to determine sample sizes and power calculations, which are derived in many cases from best estimates. When analyzing data, we look at intention to treat analyses, completers analyses, last observation carried forward, and mixed models, among other analyses.

Another challenge is that only a proportion of treated subjects respond to the treatment, and a proportion do not. In essence, the responder effect has to overcome the nonresponder effect. Ideally, we could determine responders in advance. Any drug to treat all patients is likely to have a diluted effect. Segmentation into different subtypes or novel outcome measures have been proposed and will be explored in the future.

In the meantime, mastery of statistical analysis is paramount to selecting the best analytical plan to analyze complex data.

Marwan Noel Sabbagh, MD, FAAN
Cleveland Clinic Lou Ruvo Center for Brain Health

Chapter 1

Introduction to Statistical Software and Alzheimer's Data

1.1 Introduction

This book is designed to serve as a statistical guide for data analysts, including graduate students, academic and industry scientists, and researchers who focus on Alzheimer's disease and related disorders. We present statistical techniques specific to addressing questions regarding dementia data analysis. Each chapter is motivated by a question or example that may be encountered in the evaluation of Alzheimer's disease and related disorders data. In addition, we present syntax and partial outputs obtained from four major statistical software programs (SAS, R, SPSS, and Stata) to conduct the analyses discussed in this book.

The book begins with introductory statistical techniques and then builds up to more complex and less known models for dementia data analysis. These methods are available in most statistical software. In this chapter, we provide an introduction with some basic statistical definitions as well as an overview of software programs. We also describe databases containing information on neurodegenerative diseases and the variables of interest examined in this book. Prior to starting any statistical analyses, one should understand the background of the study, including the population being investigated, the time period of the study, and the data collection methods. When utilizing any dataset, one must understand the design of the study. It is highly recommended to work with personnel of the particular study as they understand the caveats and limitations of the data.

1.2 Statistical Definitions

We define some terms central to the discipline of statistics.

WHAT IS STATISTICS?

Statistics is an interdisciplinary field focused on the study and development of methods to collect, display, test, model, analyze, and interpret data. It transcends almost every discipline. Statistics is used to measure and test differences between groups and to quantify the impact of interventions. It is used in modeling to understand associations between factors and randomness within the data. Statistics as a tool is the cornerstone of sampling and surveys and has become increasingly popular in big data analytics.

WHAT IS A PROBABILITY DISTRIBUTION?

A probability distribution is a formula that describes the possible values of a random variable and provides the probability of occurrence. Common distributions discussed in statistics include the normal, binomial, and Poisson distributions. For example, in studying a select group of participants (ranging from normal to demented), we notice that their cognitive scores, measured by the Mini-Mental State Examination (MMSE), form a bell-shaped curve (most observations lie in the center, and there are fewer observations as we move away from the center) where the mean, median, and mode of the distribution of MMSE scores coincide. The bell-shaped curve is the defining feature of the normal distribution; thus we may assume the MMSE score is normally distributed. Alternatively, consider the evaluation of whether a person has a certain allele, such as the APOE4 allele. We notice there are only two possible outcomes (APOE4 or no APOE4), and the outcomes are believed to be independent. Thus we assume the outcome of interest (whether or not an individual has the allele) follows a Bernoulli trial, and the sum of these trials follows a binomial distribution. In a study counting the number of adverse events in a defined interval of time, such as the number of cardiovascular events over the course of 10 years, we may utilize the Poisson distribution. We give a brief introduction to statistical distributions throughout the book and show how they are utilized through examples. Further background on statistical distributions can be found in Collett (2003) and Daniel and Cross (2013).

WHAT IS THE POPULATION?

The population describes the entire group of interest that we are studying. For example, if we are interested in studying the average age of onset for Alzheimer's disease (AD) in males, the population is all males with AD across the world. Since it is often not feasible to collect information from the entire population, we collect samples.

WHAT IS A SAMPLE?

A sample is a subset of the population of interest that is studied to make inferences about the whole population. We sample 1,000 men with AD and collect information to study the average age of onset in the population. The sample provides statistics, while the population provides parameters. One always should be aware of how representative their sample is compared to the entire population. There are certain biases associated with sampling, and these biases can affect the outcome, such as clinic versus community recruitment, or sampling persons in Hawaii versus Iowa. It is important to determine how generalizable the results will be to the entire population.

WHAT IS A PARAMETER?

A parameter is a value obtained based on the population of values. In the study of the age of onset of AD, the true mean age of onset among all men is the parameter value. We usually refer to the population mean as μ. In most cases, we do not know the value of the parameter, since it is usually not possible to obtain this information from every person in the population.

WHAT IS A STATISTIC?

A statistic is a value of the measurement based on the sample values. Of the sample of 1,000 men, we calculate the mean age of onset. This sample mean is a statistic, denoted as $\bar{x}$. The sample mean, among other things, is used to obtain statistical test values and evaluate statistical hypotheses.

WHAT IS A HYPOTHESIS?

A hypothesis is a research statement that is developed on the basis of some limited information or reasoning. In statistics, we often start with hypotheses as the basis for statistical tests. Suppose we wish to research whether the average age of onset of AD in males is greater than 60 years (our research hypothesis). From a sample of males with AD, we can obtain an estimate of the average age of onset (the statistic) and evaluate this hypothesis using statistical testing. The hypothesis helps frame the statistical model used on the basis of the type of outcome variable. For example, if our outcome variable is the presence/absence of AD, a binary outcome, we select statistical models appropriate for binary responses.

WHAT IS A CONFIDENCE INTERVAL?

A confidence interval is a range of values that we believe contain the parameter value (the population value). For example, after conducting our study, we believe the true mean age of onset of AD in males lies between 62 years and 66 years (having a confidence interval of width 4 and margin of error 2).

WHAT IS A LIKELIHOOD?

The likelihood is a function of model parameters given the data. The likelihood is used to estimate parameters in statistical models when we know the distribution of the responses. The likelihood function and the probability function share the same form, but what is considered known in one function is given in another, and vice versa.

WHAT IS MAXIMUM LIKELIHOOD?

Once we have the distribution, we have the likelihood. It is used to evaluate the likelihood of obtaining a certain value of the parameter given the data collected. One always wants to maximize one's chances that the sample estimates are representative of the population parameters.

1.3 Statistical Computing in SAS, R, SPSS, and Stata

In this book we make use of four statistical software programs, SAS, R, SPSS, and Stata. We provide the steps for each program to obtain the information to analyze the data. The syntax and relevant output are reported in each chapter. While the four programs can often be used to perform the same analyses, the notation and format in the output vary for each software. We encourage you to choose a program and familiarize yourself with it. We make mention of some resources for each software package in this section.

1.3.1 SAS Programming

WHAT IS SAS?

SAS is a software package used for statistics, analytics, and data management that was developed in the 1960s. It is popular with universities and companies around the world. SAS software is available on PC and Linux systems.

HOW DOES SAS PROGRAMMING WORK?

SAS programming in Base SAS is based on two primary functions, the DATA step and procedures. The DATA step is used to create, read, and prepare SAS datasets. SAS procedures (PROCs) are used to perform specific processes or statistical analyses.

There are some basic guidelines for writing syntax in SAS:

1. One can import different types of files into SAS using PROC IMPORT or the INFLIE statement in the DATA step.
2. Most syntax uses a DATA step or PROC (with the exception of setting up options, developing macros, etc.).
3. Every line of SAS syntax ends with a semicolon (;).
4. SAS data steps and procedures end with the keyword RUN or QUIT.
5. SAS syntax is not case-sensitive.

6. SAS syntax is engaged by selecting the lines to be processed and hitting the "Submit" button (a picture of a running man).

HOW ARE DATA READ INTO SAS?

If a user has a SAS dataset (.sas7bdat file) saved within a computer file, the data are accessed using a library. The library is used to reference SAS files saved in the folder (such as dataset.sas7bdat). A DATA step is used to read a data file into the working directory in SAS using the following syntax:

```
LIBNAME DTA "C:\USER\DOCUMENTS\DATA";
DATA WORKINGDATA;
     SET DTA.DATASET;
RUN;
```

Alternatively, if a user has a different file type to import, PROC IMPORT is often utilized. We consider importing an XLS file:

```
PROC IMPORT DATAFILE="C:\USER\DOCUMENTS\DATA\DATASET.XLS"
OUT=WORKINGDATA DBMS=XLS;
RUN;
```

WHAT ARE THE ADVANTAGES OF SAS?

1. SAS has the ability to handle and analyze large datasets.
2. The procedures and capabilities are rigorously tested before they are implemented in updated versions of SAS.
3. SAS provides excellent customer support to users.
4. The system is secure and is used to handle personally identifiable information.
5. The output is formatted and easy to read.
6. The log window helps users in debugging errors within the syntax.
7. There are many SAS resources to assist users in learning the SAS language (see "What Can a User Do to Learn SAS?").

WHAT ARE THE DISADVANTAGES OF SAS?

1. It is expensive to obtain a license for the SAS software package.
2. SAS may be slower to release new capabilities since it is not open source software.
3. SAS has less graphics flexibility compared to software packages such as R.
4. There is a steep curve to learning the SAS language.
5. Computing programs on SAS can require heavy computational power that may slow down a computer.

WHAT CAN A USER DO TO LEARN SAS?

SAS has many free online resources available. There are free e-learning courses on the SAS website (https://support.sas.com), and there are many online SAS support communities (https://communities .sas.com) where users can ask questions and get programming tips. SAS offers a version of their software called SAS University Edition, which is free to download and use for academic, noncommercial purposes. SAS's publishing program, SAS Press, publishes books covering many features and applications of SAS. A popular introductory SAS book is *The Little SAS Book*, by Lora Delwiche and Susan Slaughter. Each year SAS hosts the SAS Global Forum Conference, where SAS employees and users present on a variety of topics. The conference proceedings are published online and are a useful learning resource. In addition, the University of California, Los Angeles, Institute for Digital Research and Education (UCLA IDRE) has many SAS learning modules and data examples (https://stats.idre .ucla.edu/sas/).

1.3.2 R Programming

WHAT IS R?

R is a free, open source software package used for statistical computing. R is available on any platform (Mac, PC, Linux, etc.). RStudio, an integrated development environment for R, is often used as a supplement to make it easier for users to edit and debug syntax. We utilize RStudio as a tool in this book.

HOW DOES R PROGRAMMING WORK?

1. Functions in R are stored in packages. Packages are available for free through the Comprehensive R Archive Network, or CRAN (https://cran.r-project.org/), and must be installed in the R environment before being loaded using the library() function. Data manipulation and analyses in R are performed using functions.
2. Data frames are the data structures in R used to store data. The column names are referenced using the symbol $ (dataframename$columnname).
3. Values, such as calculated statistics or the output from analyses, are saved into a value by using the symbols <- or =.

HOW ARE DATA READ INTO R?

Although there are various packages to import an XLS file into R, the recommended method is to save the XLS file in a CSV format and import the CSV file using the following commands:

```
setwd("/User/Documents/Data")
dta <- read.csv("dataset.csv",header=TRUE)
```

The setwd() function is used to set the file location (a working directory), and the read.csv() function reads in the specified file (header= TRUE specifies that the first row of the CSV file contains headers, not data). The symbol <- or = is used to indicate that the data read in should be saved in the data frame called dta.

WHAT ARE THE ADVANTAGES OF R?

1. R is a free software environment that functions on all types of systems. It is available at https://www.r-project.org/.

2. R is open source, so users can write packages and contribute content in R. This gives users alternative methods for performing various statistical analyses and allows new methods to be available in R faster than other software packages.
3. R has flexible graphics and visualizations.
4. R has the capability of writing custom packages and functions.
5. R can handle large datasets and computationally intensive analyses.

WHAT ARE THE DISADVANTAGES OF R?

1. R has a steep learning curve.
2. There is no formal technical support from R, although there is a large online help community (see "What Can a User Do to Learn R?").
3. There are many available user written packages that can perform similar functions. It may take time to review and determine the best package to use for an analysis.

WHAT CAN A USER DO TO LEARN R?

Documentation for R packages, including information about the data, functions, and capabilities of the package, is available online (https://cran.r-project.org). In addition, the website R-Bloggers is a useful resource where users can ask questions and watch tutorials of analyses and data manipulation in R (https://www.r-bloggers.com). The UCLA IDRE also has many learning resources for R available on their website (https://stats.idre.ucla.edu/r/).

1.3.3 SPSS Programming

WHAT IS SPSS?

SPSS stands for Statistical Package for the Social Sciences. IBM SPSS Statistics is software for managing data and performing statistical analyses, including testing and modeling. Although it was initially intended for social sciences, SPSS is now popular in many different fields.

HOW DOES SPSS PROGRAMMING WORK?

SPSS has three main windows and a menu bar at the top. One can access:

1. The Data Editor (.sav files)

    When you open a SPSS data file, you see a working copy of your data.

    To open a different dataset, click **File <R arrow> Open <R arrow> Data.**
2. The Output Viewer (.spv files)

    The tables of the Output Viewer are saved (click **File <R arrow> Save** or **Save As**) with a file type of .spv, which can only be opened with SPSS software.
3. Syntax Editor (.sps files)

    If you are working with the SPSS programming language directly, you will also open the Syntax Editor. The Syntax Editor allows you to write, edit, and run commands in the SPSS programming language.

HOW ARE DATA READ INTO SPSS?

We encourage readers to refer to the UCLA Statistical Consulting Group website (https://stats.idrc.ucla.edu/spss/modules/how-to-read-raw-data-into-spss/) for a full accounting of methods to import data in SPSS:

1. Comma-delimited data, inline
2. Space-delimited data, inline
3. Comma-delimited data from an external file
4. Space-delimited data from an external file
5. Fixed-format data from an external file
6. Tab-delimited files and Excel files
7. Reading SAS data files into SPSS

WHAT ARE THE ADVANTAGES OF SPSS?

1. SPSS is used through the syntax editor or through the menu and dialogue boxes.
2. SPSS has an easy and intuitive user interface.
3. Multiple users can work on the same data file.
4. SPSS is often used by applied researchers for its built-in functionalities for data management, analysis, and visualization.

WHAT ARE THE DISADVANTAGES OF SPSS?

1. SPSS does not contain as many capabilities as other software programs.
2. Users may experience convergence issues (discussed in chaps. 5 and 6, for example) with more complex models.

HOW CAN A USER LEARN SPSS?

SPSS is utilized with the SPSS programming language or through menu options. The menu options can help new users get started. SPSS offers a beginner tutorial online (https://www.spss-tutorials.com /basics/), and the UCLA IDRE also has online guides to using SPSS (https://stats.idre.ucla.edu/spss/).

1.3.4 Stata Programming

WHAT IS STATA?

Stata is statistical software that offers both the use of menu options and programming. It attracts many users from diverse disciplines.

HOW DOES STATA PROGRAMMING WORK?

We encourage readers to reference https://statacommunityre sources.files.wordpress.com/2016/02/communityresource-statabasics .pdf for information on creating working directories and reading data. Stata uses the following types of files:

1. Stata-executable files contain the compiled program that is the core of Stata. These files end in .exe and are what run when you open Stata.

2. Ado files are programs that use features in the executable file to add new commands to Stata. User-written add-ons are accessed at stata.com/statalist.

HOW ARE DATA READ INTO STATA?

There are two approaches to evaluating data in Stata. The first approach is to use Stata as an interactive tool by clicking on commands. Interactive options to are available to load data, review the data, and perform the analyses of interest. This method is useful when you are trying to figure out something new because you get immediate feedback. But interactive work cannot be easily or reliably replicated or modified.

The second approach is to treat Stata as a programming language. In this approach, you write programs and call "do files." A do file contains the same commands you type in interactive Stata, but the commands are saved in a permanent file so they are debugged or modified and then rerun at will. The do files also serve as an exact record of how you obtained your results.

WHAT ARE THE ADVANTAGES OF STATA?

1. Stata has many statistical analysis capabilities available through a command prompt with Stata syntax as well as through a menu interface.
2. The documentation is well maintained and easy to reference (available through the Help option in the command prompt).

WHAT ARE THE DISADVANTAGES OF STATA?

1. It can only hold one dataset in memory at a time.
2. Graphics have limited flexibility.

WHAT CAN A USER DO TO LEARN STATA?

Stata provides links to many official and community resources to learning Stata on its website (https://www.stata.com/links/resources -for-learning-stata).

1.4 Alzheimer's and Other Neurodegenerative Databases

There are many datasets related to dementia and other neurodegenerative diseases (Bell et al. 2015). There are also Web-based resources summarizing publicly available databases, such as the National Institute on Aging Database of Longitudinal Studies (https://www.nia.nih.gov/research/dbsr/publicly-available-databases-aging-related-secondary-analyses-behavioral-and-social) as well as databases that combine independent studies such as the Global Alzheimer's Association Interactive Network (GAAIN; http://gaain.org/).

Data resources are typically available to researchers and may require compliance to data use agreements and publications policies. To verify access and to track usage, one typically submits an online application denoting institutional affiliation and scientific focus in order to gain access to data. Furthermore, all data collection needs to follow current laws and regulations as well as institutional review board (IRB) guidelines (such as sharing de-identified data that does not contain identifying information about individual deceased subjects). De-identified data do not contain protected health information (PHI) like names, social security numbers, addresses, and phone numbers. Data are typically shared with randomly generated pseudo-IDs. For the evaluation of any dataset, as stated previously, it is recommended to work directly with the study personnel to understand the design of the study, data collection process, and any caveats or limitations of the data. We briefly describe a few databases and study resources.

NATIONAL ALZHEIMER'S COORDINATING CENTER

NACC is a large relational database of standardized clinical and neuropathological research data collected over two dozen National Institute of Aging–funded sites across the United States (https://www.alz.washington.edu/) (Morris et al. 2006; Beekly et al. 2007). Standardized clinical and neuropathological assessments are performed and recorded by the 39 past and present Alzheimer's Disease Centers (ADCs), from subjects who have AD and related disorders as well as from cognitively normal subjects. Variables include cognitive measures such as the MMSE and the Clinical Dementia Rating Scale, clinical measures including mood (Geriatric Depression Scale and Neuropsychiatry Inventory Depression subscale), cardiovascular factors such as diabetes and hypertension, and neuropathological data on cases that have come to autopsy, including data on plaque and neurofibrillary tangle distributions (Thal amyloid phase and Braak NFT stage, respectively) (Braak and Braak 1991; Thal et al. 2002; Montine et al. 2012) and the Consortium to Establish a Registry for Alzheimer's Disease (CERAD) neuritic plaque density (Mirra et al. 1991). Readers may refer to the NACC online data dictionary for a complete set of variables (https://www.alz.washington.edu/WEB/dataforms_main.html).

HEALTH AND RETIREMENT STUDY

The HRS, launched in 1992, is a longitudinal study that surveyed a representative sample of approximately 20,000 people in the United States (http://hrsonline.isr.umich.edu/) (Hauser and Willis 2004). HRS is one of the largest and most comprehensive nationally represented study of Americans over 50 years of age with detailed health and economic data in the same survey. Data gleaned include but are not limited to cognitive assessments, health behaviors, linkage to Medicare claims data, earnings, employment status and history, height, weight, blood pressure, select blood-based biomarkers and genetic data.

FRAMINGHAM HEART STUDY

The FHS began in 1948 as a longitudinal study in the town of Framingham, Massachusetts, to identify common factors or characteristics that contribute to cardiovascular disease (https://www.framinghamheartstudy.org/) (Dawber et al. 1963; Splansky et al. 2007). As many persons with cardiovascular disease risk factors develop dementia, this dataset has become extremely useful to multiple disciplines. The dataset includes epidemiological data on all forms of cardiovascular disease, including arteriosclerotic and hypertensive cardiovascular disease, demographic data, alcohol and smoking status, and physical activity.

COGNITIVE FUNCTION AND AGEING STUDY

The CFAS is a multicentered, population-based study in the United Kingdom (http://www.cfas.ac.uk/) (Chadwick 1992). It was established to investigate cognitive decline and dementia in a representative population-based sample of people over 65 years of age. Questions that have been investigated include: What factors increase an individual's risk of developing dementia? What are the different underlying diseases that cause dementia? What is the degree of disability suffered by those who have dementia?

STUDY ON GLOBAL AGEING AND ADULT HEALTH

SAGE, from the World Health Organization (WHO), is a longitudinal study with a focus on data collection for adults 50 years and older from nationally representative samples in China, Ghana, India, Mexico, the Russian Federation, and South Africa (http://www.who.int/healthinfo/sage/en/). Data include but are not limited to household rosters, health expenditures, health insurance coverage, sociodemographic information, risk factors, mortality, and chronic conditions.

ROTTERDAM STUDY

The Rotterdam Elderly Study is a prospective cohort study that began recruitment in 1990 in the Netherlands, focusing on the Ommoord District in the city of Rotterdam (http://www.epib.nl/research/ergo.htm) (Hofman et al. 1991a, 1991b; Ikram et al. 2011). The main objectives were to study the risk factors of cardiovascular, neurological, endocrine, and ophthalmological diseases in elderly persons. Data gleaned include socioeconomic status, current drug use, dietary habits, physical activity, bone mineral densitometry, and data on cardiovascular, neurological, and ophthalmic diseases.

PARKINSON'S PROGRESSION MARKER INITIATIVE

Although this book mainly focuses on dementia, there are many great data resources for Parkinson's disease, another neurodegenerative disease, including PPMI (http://www.ppmi-info.org/) (Marek et al.

2011). PPMI is a longitudinal multicenter study aimed to assess the progression of clinical features, imaging, and biological markers across the Parkinson's disease spectrum, and it also includes normal controls. PPMI has clinical sites in Australia, Europe, Israel, and the United States. Data and samples acquired from study participants contribute to a comprehensive Parkinson's database and biorepository. Data include information on genetics, sleep questionnaires, the Montreal Cognitive Assessment, Geriatric Depression Scale, basic demographics, information from physical and neurological examinations (including the Unified Parkinson's Disease Rating Scale), and biomarker and imaging data, including blood samples and olfactory testing.

1.5 Data Used in This Book

1.5.1 Data Description

In this book, we analyze data from the National Alzheimer's Coordinating Center (Morris et al. 2006; Beekly et al. 2007; Weintraub et al. 2009) December 2017 data freeze. We consider 21,788 patients representing 55,626 visits to 39 ADCs. Of these patients, 9,530 have only one visit to an ADC, while the remaining patients have two or more visits (with a maximum of 10 visits). The number of patients visiting each ADC varies greatly, with a minimum of two patients (ADC 943) and a maximum of 3,496 patients (ADC 2096). We have information on subjects who have normal cognition, a primary clinical diagnosis of AD, a primary diagnosis of dementia with Lewy bodies (DLB) without Parkinson's disease, a primary diagnosis of frontotemporal dementia (FTD), or a primary diagnosis of vascular dementia (VaD) at all visits. These data were collected with visit dates between June 2005 and November 2017.

1.5.2 Variables Used in the Chapters

A summary of the variables used in one or more chapters in this book is given in table 1.1. The table contains the variable label, variable type (continuous, binary, categorical, and date), and description. We utilize various subsets of the NACC dataset. The generated variables Ch2 through Ch12 are included as indicators of which records to use in the

Table 1.1 Summary of Variables

Variable	Variable Type	Description
ADC	Categorical	Center ID
ID	Categorical	Subject ID
VISITNUM	Continuous	Visit number
VISITDATE	Date	Date of visit
MOFROMINDEX	Continuous	Time since baseline visit (months)
Diagnosis	Categorical	Diagnosis descriptors (AD, DLB, FTD, VaD, normal)
DX	Categorical	Diagnosis codes (1 = AD, 2 = DLB, 3 = FTD, 4 = VaD, 8 = normal)
DX_AD	Binary	AD diagnosis (1 = AD, 0 = no AD)
Mix_AD	Binary	Mixed diagnosis with contributing AD (1 = AD is a contributing DX, 0 = AD is not a contributing DX)
Mix_DLB	Binary	Mixed diagnosis with contributing DLB (1 = DLB is a contributing DX, 0 = DLB is not a contributing DX)
Mix_FTD	Binary	Mixed diagnosis with contributing FTD (1 = FTD is a contributing DX, 0 = FTD is not a contributing DX)
Mix_VaD	Binary	Mixed diagnosis with contributing VaD (1 = VaD is a contributing DX, 0 = VaD is not a contributing DX)
SEX	Binary	Gender (1 = male, 2 = female)
AGE	Continuous	Age (years)
AGEDEATH	Continuous	Age at death (years)
DEATHDATE	Date	Date of death
BMI	Continuous	Body mass index
NIHR	Categorical	Race (1 = white, 2 = black or African American, 3 = American Indian or Alaska Native, 4 = Native Hawaiian or Pacific Islander, 5 = Asian, 6 = multiracial)
DIABETES	Binary	Diabetes indicator (1 = recent/active, 0 = remote/inactive/absent)
HYPERTEN	Binary	Hypertension indicator (1 = recent/active, 0 = remote/inactive/absent)
HYPERCHO	Binary	Hypercholesterolemia indicator (1 = recent/active, 0 = remote/inactive/absent)
BPSYS	Continuous	Systolic blood pressure
BPDIAS	Continuous	Diastolic blood pressure
HRATE	Continuous	Heart rate
SMOKYRS	Continuous	Years smoking
CDRSUM	Continuous	Clinical Dementia Rating Scale Sum of Boxes score (0–18)
MMSE	Continuous	Mini-Mental State Examination score (0–30)
DIED	Binary	Death indicator (1 = died, 0 = censored)
SURVIVAL_TIME	Continuous	Survival time from start of study

(*continued*)

Table 1.1 (continued)

Variable	Variable Type	Description
Ch2	Binary	Indicator variable for which records to use for chapter 2 examples and exercises (1 = included, 0 = excluded)
Ch3	Binary	Indicator variable for which records to use for chapter 3 examples and exercises (1 = included, 0 = excluded)
Ch4	Binary	Indicator variable for which records to use for chapter 4 examples and exercises (1 = included, 0 = excluded)
Ch5	Binary	Indicator variable for which records to use for chapter 5 examples and exercises (1 = included, 0 = excluded)
Ch6	Binary	Indicator variable for which records to use for chapter 6 examples and exercises (1 = included, 0 = excluded)
Ch7	Binary	Indicator variable for which records to use for chapter 7 examples and exercises (1 = included, 0 = excluded)
Ch8	Binary	Indicator variable for which records to use for chapter 8 examples and exercises (1 = included, 0 = excluded)
Ch9	Binary	Indicator variable for which records to use for chapter 9 examples and exercises (1 = included, 0 = excluded)
Ch10	Binary	Indicator variable for which records to use for chapter 10 examples and exercises (1 = included, 0 = excluded)
Ch11	Binary	Indicator variable for which records to use for chapter 11 examples and exercises (1 = included, 0 = excluded)
Ch12	Binary	Indicator variable for which records to use for chapter 12 examples and exercises (1 = included, 0 = excluded)

examples and exercises for each chapter. For example, the CHAP2 dataset referenced in chapter 2 selects all observations where the variable $Ch2 = 1$.

We note in this book that we use indicator variables for the cardiovascular risk factors diabetes (DIABETES), hypertension (HYPERTEN), and hypercholesterolemia (HYPERCHO). While we define these variables as binary variables (collapsing the absent category with remote/inactive), the reader should be aware that the NACC's *Researcher's Data Dictionary—Uniform Data Set* defines DIABETES,

HYPERTEN, and HYPERCHO as categorical variables where 0 = Absent, 1 = Recent/Active, and 2 = Remote/Inactive.

1.5.3 Accessing the Data

The data for this book constitute a limited excerpt from NACC and should only be utilized for educational purposes. To access these data, please visit http://www.public.asu.edu/~jeffreyw/. Further distribution or reproduction of these data, research analysis for publication, or any other purpose beyond the specific examples provided in *Fundamental Statistical Methods for Analysis of Alzheimer's and Other Neurodegenerative Diseases* are strictly prohibited. Persons wishing to access the NACC database for scientific research must visit the NACC website, www.alz.washington.edu, to apply for access.

1.6 Statistical Models for Other Diseases

While this book concentrates on statistical models for the analysis of Alzheimer's disease and related disorders data, the models are by no means unique to these kinds of data. These models are applicable for other conditions such as diabetes, stroke, cancer, hypertension, and obesity. The models in this book are fitted to either cross-sectional data or longitudinal data.

CROSS-SECTIONAL DATA (CHAPTERS 2, 3, 8, AND 11)

In cross-sectional data, each patient is measured at one time-point. We ask questions such as:

1. Is the random component following a distribution from the exponential family?
2. Are the observations independent?
3. Which covariates and factors does one want to use to explain the mean of the specified distribution?

LONGITUDINAL DATA (CHAPTERS 4, 5, 6, 7, 9, 10, AND 12)

Similarly, in longitudinal data with repeated measures, we ask questions such as:

1. Are the distribution and conditional distribution of the random component from the exponential family?
2. How are the observations correlated?
3. Which covariates and factors does one want to use to explain the mean of the specified distribution? Which ones are fixed and which ones are random?

While the researcher interested in studying dementia will be happy to see familiar variables, one can easily replace the variables to applications in other fields and continue with any of the models in chapters 2 through 12.

1.7 Book Structure

This book has 12 chapters. The remainder of this book is structured as follows:

Chapter 2 reviews statistical topics that one may have learned in an introductory course in statistics. We cover one-sample tests, two-sample tests, one-way analysis of variance, simple linear regression, multiple regression analysis, and logistic regression analysis. We provide references to help with one's familiarity of the material.

Chapter 3 discusses generalized linear models. This class of models is a generalization of the models discussed in chapter 2. These models assume that the observations are independent.

Chapter 4 presents methods to model continuous correlated data in a longitudinal or clustered structure. We use generalized estimating equations and random effects models to analyze continuous outcomes.

Chapter 5 addresses the analysis of hierarchical binary data. We use generalized estimating equations and random effects models to analyze continuous outcomes.

Chapter 6 introduces Bayesian modeling as an alternative to the frequentist modeling approaches for binary data.

Chapter 7 introduces multiple-membership, multiple-classification models used in hierarchical structures that are not completely nested.

Chapter 8 addresses survival models to model the time to an event. We present Kaplan Meier and Cox regression models and Bayesian modeling.

Chapter 9 fits marginal models with time-dependent covariates. We introduce generalized method of moments models to analyze such data and to address the time-dependent covariates.

Chapter 10 introduces the joint modeling of the mean and dispersion to address extra variation found in the data.

Chapter 11 discusses big data analytics and machine learning methods. We provide an overview of a number of approaches, in particular, neural networks.

Chapter 12 presents a case study. We start with the raw data and walk through the model-building process.

Exercises are included at the end of most chapters as a means of reinforcing the material covered.

STATISTICAL SOFTWARE

We demonstrate the statistical methods throughout this book using SAS, R, SPSS, and Stata. There are instances when we focus on less than this full complement of software programs. In some examples, we ran into nonconvergence (discussed in chaps. 4, 5, and 6) and so were not able to provide useable output. In these cases, however, we provide the syntax for reference so readers can apply these methods to different datasets. In addition, some software programs do not have the capabilities to perform all analyses discussed in this book, which are mentioned in the corresponding section.

1.8 Summary

This chapter introduces the reader to statistical terms, neurodegenerative disease databases, information on accessing the data, a summary of variables, and an overview of the topics discussed in this book. It also provides the reader with an introduction to the software packages SAS, R, SPSS, and Stata and useful references to become familiar with these programs and to apply them in the exercises throughout this book.

Chapter 2

Review of Introductory Statistical Methods

2.1 Introduction

In this chapter, we review descriptive statistics as well as basic statistical tests and models for continuous, binary, and categorical response data. We refer to types of data based on the characteristics of the response or outcome variable. To demonstrate these methods, we analyze a subset of data from the National Alzheimer's Coordinating Center (NACC) (Morris et al. 2006; Beekly et al. 2007; Weintraub et al. 2009). These data contain information from the baseline visit of 2,031 patients from 33 Alzheimer's Disease Centers (ADCs), with visits between September 2005 and November 2016. Of these patients, 1,681 were clinically diagnosed with Alzheimer's disease (AD) and 350 were considered nondemented individuals (normal). A subset of the data analyzed in this chapter is given in table 2.1. We analyze these data using the statistical software SAS, R, SPSS, and Stata.

The data consist of several types of variables, including continuous, binary, and categorical:

Continuous variables are measured on a continuum and take on many or an infinite number of possible values. Examples of continuous variables are age, weight, height, and blood pressure (table 2.2). Continuous variables are often visualized using a histogram, such as a plot examining the frequencies of weight for the 2,031 normal and AD subjects (fig. 2.1).

Binary variables describe information that takes one of two possible outcomes (e.g., yes/no or present/absent). Its mean is called a proportion or probability, which lies on a scale between 0 and 1. Binary variables are common in dementia studies, such as whether or not

Table 2.1 A Subset of Data Used in Chapter 2

ADC	ID	Diagnosis	AGEDEATH	SEX	BMI	DIABETES	HYPERTEN	HYERCHO
8646	731	1	84	2	33.8	0	1	1
1416	4864	1	81	1	33.5	0	0	0
8658	5734	2	77	1	24.9	1	1	0
6713	6109	2	75	1	27.2	0	1	1
4967	6556	1	63	1	25.6	0	0	1
8658	7556	2	76	2	25.5	0	1	1
490	7791	1	84	2	25.9	0	1	0
289	9523	1	86	1	22.2	1	1	0
6518	12692	1	91	2	24.8	0	1	1
4967	14469	1	77	1	27.1	0	0	0

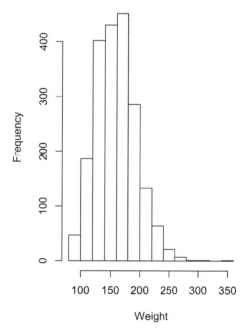

Figure 2.1 Histogram of weight.

the patient received a particular diagnosis, had a heart attack, or is still active during the study (table 2.2). The frequency of each outcome for a binary variable can be quickly visualized using a bar chart. We demonstrate this by evaluating the frequency of gender (1 = male,

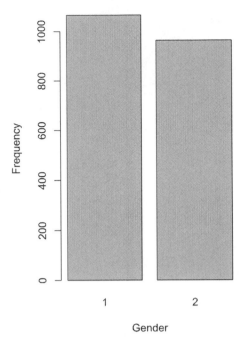

Figure 2.2 Bar chart of gender.

2 = female) of our subjects. From the bar chart, we see that there are more males in our subset than females (fig. 2.2).

Categorical variables consist of several categories, such as a scale of severity or a temporal aspect, which may have the options *none, sparse, moderate,* or *frequent*; or *none, recent/active,* or *remote/inactive*. Variables with more than two categories are referred to as categorical. Examples include race and state of residence (table 2.2). Bar charts can also be used to visualize the number of categories and frequency of each possible outcome. Figure 2.3 displays a frequency chart of the reported races of the subjects. We see there are six races represented in our data (1 = white, 2 = black or African American, 3 = American Indian or Alaska Native, 4 = Native Hawaiian or Pacific Islander, 5 = Asian, and 6 = multiracial). We see that the vast majority of subjects in our dataset are white, followed by black or African American, and multiracial.

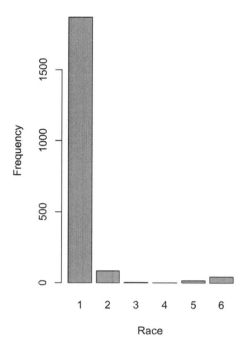

Figure 2.3 Bar chart of race.

Table 2.2 Examples of Variable Types

Data Type	Examples
Continuous	Age, weight, height, blood pressure
Binary	Gender, presence/absence of a diagnosis, previous heart attack, history of diabetes
Categorical	Race, state of residence, dementia type

2.2 Statistical Measures

A statistic is an estimate of some feature of the population of observations. There are two types of statistics, *descriptive* and *inferential* statistics. Descriptive statistics provide an initial insight into the data, including where the data are centered. These statistics also describe how the values are spread and the presence of outlying observations. Such information is included in measures of central tendency (*mean, median,* and *mode*), measures of spread (*standard deviation, variance, range*), or measures of relative standing (*z-values, percentiles, median, quartiles, interquartile range*).

2.2.1 Measures of Central Tendency

One measure of central tendency is the mean, or the arithmetic average. The mean describes the center of the data and is one type of average of the observations. For a set of observations y_i where $i = 1, 2, \ldots, n$ (such that there are a total n observations), the sample mean (called a statistic, as it is obtained from the sample) is defined as

$$\bar{y} = \frac{\sum_{i=1}^{n} y_i}{n}.$$

This is an average of the sample of observations with a sample size of n. It estimates the population mean, referred to as μ.

The variable AGEDEATH indicates the age of the patient at death (if applicable). Using a sample of 1,681 AD patients, we estimate that the mean *age at death* for patients diagnosed with AD as 80.8 years. In this computation, we allow each patient to have equal importance. But there are times when equal importance is not advisable, as in the case of skewed data. In such cases, we obtain a weighted average. For each observation, there is a weight w_i, $i = 1, 2, \ldots, n$, such that the weighted average is calculated as

$$\bar{y}_w = \frac{\sum_{i=1}^{n} w_i \times y_i}{\sum_{i=1}^{n} w_i}.$$

The median is another measure of central tendency. It is the center value of the ordered observations. While both the mean and median address centrality, the mean is influenced by extreme values because it uses the magnitude of observations. But the median depends on the order, rather than the magnitude of the observations, and thus it is not influenced by extreme values. The median is more useful in describing the center of skewed data or when data are rank ordered (such as when reporting Braak Neurofibrillary Tangle Stage, a pathological measure of AD progression).

When the mean and median are close in value, the data are symmetric with the median at its center. If the mean is much larger than the median, the data are *skewed to the right* (a few relatively large observations). If the mean is much smaller than the median, then the data are *skewed to the left* (a few relatively small observations). In the example of age at death, the median is 83 years, which is slightly larger than the mean of 80.8 and indicates that there are a few observations with early ages of death. From figure 2.4, we can see that the age at death data are left skewed. Most subjects had ages of death in later years; however, there were a few subjects who died at younger ages.

The mode is a useful measure of central tendency. It indicates the most frequently occurring value in the data. When there is more than one mode, we refer to the data as *bimodal* (two modes) or *multimodal*

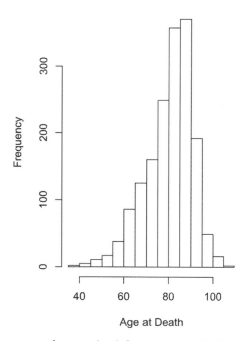

Figure 2.4 Histogram of age at death for patients with Alzheimer's disease.

(more than two modes). It is possible for the data not to have a mode. In our data, the mode of the age at death is 90 years, which occurs 106 times, or for 6.3% of AD subjects.

2.2.2 Measures of Spread

Measures of spread (also referred to as *variation, deviation,* or *dispersion*) describe the differences in values among the observations in the data. A common measure of spread used with continuous variables is the variance. The sample variance is defined as

$$s^2 = \frac{1}{(n-1)} \sum_{i=1}^{n} (y_i - \bar{y})^2,$$

where y_i is the value of the ith observation in the sample and $\bar{y}$ is the mean of the n observations in the sample. Thus the variance is an average of the squared distances between each observation value and the mean. Data with more extreme values will have more cases where the distances are further from the mean, and thus the variance will be larger. If one had the opportunity to have the entire population with population size N, y_i is replaced with Y_i, $\bar{y}$ is replaced with μ, and $(n-1)$ with N, resulting in the population variance of

$$\sigma^2 = \frac{1}{N} \sum_{i=1}^{N} (Y_i - \mu)^2.$$

Another common measure of spread is the standard deviation s, which is the square root of the variance. The sample standard deviation is defined as

$$s = \sqrt{s^2} = \sqrt{\frac{1}{(n-1)} \sum_{i=1}^{n} (y_i - \bar{y})^2}.$$

In examining the spread of the age at death for AD patients, we find that the variance and standard deviation are 110.4 years^2 and 10.5 years, respectively.

The range is another measure of spread. It is the difference between the minimum value and maximum value. This is a single value and not a set of values, as is often mistaken. In the case of the subset of NACC data, the minimum age at death is 39 years, while the maximum age at death is 106 years. Thus the range for age at death is 67 years. In practice, an age at death of 39 years is unusual for Alzheimer's-related patient deaths. One would want to investigate this record to determine whether it was recorded incorrectly or whether there is some other information worthy of note.

2.2.3 Measures of Relative Standing

Percentiles are measures of relative standing. The percentile indicates where the observation lies in relation to the other observations. It is based on the ordered data segmented into 100 parts. The median is the 50th percentile and describes the center of the data. The 25th percentile (Q_1) and 75th percentile (Q_3), called the first and third quartiles, respectively, are key measures of relative standing. In our ongoing example, the second quartile, or the median, of the age at death is 83 years. The first quartile, or 25th percentile, is 75 years, and the third quartile, or 75th percentile, is 88 years. The interquartile range (IQR) describes the distance between the first and third quartiles, such that $IQR = Q_3 - Q_1$. For the variable age at death, the interquartile range is $IQR = 88 - 75 = 13$ years.

A key measure of relative standing is the z-value. The z-value is calculated by taking the difference between the observation and its mean and dividing the result by the standard deviation. The z-value is a measure of the number of standard deviations that an observation lies from the mean. A z-value of 0 signifies that the observation is equal to the mean. When a z-value is less than two standard deviations below the mean or more than two standard deviations above the mean, we refer to such an observation as an outlier. In other words, it is customary for an observation that lies more than two standard deviations from the mean to be considered as extreme. Throughout the text, we will either refer to or make use of this value of 2. The 2 is an approximate value of 1.96, which is derived from the standard normal distribution.

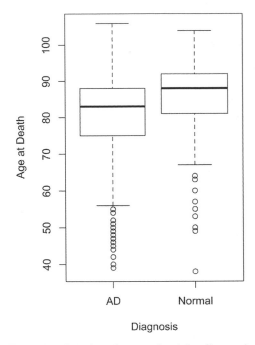

Figure 2.5 Boxplot of age at death by diagnosis.

Box and whisker plots (fig. 2.5) are typically utilized to visualize the spread and standings of observations in the data. We compare the spread of the age at death for AD patients and normal patients. The IQR for normal patients is 11 years, as the first and third quartiles for age at death for normal patients are 81 and 92 years, respectively. The box and whisker plot shows the spread of the age at death (y-axis) for AD patients and normal patients (x-axis). The bold line in the middle of each box indicates the median for each group. The plots show that the median age at death for normal patients is higher than the median age at death for AD patients. The edges of the box represent the first and third quartiles, while the edges of the whiskers denote the smallest and largest observations in the data (excluding outliers).

Problem: What are the measures of spread and measures of central tendency for the variable *age at death* for AD patients in the dataset?

Solution: For AD patients, we obtain a mean age at death of 80.813 years and median age at death of 83.00 years.

The MEANS Procedure

Analysis Variable: AGEDEATH

Mean	Median	Mode	Min	Max	Variance	Std Dev	Lower Quartile	Upper Quartile
80.813	83.00	90.00	39.000	106.00	110.395	10.507	75.000	88.000

2.2.4 SAS Syntax and Output for Descriptive Statistics

The SAS syntax follows:

```
¹PROC MEANS DATA=CHAP2 MEAN MEDIAN MODE MIN MAX VAR STD Q1 Q3;
²VAR AGEDEATH;
³WHERE DX = 1;
⁴RUN;
```

[1]Denotes the SAS procedure to the dataset called CHAP2 requesting mean, median, mode, minimum (MIN), maximum (MAX), variance (VAR), standard deviation (STD), first quartile (Q1) and third quartile (Q3).
[2]The VAR statement specifies the variable of interest, AGEDEATH.
[3]The results are requested for DX = 1, patients diagnosed with Alzheimer's disease.
[4]All SAS procedure calls are terminated with RUN.

SAS OUTPUT

The MEANS Procedure

Analysis Variable: AGEDEATH

Mean	Median	Mode	Min	Max	Variance	Std Dev	Lower Quartile	Upper Quartile
80.813	83.00	90.00	39.000	106.00	110.395	10.507	75.000	88.000

Comments: For the variable age at death (AGEDEATH), the mean is 80.813 years, the median is 83 years, the mode is 90 years, the minimum is 39 years, and the maximum is 106 years. The variance is 110.395 years[2]. The standard deviation is 10.507 years. The 25th percentile (lower quartile) of age at death for AD patients is 75 years, and the 75th percentile (upper quartile) is 88 years.

2.2.5 R Syntax and Output for Descriptive Statistics

The R syntax follows:

```
¹AD_dta <- chap2[chap2$DX==1,]
¹normal_dta <- chap2[chap2$DX==8,]
²#Descriptive statistics: mean, median, mode, variance, sd,
quantiles, correlation
³mean(AD_dta$AGEDEATH)
³median(AD_dta$AGEDEATH)
³min(AD_dta$AGEDEATH)
³max(AD_dta$AGEDEATH)
³var(AD_dta$AGEDEATH)
³sd(AD_dta$AGEDEATH)
³quantile(AD_dta$AGEDEATH,probs=c(0.25,0.5,0.75))
³quantile(normal_dta$AGEDEATH,probs=c(0.25,0.5,0.75))
#Histogram
⁴hist(AD_dta$AGEDEATH,xlab="Age At Death",main=NULL)
#Box and whisker plot:
⁵boxplot(AGEDEATH~Diagnosis,data=chap2, xlab="Diagnosis",
ylab="Age of Death")
```

[1]Using two datasets, data for AD (DX = 1) and normal patients (DX = 8), select the records in chap2 where chap2$DX is the diagnosis of interest. The symbol $ is used to select columns/variables from within the data frame chap2.

[2]Comments are denoted using the symbol #.

[3]Descriptive statistics are obtained using built-in functions, mean() or median(). R does *not* have a built-in function to determine the mode of the data.

[4]A histogram is created using the hist() function. The option xlab= sets the label for the *x*-axis, and main=NULL produces a plot with no title. [5]A simple boxplot is generated with the boxplot() function. The options specify the variables to plot, the data frame the variables are saved in (data=), the *x*-axis title (xlab=), and the *y*-axis title (ylab=). A title is added to the boxplot using the option main=.

R OUTPUT

```
mean(AD_dta$AGEDEATH)
## [1] 80.81261
median(AD_dta$AGEDEATH)
## [1] 83
> min(AD_dta$AGEDEATH)
[1] 39
> max(AD_dta$AGEDEATH)
[1] 106
var(AD_dta$AGEDEATH)
## [1] 110.3952
sd(AD_dta$AGEDEATH)
## [1] 10.50691
quantile(AD_dta$AGEDEATH,probs=c(0.25,0.5,0.75))
## 25% 50% 75%
##  75  83  88
quantile(normal_dta$AGEDEATH,probs=c(0.25,0.5,0.75))
## 25% 50% 75%
##  81  88  92
```

Comments: For the variable age at death (AGEDEATH), the mean is 80.813 years, the median is 83 years, the minimum is 39 years, and the maximum is 106 years. The variance is 110.395 years^2. The standard deviation is 10.507 years. The 25th percentile (lower quartile) of age at death for AD patients is 75 years, and the 75th percentile (upper quartile) is 88 years. For normal subjects, the 25th percentile is 81 years, and the 75th percentile is 92 years.

2.2.6 SPSS Syntax and Output for Descriptive Statistics

The SPSS syntax follows:

```
FREQUENCIES VARIABLES=AGEDEATH
  /NTILES=4
  /PERCENTILES=25.0 75.0
  /STATISTICS=STDDEV VARIANCE RANGE MINIMUM MAXIMUM MEAN MEDIAN
MODE SUM SKEWNESS SESKEW KURTOSIS
    SEKURT
  /ORDER=ANALYSIS.
Or by pull down menu we use
ANALYZE → DESCRIPTIVE STATISTICS → FREQUENCIES → STATISTICS
```

SPSS OUTPUT

Statistics

AGEDEATH	N	Valid	1681
		Missing	0
	Mean		80.81
	Std. Error of Mean		.256
	Median		83.00
	Mode		90
	Std. Deviation		10.507
	Variance		110.395
	Skewness		−.795
	Std. Error of Skewness		.060
	Kurtosis		.677
	Std. Error of Kurtosis		.119
	Range		67
	Minimum		39
	Maximum		106
	Sum		135846
	Percentiles	25	75.00
		50	83.00
		75	88.00

Comments: For the variable age at death (AGEDEATH), the mean is 80.81 years, the median is 83 years, the mode is 90 years, the minimum is 39 years, and the maximum is 106 years. The variance is 110.395 years^2. The standard deviation is 10.507 years. The 25th percentile (lower quartile) of age at death for AD patients is 75 years, and the 75th percentile (upper quartile) is 88 years.

2.2.7 Stata Syntax and Output for Descriptive Statistics

The Stata syntax follows:

```
. SUMMARIZE AGEDEATH, DETAIL
```

STATA OUTPUT

			AGEDEATH	
AGEDEATH				
Percentiles		Smallest		
1%	49	39		
5%	62	40		
10%	66	42	Obs	1,681
25%	75	44	Sum of Weight	1,681
50%	83		Mean	80.81261
		Largest	Std Dev	10.50691
75%	88	104		
90%	92	104	Variance	110.3952
95%	95	106	Skewness	-.7947503
99%	101	106	Kurtosis	3.67105

Comments: For the variable age at death (AGEDEATH), the mean is 80.813 years, the median is 83 years (50th percentile), the minimum is 39 years (smallest), and the maximum is 106 years (largest). The variance is 110.395 years^2. The standard deviation is 10.507 years. The 25th percentile (lower quartile) of age at death for AD patients is 75 years, and the 75th percentile (upper quartile) is 88 years.

2.3 Measures of Association

In statistics and biostatistics, identifying and understanding relationships between variables are important. We consider two measures of association, the covariance and the correlation. These two measures are related to one another, although their scales of measurement differ.

The covariance between two variables describes a linear relationship. This measure lies between negative infinity ($-\infty$) and positive infinity (∞) in values. The sample covariance between the two variables x and y is

$$S_{xy} = \frac{1}{n-1} \sum_{i=1}^{n}(x_i - \bar{x})(y_i - \bar{y}),$$

where these values (x_i, y_i) are ordered pairs. When s_{xy} takes on a negative value, it means that as one variable increases, the other decreases. A positive value indicates that as one variable increases, the other also increases, and as one decreases, the other decreases. A value of 0 means there is no association, and so as one variable increases or decreases, the other is not affected. Although the covariance describes the association between two variables, it is difficult to determine the relative strength of the association on a scale of $-\infty$ to ∞.

A standardization of the covariance is the correlation, however, which is much easier to interpret. The sample correlation (r_{yx}), an estimate of the true population correlation coefficient ρ_{yx}, is

$$r_{yx} = \frac{s_{yx}}{s_y\,s_x},$$

where s_{yx} is the covariance between y and x and s_y and s_x are the sample standard deviations of y and x, respectively. The sample correlation r_{yx} ranges between -1 and 1, where values of r_{yx} close to 0 indicate little to no association between the two variables (Y and X). Values of r_{yx} close to 1 indicate a strong positive association. Thus as one variable increases, the second variable increases. Alternatively, values of

r_{yx} close to -1 indicate a strong negative association, in which one variable increases as the second variables decreases. Scatterplots are often used to visualize the relationship between two variables and can be used to understand the strength of the association. Figure 2.6 contains sample scatterplots between two variables, X and Y. Figure 2.6a has weak positive correlation ($r = 0.3688$), 2.6b has strong positive correlation ($r = 0.9067$), 2.6c has moderate negative correlation ($r = -0.5738$), and 2.6d has zero correlation ($r = 0.0389$).

The correlation provides a quick glimpse of the basic linear relationship between the two covariates. But one shortcoming or caution to note is that this correlation assumes that the two covariates are the only two variables of interest. There are two types of correlation, the parametric such as the Pearson correlation coefficient or the nonparametric such as the Kendall correlation or the Spearman correlation. By parametric, we mean that the variables have an underlying distribution, whereas nonparametric means that there is no distributional assumption. We show later in model fitting (Y vs. $X1$) that the addition of additional variables (Y vs. $X1$, $X2$, and $X3$) affects the association between the two variables (Y and $X1$).

Problem: What is the correlation between age at death and body mass index?

Solution: In our study of AD patients, the correlation between age at death and body mass index (BMI) is -0.09. This is a negative correlation, which indicates that as a patient's BMI increases, the age at death decreases. Thus patients with higher BMI tend to die at an earlier age; in other words, patients with lower BMI tend to die at older ages. But the magnitude of the correlation is 0.09, which is close to 0, and so the association is not considered to be strong. We may not have a large data spread as it relates to age, given that AD patients tend to have a limited age range of death; hence in our model we examine the range, median, and average of variables in addition to relying on correlations. The covariance between age at death and BMI is -4.03, which indicates

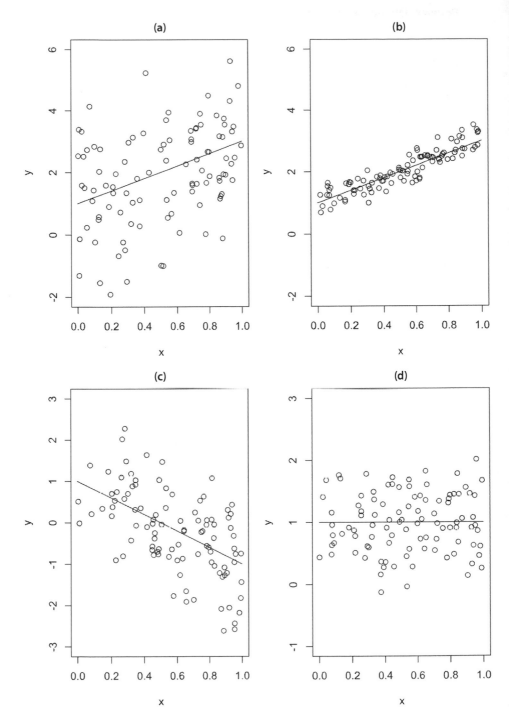

Figure 2.6 Scatterplots with varying associations.

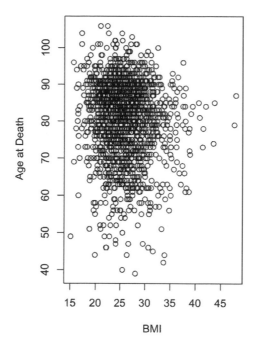

Figure 2.7 Scatterplot of BMI versus age at death for patients with Alzheimer's disease.

the same negative association, but the relative strength cannot be easily interpreted since it is not scaled. We use each of SAS, R, SPSS, and Stata. A scatterplot of BMI and age at death for AD patients is shown in figure 2.7.

2.3.1 SAS Syntax and Output for Correlation

The SAS syntax follows:

```
¹PROC CORR DATA=CHAP2 COV;
²VAR AGEDEATH BMI;
³WHERE DX = 1;
RUN;
```

[1]SAS procedure for obtaining the correlation. To view the covariance, the option COV is added.

[2]The variables for correlation are AGEDEATH and BMI.

[3]We are only interested in AD patients, so we specify DX = 1.

SAS OUTPUT

			The CORR Procedure			
			Simple Statistics			
Variable	N	Mean	Std Dev	Sum	Minimum	Maximum
AGEDEATH	1681	80.813	10.507	135846.000	39.000	106.000
BMI	1681	25.799	4.365	43369.000	15.100	48.000

Comments: The variance of AGEDEATH is $10.51^2 = 110.40$, and for BMI it is $4.36^2 = 19.01$.

Pearson Correlation Coefficients, N = 1681		
Prob > |r| under H0: Rho=0		
	AGEDEATH	BMI
AGEDEATH		−0.089
	1.000	0.003
BMI	−0.089	
	0.003	1.000

Comments: The correlation between AGEDEATH and BMI is −0.089, with a p-value of 0.0003. The p-value tells that the correlation is significant.

2.3.2 R Syntax and Output for Correlation

The R syntax follows:

```
[1]cor(AD_dta$AGEDEATH,AD_dta$BMI)
```

[1]The command cor() calculates the correlation between the two specified variables.

R OUTPUT

```
cor(AD_dta$AGEDEATH,AD_dta$BMI)
## [1] -0.088
```

Comments: The correlation between AGEDEATH and BMI is −0.088, with a *p*-value of 0.003. The *p*-value indicates that the correlation is significant.

2.3.3 SPSS Syntax and Output for Correlation

The SPSS syntax for parametric correlation follows:

```
CORRELATIONS
    /VARIABLES=AGEDEATH BMI
    /PRINT=TWOTAIL NOSIG
    /MISSING=PAIRWISE.
```

SPSS OUTPUT

| Variable | Variable2 | Statistic | | | | |
		Correlation	Count	Lower C.I.	Upper C.I.	Notes
AGEDEATH	AGEDEATH	1.000	1681	—	—	
	BMI	−.088	1681	−.135	−.040	
BMI	AGEDEATH	−.088	1681	−.135	−.040	
	BMI	1.000	1681	—	—	

Comments: The correlation between is −0.088, with a 95% confidence interval (−0.135, −0.040).

The SPSS syntax for nonparametric correlation follows:

```
NONPAR CORR
    /VARIABLES=AGEDEATH BMI
    /PRINT=BOTH TWOTAIL NOSIG
    /MISSING=PAIRWISE.
```

SPSS OUTPUT

```
                        Nonparametric Correlations

                                                    AGEDEATH        BMI

Kendall's tau_b  AGEDEATH  Correlation Coefficient    1.000      -.060**
                           Sig. (2-tailed)                .         .000
                           N                            1681        1681

                 BMI       Correlation Coefficient   -.060**      1.000
                           Sig. (2-tailed)             .000          .
                           N                            1681        1681

Spearman's rho   AGEDEATH  Correlation Coefficient    1.000      -.088**
                           Sig. (2-tailed)                .         .000
                           N                            1681        1681

                 BMI       Correlation Coefficient   -.088**      1.000
                           Sig. (2-tailed)             .000          .
                           N                            1681        1681
```

**. Correlation is significant at the 0.01 level (2-tailed).

Comments: The correlation between AGEDEATH and BMI is −0.088, with a 95% confidence interval (−0.144, −0.058). The confidence interval does not contain zero, so we conclude the correlation is significantly different from zero.

2.3.4 Stata Syntax and Output for Correlation

The Stata syntax follows:

```
. PWCORR AGEDEATH BMI, OBS SIG
```

STATA OUTPUT

```
(Obs = 1,681)
                  AGEDEATH       BMI

AGEDEATH          1.0000

BMI              -0.088       1.0000
```

Comments: The correlation between age at death and BMI is −0.1015, with a p-value of 0.000. This suggests that the correlation is significant. As BMI increases, age at death decreases for AD patients.

2.4 Statistical Test for Continuous Data

When conducting statistical tests for continuous response data, it is important to decipher the type of response variable (binary, categorical, and continuous). We begin by discussing cases when the response variable is continuous. Such variables are common in dementia data, as many studies are often interested in evaluating quantitative measurements for cognitive or daily functioning. When fitting models, we are often interested in the mean parameter of the distribution. The aim is to model the mean by identifying covariates or factors that may affect it. We begin by asking questions about the population mean, as that is the parameter of paramount importance. The question is never about the statistic, as we have the sample values and therefore we know the statistic. The question is about the parameter. The interest is usually presented in the form of a hypothesis.

Consider the null hypothesis that you believe the mean has a certain value, $H_0: \mu = \mu_0$, where μ_0 is a hypothesized population mean. Using the alternative hypothesis, we may ask if the mean is less than, greater than, or different from the hypothesized value. The corresponding alternative hypothesis for each of these scenarios in statistical form is

$$H_a: \mu < \mu_0, \; H_a: \mu > \mu_0 \text{ or } H_a: \mu \neq \mu_0.$$

One-sided tests include testing if the mean is less than the hypothesized value or greater than the hypothesized value. A two-sided test assesses whether the mean is different from the hypothesized value (either greater than or less than). As a means of testing the hypothesis, we use a test statistic or construct a confidence interval. There is ongoing debate as to the real advantage of relying on confidence intervals. But because this textbook has the sole purpose of introducing many of the common approaches and sometimes the not-so-common but useful approaches, we will present both sides.

The test statistic is a random variable calculated from the information in the sample. It relies on mirroring a certain distribution to determine whether the data support the null or its alternative. In testing about the mean under the conditions of a small sample or when the population variance is unknown (as is usually the case), we use the test statistic

$$t = \frac{\bar{y} - \mu_0}{s/\sqrt{n}},$$

where μ_0 is the hypothesized mean being tested, $\bar{y}$ is the sample mean, s is the standard deviation of the sample of observations, and n is the sample size. The calculated test statistic is compared to the critical value t_α^*, which is determined by the allowable type I error rate (α). Type I error is the probability that one decides to reject the null hypothesis but later finds the hypothesis should not be rejected. This type of error occurs when we falsely conclude statistical significance. We set the type I error rate—also referred to as alpha, the significance level, or the error level. This rate represents the probability that we reject the null hypothesis when we should not have. The error rate is typically set as $\alpha = 0.05$. Alternatively, type II error is the probability that we do not reject the null hypothesis when it is false (we should have rejected the null). This value is related to the power of a test (type II error $= 1 -$ power) and is usually controlled to be around 20%.

In the test statistic, one uses the calculated value and finds the probability of obtaining values larger than the test statistic value under a t-distribution (or the distribution we believe the test statistic follows). That probability is referred to as the p-value. The p-value is compared to the significance level, α. If the p-value is less than α, one rejects the null hypothesis and declares that based on the sample data there is sufficient evidence to believe that the research hypothesis is supported. In general, when we rely on hypothesis testing to address the research question, we reject the null hypothesis and believe that the state of nature has changed when the p-value is less than α. But one should look at the magnitude, as a p-value close to α (such as $p = 0.049$ for $\alpha = 0.05$) does not necessarily indicate significance and should be further evaluated. The American Statistical Association released a statement on statistical significance and p-values with principles for the underlying use and interpretation of the p-value (Wasserstein and Lazar 2016).

For example, the average age at death for AD patients in our sample is 80.8 years. The 2017 average life expectancy in the United States is approximately 78.8 years. We are interested in determining whether the average lifespan of patients with AD is significantly different than the average lifespan reported in the United States for 2017 (78.8 years). Thus we are interested in the hypotheses H_0: $\mu = 78.8$ and H_a: $\mu \neq 78.8$.

Using statistical software, we perform a one-sample t-test. We obtain a test statistic of 7.85, with a p-value < 0.0001. This is highly statistically significant (as $p < \alpha$), and so we reject the null hypothesis. We conclude that the average life expectancy of AD patients in our sample is significantly different from the 2017 US national average life expectancy ($p < 0.0001$). An alternative approach is to obtain the two-sided confidence interval for the mean. The confidence interval states the degree of belief in a set of possible values. Any of the values within the interval are believed to be probable solutions. If that range contains the contested hypothesize value, then we declare that the evidence does not conflict with the statement presented under the null. If the range does not contain the null hypothesis value, however, we conclude that the evidence contradicts the statement made under the null.

Problem: In the Alzheimer's patient data we analyzed previously, is the mean age at death different from age 78.8?

Solution: We obtained the confidence interval for age at death as (80.31, 81.315). Since the confidence interval does not include 78.8 years, we conclude that the true population mean is different from 78.8 years.

Mean	95% CL Mean	
80.813	80.310	81.315

We obtain these values from SAS, R, SPSS, and Stata.

2.4.1 SAS Syntax and Output for a One-Sample t-Test

The SAS syntax follows:

```
¹PROC TTEST DATA=CHAP2 H0 = 78.8 SIDES=2 ALPHA=0.05;
²VAR AGEDEATH;
³WHERE DX = 1;
RUN;
```

[1]We use the TTEST procedure to perform a one-sample t-test.
[2]The VAR statement indicates the variable under testing.
[3]The WHERE statement allows us to analyze DX=1 (Alzheimer's patients).

SAS OUTPUT

The TTEST Procedure

Variable: AGEDEATH

N	Mean	Std Dev	Std Err	Minimum	Maximum
1681	80.813	10.507	0.256	39.000	106.0

Mean	95% CL Mean		Std Dev	95% CL Std Dev	
80.813	80.310	81.315	10.507	10.163	10.875

Comments: There are 1,681 cases with mean of 80.813 and standard deviation of 10.507, and the values ranged from 39 to 106. The confidence interval lies between (80.310, 81.315). Since this range does not contain 78.8, we declare that they are different.

DF	t Value	Pr > |t|
1680	7.85	<.0001

Comments: The test statistic for the t-test is 7.85. A p-value for this test assuming a two-tailed test gives a p-value of <.0001. Thus the data show that age at death is significantly different from a value of 78.8.

2.4.2 R Syntax and Output for a One-Sample t-Test

The R syntax follows:

```
¹t.test(AD_dta$AGEDEATH,mu=78.8,alternative=c("two.sided"))
```

[1]The R function t.test() performs *t*-tests. The inputs include the variable being evaluated, the mean value being tested (mu=), as well as the specification of the alternative hypothesis (alternative=), which has the options "two.sided," "less," or "greater."

R OUTPUT

```
t.test(AD_dta$AGEDEATH,mu=78.8,alternative=c("two.sided"))
##
##   One Sample t-test
##
## data:   AD_dta$AGEDEATH
## t = 7.8536, df = 1680, p-value = 7.152e-15
## alternative hypothesis: true mean is not equal to 78.8
## 95 percent confidence interval:
##   80.30998 81.31525
## sample estimates:
## mean of x
##   80.81261
```

Comments: The test statistic is 7.85, and the *p*-value is <0.0001. The 95% confidence interval for the age at death for AD patients is (80.31, 81.32), and because the average age of death of the US population is 78.8 and outside of this mean, the age at death for AD patients in our sample is significantly different.

2.4.3 SPSS Syntax and Output for a One-Sample t-Test

The SPSS syntax follows:

```
T-TEST
  /TESTVAL=78.8
  /MISSING=ANALYSIS
  /VARIABLES=AGEDEATH
  /CRITERIA=CI(.95).
```

SPSS OUTPUT

One-Sample Statistics				
	N	Mean	Std. Deviation	Std. Error Mean
AGEDEATH	1681	80.81	10.507	.256

One-Sample Test

	Test Value = 78.8					
					95% Confidence Interval of the Difference	
	t	df	Sig. (2-tailed)	Mean Difference	Lower	Upper
AGEDEATH	7.854	1681	.000	2.013	1.51	2.52

Comments: The sample mean is 80.81, with standard error of 0.256. This gives a t-test statistic value of $t = (80.81 - 78.8)/0.256 = 7.854$. The p-value for testing is 0.000. Thus the mean of our sample is different from the national average. The confidence interval of the difference is (1.51, 2.52), which does not contain zero. The confidence interval for age at death is (81.32, 83.16), and it does not contain 78.8.

2.4.4 Stata Syntax and Output for a One-Sample t-Test

The Stata syntax follows:

```
. ttest agedeath == 78.8
```

STATA OUTPUT

One-Sample T Test

Variable	Obs	Mean	Std. Err.	Std. Dev.	[95% Conf. Interval]	
agedeath	1,681	80.812	.256	10.507	80.310	81.315

mean = mean (agedeath)   t = 7.854

Ho: mean = 78.8   degrees of freedom = 1680

Ha: mean < 78.8   Ha: mean != 78.8   Ha: mean > 78.8
Pr(T < t) = 1.000   Pr(|T| > |t|) = 0.000   Pr(T > t) = 0.00

Comments: The sample mean is 80.812, with standard error of 0.256. This gives a t-test statistic value of $t = (80.81-78.8)/0.256 = 7.854$. Since we are interested in the two-sided t-test, we look at the column where the alternative hypothesis (H_a) is the mean and is not equal to (!=) 78.8. The p-value for testing this hypothesis is 0.000. Thus the mean is different from the national average. The confidence interval for the mean is (80.310, 80.315), which does not contain 78.8 years.

2.5 Statistical Test for Comparing Continuous Population Means

The comparison of two population means is common. The null hypothesis of this test is written in statistical form as

$$H_0: \mu_1 = \mu_2 \text{ or } H_0: \mu_1 - \mu_2 = 0.$$

The research goal, or alternative hypothesis, is one of these:

$$H_a: \mu_1 \neq \mu_2 \text{ or } H_a: \mu_1 > \mu_2 \text{ or } H_a: \mu_1 < \mu_2.$$

The test statistic is calculated as

$$t = \frac{(\bar{y}_1 - \bar{y}_2) - (\mu_1 - \mu_2)}{\sqrt{\dfrac{s_1^2}{n_1} + \dfrac{s_2^2}{n_2}}}.$$

Its value is compared to the critical value t_α^* based on the significance level α.

For example, we consider the life expectancies of AD and normal patients. The average lifespan of AD patients in our sample is 80.8 years, while the average lifespan for normal patients is 86.2 years within the data. These are sample values, however. Our interest is in the population. In our example, we are interested in testing if on average the lifespan of normal patients is significantly higher than the lifespan of AD patients. This is our research or alternative hypothesis, H_a: $\mu_N > \mu_{AD}$, which is also written as H_a: $\mu_N - \mu_{AD} > 0$. We use statistical software to perform a two-sample t-test and find that the age at death for normal patients is significantly higher for AD patients within our cohort of data (t-value = 8.88, p-value < 0.0001).

When we perform statistical tests or obtain confidence intervals, we make certain distributional assumptions. One of these assumptions is to believe that there are equal variances across the subpopulations, which is known as homoscedascity. Welch's t-test allows one to move forward regardless of whether there is homoscedascity or heteroscedascity (nonconstant variance). Welch's t-test, also known as the unequal variances t-test, is an adjustment of the two-sample t-test, which allows for unequal variances between the two groups. For this method, the degrees of freedom (DF) is approximated using the Satterthwaite equation

$$DF = \frac{\left(\dfrac{s_1^2}{n_1} + \dfrac{s_2^2}{n_2} \right)^2}{\dfrac{s_1^4}{n_1^2(n_1-1)} + \dfrac{s_2^4}{n_2^2(n_2-1)}},$$

where s_1 and s_2 are the standard deviations and n_1 and n_2 are the sample sizes of groups 1 and 2, respectively. After adjusting for unequal variances in the two groups, we perform a Welch's t-test to obtain a comparison of the means between the two groups.

Returning to the previous example, we evaluate the variances of the lifespans of normal and AD patients. The null hypothesis for the equality of variances test is that the variances between the two groups are equal,

$$H_0: \sigma_1^2 = \sigma_2^2.$$

From the equality of variances test shown in the statistical output below, the p-value is 0.0174. Since this p-value is less than $\alpha = 0.05$, it suggests that there are unequal variances, or that is heteroscedasticity, between the two groups. We use the Satterthwaite adjustment for unequal variances, and although we obtain the same conclusion, the t-statistic is found to be 9.50 with a p-value < 0.0001. We conclude that the age at death for normal patients is significantly higher than the age of patients diagnosed with AD in our cohort.

Problem: We wish to compare the means of AD patients to normal patients as it pertains to the age at death. Do the means differ?

Solution: We have evidence of differences between those with AD diagnosis and those without.

t	df	Sig. (2-tailed)	Mean Difference	Std. Error Difference	95% Confidence Interval of the Difference	
					Lower	Upper
−8.883	2029	.000	−5.396	.607	−6.587	−4.205

The differences between the groups is 8.883, the p-value is .000, and 95% confidence interval is $(-6.587, -4.205)$.

2.5.1 SAS Syntax and Output for a Two-Sample t-Test

The SAS syntax follows:

```
¹PROC TTEST DATA=CHAP2 ALPHA=0.05;
²CLASS DIAGNOSIS;
³VAR AGEDEATH;
RUN;
```

[1]The SAS procedure PROC TTEST is used to conduct the two-sample *t*-test.

[2]CLASS is a SAS word that indicates which variables are categorical or binary.

[3]The response variable is age at death.

SAS OUTPUT

```
                    The TTEST Procedure
                    Variable: AGEDEATH
```

Diagnosis	N	Mean	Std Dev	Std Err	Minimum	Maximum
AD	1681	80.813	10.507	0.256	39.000	106.0
Normal	350	86.209	9.489	0.507	38.000	104.0
Diff (1 − 2)		−5.396	10.339	0.608		

Comments: The mean age at death for the AD group (80.81 years) is compared to the mean age at death of the normal group (86.21 years). The statistical difference is −5.396.

Diagnosis	Method	Mean	95% CL Mean		Std Dev	95% CL Std Dev	
AD		80.813	80.310	81.315	10.507	10.163	10.875
Normal		86.209	85.211	87.206	9.489	8.834	10.249
Diff (1 − 2)	Pooled	−5.396	−6.587	−4.205	10.339	10.030	10.667
Diff (1 − 2)	Satterthwaite	−5.396	−6.512	−4.280			

Comments: The confidence interval for each group is given above in the 95% CL Mean column. Our interest is in the confidence interval for the difference, however. The pooled (−6.587, −4.205) and the Satterthwaite (−6.512, −4.280) confidence intervals are the 95% confidence interval estimates for the differences. These intervals do not contain zero. The *p*-values are less than 0.0001 for equal variance or unequal variances. The *p*-value for checking the equality of variances was 0.0174.

Method	Variances	DF	t Value	Pr > |t|
Pooled	Equal	2029	−8.88	<.0001
Satterthwaite	Unequal	542.6	−9.50	<.0001
	Equality of Variances			
Method	Num DF	Den DF	F Value	Pr > F
Folded F	1680	349	1.23	0.017

Comments: The equality of variances test is used to determine whether the two groups have equal variances. Since $p = 0.017 < 0.05$, there is evidence that the variances between the two groups are not equal, and thus the Satterthwaite confidence interval should be used. This is determined by using an F-test with numerator degrees of freedom (Num DF) 1,680 and denominator degrees of freedom (Den DF) 349.

2.5.2 R Syntax and Output for a Two-Sample t-Test

The R syntax follows:

```
#Two group t-test
¹t.test(normal_dta$AGEDEATH,AD_dta$AGEDEATH,alternative=c
("greater"),var.equal=TRUE)
#Welch's t-test
²t.test(normal_dta$AGEDEATH,AD_dta$AGEDEATH,alternative=c("great
er"),var.equal=FALSE)
```

[1]The t.test() function performs the two-sample t-test. When the option var.equal=TRUE, it indicates equal variances between the two groups and that the two-sample t-test should be used.
[2]To perform a Welch's t-test for unequal variances, specify the option var.equal=FALSE.

R OUTPUT

```
#Two group t-test
t.test(normal_dta$AGEDEATH,AD_dta$AGEDEATH,alternative=c("greater"),var.
equal=TRUE)
##
##   Two Sample t-test
##
## data:  normal_dta$AGEDEATH and AD_dta$AGEDEATH
## t = 8.8829, df = 2029, p-value < 2.2e-16
## alternative hypothesis: true difference in means is greater than 0
## 95 percent confidence interval:
##   4.396335       Inf
## sample estimates:
## mean of x mean of y
##   86.20857   80.81261
#Welch's t-test
t.test(normal_dta$AGEDEATH,AD_dta$AGEDEATH,alternative=c("greater"),var.
equal=FALSE)
##
##   Welch Two Sample t-test
##
## data:  normal_dta$AGEDEATH and AD_dta$AGEDEATH
## t = 9.4957, df = 542.6, p-value < 2.2e-16
## alternative hypothesis: true difference in means is greater than 0
## 95 percent confidence interval:
##   4.459668       Inf
## sample estimates:
## mean of x mean of y
##   86.20857   80.81261
```

Comments: For the two-sample t-test, we obtain a t-statistic of 8.883 and a p-value < 0.0001. For the Welch's two-sample t-test, the test statistic is 9.496, and the p-value is < 0.0001. Both confidence intervals report the 95% confidence interval for difference in age at death between normal and AD groups. Using both methods, we find that the mean of ages at death for the normal and AD groups are significantly different.

2.5.3 SPSS Syntax and Output for a Two-Sample t-Test

The SPSS syntax follows:

```
T-TEST GROUPS=Diagnosis('AD' 'Normal')
   /MISSING=ANALYSIS
   /VARIABLES=AGEDEATH
   /CRITERIA=CI(.95).
```

SPSS OUTPUT

Group Statistics

	Diagnosis	N	Mean	Std. Deviation	Std. Error Mean
AGEDEATH	AD	1681	80.81	10.507	.256
	Normal	350	86.21	9.489	.507

Comments: Two-sample t-test: t-statistic (-5.396) and p-value (0.000). Means of age at death for the normal and AD groups are different. A 95% confidence interval for difference in age at death between normal and AD groups is (-6.512, -4.280).

Independent Samples Test

		Levene's Test for Equality of Variances		t-test for Equality of Means						
		F	Sig.	t	df	Sig. (2-tailed)	Mean Difference	Std. Error Difference	95% Confidence Interval of the Difference	
									Lower	Upper
AGEDEATH	Equal variances assumed	7.569	.006	-8.883	2029	.000	-5.396	.607	-6.587	-4.205
	Equal variances not assumed			-9.496	542.60	.000	-5.396	.568	-6.512	-4.280

2.5.4 Stata Syntax and Output for a Two-Sample t-Test

The Stata syntax follows:

```
. ttest agedeath, by(diagnosis) unequal welch
```

STATA OUTPUT

Two-sample t-test with unequal variances

```
Group |    Obs     Mean   Std. Err.  Std. Dev. [95% Conf. Interval]
  AD |   1,681   80.813    .256       10.507   [80.310   81.315]
Normal|    350   86.209    .508        9.489   [85.211   87.206]
combined| 2,031  81.742    .234       10.535   [81.284   82.201]
 diff |         -5.396     .568                [-6.512   -4.280]
diff = mean(AD) - mean(Normal)                     t = -9.4957
Ho: diff = 0          Welch's degrees of freedom = 543.674
Ha: diff < 0       Ha: diff != 0    Ha: diff > 0
Pr(T<t) = 0.0000   Pr(|T| > |t|) = 0.0000       Pr(T>t) = 1.000
```

Comments: The confidence interval for the difference is (−6.512, −4.280). These intervals do not contain zero. The p-value is 0.0000 for the test of equal variances, which suggests unequal variances.

2.6 Simple Linear Regression

In the one-sample t-test, we consider one variable of interest, the response, and do not account for any input variables. In the two-sample t-test, we consider one variable of interest (or the response) and account for one binary predictor. We now consider the simple linear regression model where there is one continuous response and one continuous predictor. It describes the impact of covariate (X) on the outcome (Y) through some parameter (β). Simple linear regression refers to the special case when the impact of one predictor is being evaluated on the outcome variable. It is called a marginal mean or population averaged model. It tells about the mean of a continuous distribution.

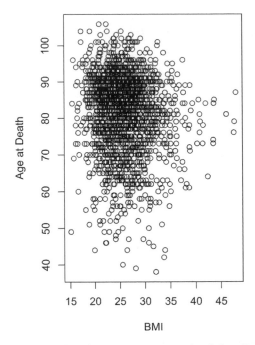

Figure 2.8 Scatterplot of BMI versus age at death for all patients.

Consider a scatterplot of BMI versus age at death for 2,031 patients (fig. 2.8). The scatterplot provides a visualization of the relationship between BMI and age at death. It appears that, in general, as BMI increases, the age at death tends to decrease, but it appears this only happens up to a certain age. This is referred to as the anorexia of aging.

We quantify and describe the relationship between these two variables in terms of the parameters, the intercept β_0 and the slope β_1, such that for each observation

$$Y_i = \beta_0 + \beta_1 X_{i1} + \varepsilon_i,$$

where X_{i1} is the value of the predictor and ε_i is the random variation. In this case, for one predictor (denoted as X), we would like to estimate the parameters β_0 and β_1. In particular, we wish to evaluate the relationship between BMI and age at death for all subjects in our sample (normal and AD diagnoses). We fit the simple linear regression model

$$\text{expected (age at death)} = \hat{\beta}_0 + \hat{\beta}_1 \text{ BMI.}$$

We seek to identify the relationship between these two variables using a linear model. If this relationship holds, we describe it in a few different ways. We may say that BMI drives age at death, or that there is a relationship between age at death and BMI. Moreover, we may say that BMI is a significant predictor of age at death. The strength of this model lies in its ability to identify linear relationships to some degree of accuracy.

In linear modeling, there are a few key assumptions. First, we assume that the outcome Y follows a normal distribution for any values of the predictor X. Thus there is a range of possible outcomes we may see for a particular value of X, which is described by the normal distribution. The second assumption, as mentioned previously, is that for each subpopulation of X, we have constant variance or homoscedasticity. The third key assumption is that the observations are independent. This is crucial and often overlooked. By independence, we mean that the mechanism that gives rise to this observation has nothing to do with the other observation. In chapters 4 and 5, we consider the case when this assumption is not met.

Problem: Does BMI affect the age at death for these Alzheimer's patients based on the data?

Solution: For now, we want to highlight the facts once you obtain the model.

		Parameter Estimates			
Variable	DF	Parameter Estimate	Standard Error	t Value	Pr > |t|
Intercept	1	87.945	1.370	64.20	<.0001
BMI	1	−0.240	0.052	−4.59	<.0001

The parameter estimates, based on the data, are given as the equation

$$\widehat{\text{age at death}} = 87.95 - 0.24\,\text{BMI}.$$

The hat symbol $(\char`\^)$ over the outcome indicates a predicted value or a model-estimated value. The slope parameter estimate for BMI, $\hat{\beta}_1 = -0.24$, has a p-value < 0.0001, which indicates that BMI is a statistically significant predictor of age at death. The negative sign indicates that age at death and BMI are negatively associated. As BMI increases, the predicted age at death decreases. The fitted regression line for this data is overlaid on the scatterplot of age at death versus BMI (fig. 2.9).

For a given BMI value, we provide a prediction of the average patient's age at death. For example, for a patient from a subpopulation of BMI of 30 at the baseline visit, we predict the age at death as $87.95 - 0.24(30) = 80.75$ years. The intercept parameter β_0 is estimated

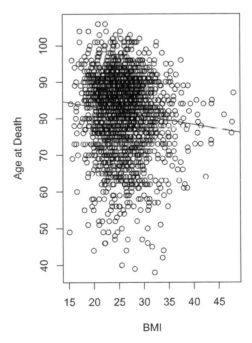

Figure 2.9 Scatterplot of BMI versus age at death with regression line.

to be 87.95. The interpretation of the intercept is that when BMI is zero, we expect age at death to be 87.95 years, although it does not make sense in this case. Moreover, when making predictions from a linear regression equation, it is advised not to go beyond the scope of the data. For example, in the data, the BMI ranges from 15.1 to 48. Thus it is only appropriate to predict the age at death for patients with BMI values in this range. To talk about age at death at 87.95 years, we would need BMI to be zero, and zero is beyond the scope of the data. We show how to obtain linear regression results in SAS, R, SPSS, and Stata.

2.6.1 SAS Syntax and Output for Simple Linear Regression

The SAS syntax follows:

```
¹PROC REG DATA=CHAP2;
²MODEL AGEDEATH=BMI;
RUN;
```

[1]PROC REG is used for linear regression.
[2]Fits a linear model. The output variable is listed on the left, and the predictor is on the right.

SAS OUTPUT

The REG Procedure

Dependent Variable: AGEDEATH

Source	DF	Sum of Squares	Mean Square	F Value	Pr > F
Model	1	2320.426	2320.426	21.11	<.0001
Error	2029	223000	109.906		
Corrected Total	2030	225320			

Comments: This model consists of BMI as a predictor and returns a model that reveals a p-value of <0.0001. It tells us that BMI is a significant predictor in modeling age at death within our dataset. The F-value for $H_0: \beta_1 = 0$ versus $H_a: \beta_1 \neq 0$ is 21.11, with a p-value of <0.0001.

There are 225,320 variation units to be explained by BMI. BMI only explained 2,320.426, or 1.03%, however.

Root MSE	10.484	R-Square	0.0103
Dependent Mean	81.742	Adj R-Sq	0.010
Coeff Var	12.825		

Comments: Though the BMI is significant in modeling age at death, it only explains (2,320.425/225,320) = 1.03% of the variation in age at death. There are other predictors of importance that we should consider. While BMI is a statistically significant predictor, we may not want to rely on a model with only one variable.

		Parameter Estimates			
Variable	DF	Parameter Estimate	Standard Error	t Value	Pr > |t|
Intercept	1	87.945	1.370	64.20	<.0001
BMI	1	−0.240	0.052	−4.59	<.0001

Comments: The model is written as: $\overline{\text{age at death}} = 87.95 - 0.24 \text{ BMI}$. The negative association between BMI and age at death (−0.240) is significant (p-value < 0.0001). The negative slope indicates that higher BMI is associated with a younger age at death.

Comments: Figures 2.10 and 2.11 display plots that evaluate the fit of the data. Residual plots are important diagnostics that identify what is wrong or need attention in the model. We look for patterns in residual plots to help identify possible problems.

2.6.2 R Syntax and Output for Simple Linear Regression

The R syntax follows:

```
#Simple linear regression
¹reg <- lm(AGEDEATH~BMI,data=chap2)
²summary(reg)
```

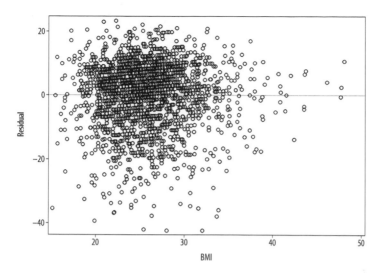

Figure 2.10 Residual plot for age at death.

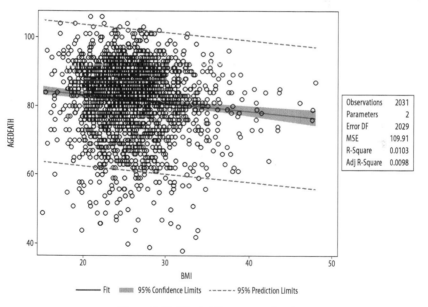

Observations	2031
Parameters	2
Error DF	2029
MSE	109.91
R-Square	0.0103
Adj R-Square	0.0098

——— Fit ▨▨▨ 95% Confidence Limits ‒‒‒‒‒ 95% Prediction Limits

Figure 2.11 Fit plot for age at death.

```
#scatterplot
³plot(dta$BMI,dta$AGEDEATH,main="Scatterplot of BMI vs Age of
Death",
     xlab="BMI",ylab="Age of Death")
```

[1]The function lm() fits linear models. It requires the outcome variable to be specified first, followed by ~ and the predictor's name. The model fit and output are saved to reg1.

[2]The summary statement provides an output of the regression model (reg1).

[3]The scatterplot is generated using the plot() statement in R.

R OUTPUT

```
summary(reg)
##
## Call:
## lm(formula = AGEDEATH ~ BMI, data = chap2)
##
## Residuals:
##     Min      1Q  Median      3Q     Max
## -42.241  -5.957   1.911   7.483  23.407
##
## Coefficients:
##              Estimate Std. Error t value Pr(>|t|)
## (Intercept) 87.94521    1.36982  64.202  < 2e-16 ***
## BMI         -0.24000    0.05223  -4.595 4.6e-06 ***
## ---
## Signif. syntaxs:  0 '***' 0.001 '**' 0.01 '*' 0.05 '.' 0.1 ' ' 1
##
## Residual standard error: 10.48 on 2029 degrees of freedom
## Multiple R-squared:  0.0103, Adjusted R-squared:  0.009811
## F-statistic: 21.11 on 1 and 2029 DF,  p-value: 4.596e-06
```

Comments: This model consists of BMI and returns a model that reveals a p-value of <0.0001. It tells us that BMI is a significant predictor in modeling age at death within our dataset. Though the BMI is significant in modeling age at death, it only explained 1.03% of the variation in age at death. The model is written as:

$$\overline{\text{age at death}} = 87.95 - 0.24\,\text{BMI}.$$

The negative impact of BMI on age at death (-0.24) is significant (<0.0001).

2.6.3 SPSS Syntax and Output for Simple Linear Regression

The SPSS syntax follows:

```
REGRESSION
  /MISSING LISTWISE
  /STATISTICS COEFF OUTS CI(95) R ANOVA
  /CRITERIA=PIN(.05) POUT(.10)
  /NOORIGIN
  /DEPENDENT AGEDEATH
  /METHOD=ENTER BMI.
```

SPSS OUTPUT

Model Summary

Model	R	R Square	Adjusted R Square	Std. Error of the Estimate
1	.101	.010	.010	10.484

a. Predictors: (Constant), BMI

Comments: The model, which includes an intercept term (constant) and BMI, only explains 1.0% of the variation in age at death. An estimate of the constant variance in the model is $10.48^2 = 109.83$. A measure of the correlation between the age at death and the model value for the age at death is 0.101.

ANOVA

Model	Sum of Squares	df	Mean Square	F	Sig.
1 Regression	2320.426	1	2320.426	21.113	.000
Residual	222999.897	2029	109.906		
Total	225320.323	2030			

a. Dependent Variable: AGEDEATH
b. Predictors: (Constant), BMI

Comments: This model consists of BMI and returns a model that reveals a p-value of .000. This result indicates that BMI is a significant predictor for modeling age at death in our data.

Coefficients

Model	Unstandardized Coefficients B	Std. Error	Standardized Coefficients Beta	t	Sig.	95.0% Confidence Interval for B Lower Bound	Upper Bound
1 (Constant)	87.945	1.370		64.202	.000	85.259	90.632
BMI	-.240	.052	-.101	-4.595	.000	-.342	-.138

a. Dependent Variable: AGEDEATH

Comments: The model is $\overline{\text{age at death}} = 87.95 - 0.24$ BMI.
The negative association between BMI and age at death (-0.240) is significant (p-value < 0.0001). While BMI is significant in modeling age at death, previous output showed that BMI only explains 1.03% of the variation in age at death. Thus other predictors should be considered.

2.6.4 Stata Syntax and Output for Simple Linear Regression

The Stata syntax follows:

```
.regress agedeath bmi, beta
```

STATA OUTPUT

Source	SS	df	MS				
				Number of obs	=	2,031	
				F(1, 2029)	=	21.11	
Model	2320.426	1	2320.426	Prob > F	=	0.000	
Residual	222999.897	2,029	109.906	R-squared	=	0.010	
				Adj R-squared	=	0.010	
Total	225320.323	2,030	110.995	Root MSE	=	10.484	

AGEDEATH	Coef.	Std. Err.	t	P>t	Beta
bmi	-.240	.0522	-4.59	0.000	-.101
_cons	87.945	1.370	64.20	0.000	.

Comments: Though the BMI is significant in modeling age at death, it only explains 1.0% of the variation in age at death. The model is age at death $= 87.95 - 0.24$ BMI. The negative association between BMI and age at death (-0.240) is significant (p-value < 0.0001).

2.7 Multiple Linear Regression

In section 2.6, we discussed simple linear regression, which has one predictor. In practice, it is common to see a regression analysis with more than one predictor. We refer to such as multiple regression. For example, we may wish to predict a patient's age at death based on numerous predictors, including BMI, diagnosis (DX, AD vs. normal), hypertension, hypercholesterolemia, or diabetes). There are now six regression parameters of interest, one for the intercept (β_0) and one each for the five predictors (β_1 through β_5) such that

$$E \text{ (age at death)} = \beta_0 + \beta_1 \text{BMI} + \beta_2 \text{DX} + \beta_3 \text{hypertenison} + \beta_4 \text{hyperglocermia} + \beta_5 \text{diabetes}.$$

This model is not complete until we provide the assumptions. As was discussed with simple linear regression, there are three primary assumptions. We assume that each subpopulation provides a population of responses that if plotted will look like a normal distribution (bell-shaped curve, with equal variance around the mean). In addition, we assume that the variance of the responses at each subpopulation is the same and that the outcomes are produced on the basis of a mechanism, which is different from other cases. Note that in simple linear regression we used a scatterplot to visualize the relationship between the predictor and the outcome. Although evaluating scatterplots can help us to understand the impact of one covariate on the outcome, it does not account for correlation among the predictors. This phenomenon, known as multicollinearity, may exist in the data and can create contradictory results in a multivariable setting. Some programs will report multicollinearity statistics if you ask for it, while others produce multicollinearity statistics by default. We measure multicollinearity with the variance inflation factor (VIF) and tolerance. If VIF > 10 or tolerance < 0.01, then we declare that multicollinearity is present. Multicollinearity is only a problem if you are interested in determining which of the covariates affect the model best on a differential basis. If one is interested in prediction, then multicollinearity is not a factor.

Problem: Do BMI, diagnosis (AD vs. normal), hypertension, diabetes, and hypercholesterolemia affect the age at death?

Solution: For now, we concentrate on explaining the results obtained. In the example data, we obtain the following fitted multiple linear regression model:

$$\overline{\text{age at death}} = 92.07 - 0.30\,\text{BMI} - 5.03(\text{DX} = \text{AD}) \\ + 3.89\,\text{HT} + 0.01\,\text{HC} - 1.01\,\text{DB}$$

where BMI, Alzheimer's diagnosis (as opposed to normal), hypertension (HT), hypercholesterolemia (HC), and diabetes (DB) are predictors. Table 2.3 summarizes the parameter estimates, standard errors, and the p-values for each covariate.

Table 2.3 Multiple Linear Regression Model Fit

Covariate	Parameter Estimate	Std Err	p-Value
Intercept	92.07	1.43	<0.0001
BMI	−0.30	0.05	<0.0001
DX = AD	−5.03	0.60	<0.0001
Hypertension	3.89	0.48	<0.0001
Hypercholesterolemia	0.01	0.47	0.991
Diabetes	−1.01	0.81	0.211

We find that BMI, diagnosis, and hypertension are statistically significantly associated with age at death. The p-value for each of these covariates is <0.05. When we fit the simple regression model, we found that BMI was significantly negatively associated with age at death. In this multivariable setting, BMI still has a negative association with age at death. While this is comforting, we do not always expect to see this trend owing to multicollinearity.

We started the regression section with a continuous variable as the predictor. But in our multivariable setting we included several predictors, of which some are binary. Because a binary variable does not have a numeric ordering, we cannot interpret the parameter estimate in the same way we did with a continuous covariate. Binary variables have values such as present or absent, and they cannot be discussed in terms of increasing or decreasing. We begin with identifying which of the two categories of the binary variable is coded as the reference category. The reference category takes on the value 0. For example, for the binary variable DX, the parameter estimate is −5.03 and the reference category (DX = 0) is a normal diagnosis. This suggests that, on average, if we compare two patients and the only difference is the diagnosis (normal vs. AD), the patient diagnosed with AD is expected to live 5.03 years less than the patient with a normal diagnosis based on the data analyzed. The p-value of <0.0001 shows that it is significant difference. Similarly, patients with hypertension are found to be associated with a higher age at death compared to patients with no such diagnosis. Nonintuitive results such as these require further in-depth assessment. For example, we may have survival bias present in our data, as we are only evaluating patients that have lived long enough to be evaluated at an ADC, as well as understanding recruitment bias within each center.

We can fit a multiple linear regression model using any of the four statistical software programs, SAS, R, SPSS, and Stata.

2.7.1 SAS Syntax and Output for Multiple Linear Regression

The SAS syntax follows:

```
/*METHOD 1: USING PROC REG*/
¹DATA CHAP2;
SET CHAP2;
IF DX = 8 THEN DX_RECODE = 0;
ELSE IF DX = 1 THEN DX_RECODE = 1;
RUN;
```

DX is a binary variable, recoded so that $0 =$ normal and $1 =$ AD. PROC GLM also performs regression. We demonstrate both.

```
²PROC REG DATA=CHAP2;
MODEL AGEDEATH=BMI DX HYPERTEN HYPERCHO DIABETES;
RUN;
/*METHOD 2: USING PROC GLM*/
³PROC GLM DATA=CHAP2;
CLASS DX(REF="8");
MODEL AGEDEATH=BMI DX HYPERTEN HYPERCHO DIABETES /SOLUTION;
RUN;
```

[1]In the DATA step, we recode DX to 0 (normal) and 1 (AD).
[2]PROC REG does not support categorical variables.
[3]PROC GLM is another procedure that fits the regression model. It uses the CLASS statement. The SOLUTION option in the MODEL statement allows the parameter estimates in the output.

SAS OUTPUT

Dependent Variable: AGEDEATH					
Analysis of Variance					
Source	DF	Sum of Squares	Mean Square	F Value	Pr > F
Model	5	18078	3615.693	35.33	<.0001
Error	2025	207242	102.342		
Corrected Total	2030	225320			

Comments: The five covariates jointly affect the age at death. The analysis of variance *p*-value is <0.0001, which indicates that one or more covariates significantly affect the outcome.

Root MSE	10.116	R-Square	0.080
Dependent Mean	81.742	Adj R-Sq	0.078
Coeff Var	12.376		

Comments: The five predictors provide 8% of the variation in age at death.

Parameter Estimates					
Variable	DF	Parameter Estimate	Standard Error	t Value	Pr > |t|
Intercept	1	92.073	1.428	64.49	<.0001
BMI	1	-0.304	0.052	-5.89	<.0001
DX	1	-5.025	0.599	-8.39	<.0001
HYPERTEN	1	3.892	0.483	8.06	<.0001
HYPERCHO	1	0.006	0.474	0.01	0.991
DIABETES	1	-1.010	0.807	-1.25	0.211

Comments: The five covariates simultaneously showed significance. The extra effect is only realized by BMI, DX, and hypertension, however. All

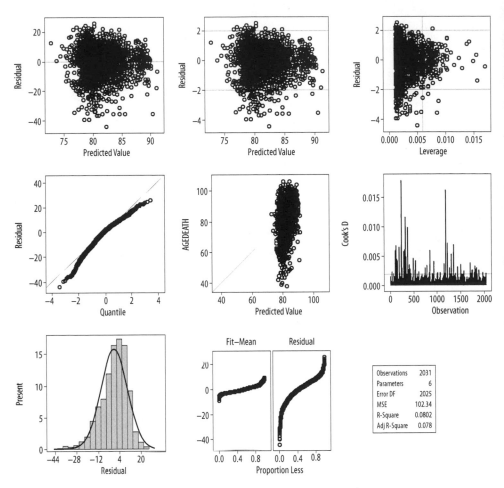

Figure 2.12 Fit diagnostics for age at death.

had p-values <0.0001. Regression parameter estimates for the model p-values for impact of the covariate on the outcome show significance for BMI, DX, and hypertension.

Comments: The residual plots in figure 2.12 give us glimpses of how the model fits. Moving across horizontally, plot 1 tells about the residual and predicted. Plot 2 tells about the residual studentized. Plot 3 is about the leverages. They tell how close the covariates are from the average. Plot 4 tells about the residuals and whether they are on a straight line to tell about normality. Plot 5 tells about the observed and predicted values. They tell how well the fit is. Plot 6 is Cook's D. These tell how influential points are to the fit. Plot 7 tells about normality for the observed Y-values. Plot 8 tells about the mean fit and the residual. We look at this to tell us how we improve.

The GLM Procedure

Dependent Variable: AGEDEATH

Source	DF	Sum of Squares	Mean Square	F Value	Pr > F
Model	5	18078.464	3615.693	35.33	<.0001
Error	2025	207241.859	102.342		
Corrected Total	2030	225320.323			

Comments: The analysis of variance p-value is <0.0001, which indicates that one or more covariates significantly affect the outcome.

R-Square	Coeff Var	Root MSE	AGEDEATH Mean
0.080	12.376	10.116	81.742

Source	DF	Type III SS	Mean Square	F Value	Pr > F
BMI	1	3550.885	3550.885	34.700	<.0001
DX	1	7206.746	7206.746	70.420	<.0001
HYPERTEN	1	6654.225	6654.225	65.020	<.0001
HYPERCHO	1	0.014	0.014	0.000	0.991
DIABETES	1	160.306	160.306	1.570	0.211

Comments: Regression parameter estimates' impact of the covariate on the outcome shows significance for BMI, DX, and hypertension. Regression parameter estimates for the model p-values for the impact of the covariate on the outcome show significance for BMI, DX, and hypertension in our cohort. This frame gives us the same results as the Analysis of Parameters table below. They both describe the residual effects.

Analysis of Parameters

Parameter		Estimate		Standard Error	t Value	Pr > |t|
Intercept		92.073	B	1.428	64.490	<.0001
BMI		-0.304		0.052	-5.890	<.0001
DX	1	-5.025	B	0.599	-8.390	<.0001
DX	8	0.000	B	.	.	.
HYPERTEN		3.892		0.483	8.060	<.0001
HYPERCHO		0.006		0.474	0.010	0.991
DIABETES		-1.010		0.807	-1.250	0.211

Comments: Regression parameter estimates' impact of the covariate on the outcome shows significance for BMI, DX, and hypertension. Regression parameter estimates for the model p-values for the impact of the covariate on the outcome show significance for BMI, DX, and hypertension. B stands for biased estimates.

2.7.2 R Syntax and Output for Multiple Linear Regression

The R syntax follows:

```
#Multiple linear regression
1chap2$DX <- as.factor(chap2$DX)
2chap2 <- within(chap2, DX <- relevel(DX, ref = "8"))
3 reg <- lm(AGEDEATH~BMI+DX+HYPERTEN+HYPERCHO+DIABETES,data=chap2)
summary(reg)
```

[1]By default, DX was defined as a numeric variable in R. DX is set as a factor variable (categorical) using the as.factor() function.
[2]The relevel function selects the reference category for a categorical variable.
[3]The lm() function is used for linear regression. The regression output is saved in reg.

R OUTPUT

```
summary(reg)
##
## Call:
```

```
## lm(formula = AGEDEATH ~ BMI + DX + HYPERTEN + HYPERCHO + DIABETES,
##     data = chap2)
##
## Residuals:
##     Min      1Q  Median      3Q     Max
## -44.302  -5.604   1.512   6.935  25.740
##
## Coefficients:
##               Estimate Std.   Error    t value  Pr(>|t|)
## (Intercept) 92.073450      1.427666   64.492   < 2e-16 ***
## BMI         -0.304408      0.051679   -5.890   4.50e-09 ***
## DX1         -5.025121      0.598829   -8.392    < 2e-16 ***
## HYPERTEN     3.892100      0.482682    8.063   1.26e-15 ***
## HYPERCHO     0.005503      0.473971    0.012      0.991
## DIABETES    -1.010091      0.807070   -1.252      0.211
## ---
## Signif. codes:  0 '***' 0.001 '**' 0.01 '*' 0.05 '.' 0.1 ' ' 1
##
## Residual standard error: 10.12 on 2025 degrees of freedom
## Multiple R-squared:  0.08023,    Adjusted R-squared:  0.07796
## F-statistic: 35.33 on 5 and 2025 DF,  p-value: < 2.2e-16
```

Comments: The analysis of variance p-value is <0.0001, which indicates that one or more covariates significantly affect the outcome. Regression parameter estimates for the model show significance. The p-values for the impact of the covariate on the outcome show significance for BMI, DX, and hypertension.

2.7.3 SPSS Syntax and Output for Multiple Linear Regression

The SPSS syntax follows:

```
REGRESSION
  /MISSING LISTWISE
  /STATISTICS COEFF OUTS CI(95) R ANOVA COLLIN TOL
  /CRITERIA=PIN(.05) POUT(.10)
```

```
/NOORIGIN

/DEPENDENT AGEDEATH

/METHOD=ENTER BMI DX HYPERTEN HYPERCHO DIABETES

/RESIDUALS DURBIN.
```

SPSS OUTPUT

Model Summary

Model	R	R Square	Adjusted R Square	Std. Error of the Estimate	Durbin-Watson
1	.284	.080	.078	10.115	1.934

Comments: The dependent variable is AGEDEATH with predictors: DIABETES, DX, HYPERCHO, BMI, and HYPERTEN. The variation explained by the predictors is 8%. An estimate of the assumed constant variance of the model is $10.12^2 = 109.38$. The Durbin-Watson (DW) value is given to check the assumption of certain type of serial correlation among the outcomes. If DW is less than d_L, conclude significance, or if DW is larger than d_u, do not conclude significance. Otherwise, we are inconclusive. We obtain d_L and d_u by looking up the Durbin-Watson tables. The DW value is 1.934. The $d_L = 1.57$, and $d_u = 1.78$. We conclude that autocorrelation is not significant.

ANOVA

	Model	Sum of Squares	df	Mean Square	F	Sig.
1	Regression	18115.635	5	3623.127	35.409	.000
	Residual	207204.688	2025	102.323		
	Total	225320.323	2030			

Comments: The analysis of variance p-value is <0.0001, which indicates that one or more covariates significantly affect the outcome. It tests the hypothesis $H_0 = \beta_1 = \ldots = \beta_5 = 0$.

Coefficients

| Model | Unstandardized Coefficients | | Standardized Coefficients | t | Sig. | 95.0% Confidence Interval for B | | Collinearity Statistics | |
	B	Std. Error	Beta			Lower Bound	Upper Bound	Tolerance	VIF
1 (Constant)	86.313	1.341		64.386	.000	83.684	88.942		
BMI									
DX	-.303	.052	-.128	-5.867	.000	-.405	-.202	.950	1.052
HYPERTEN	.717	.086	.180	8.389	.000	.550	.885	.986	1.014
HYPERCHO	3.898	.482	.184	8.089	.000	2.953	4.843	.874	1.144
DIABETES	-.001	.473	.000	-.002	.999	-.929	.928	.908	1.101
	-1.023	.736	-.031	-1.389	.165	-2.466	.421	.933	1.071

a. Dependent Variable: AGEDEATH

Comments: The dependent variable is AGEDEATH (see note a from the SPSS output) with predictors: DIABETES, DX (diagnosis), HYPERCHO (hypercholesterolemia), BMI, and HYPERTEN (hypertension). The variation explained by the predictors is 8%. BMI, diagnosis, and hypertension are significant predictors. SPSS also provides collinearity estimates, which allow one to check for multicollinearity (correlation among the predictors). Multicollinearity is only a problem if the interest is in determining which covariate best affects the model. If one is interested in prediction, then multicollinearity is not a factor. We measure multicollinearity with the variance inflation factor (VIF) and tolerance. If VIF > 10 or tolerance < .01, then we declare that multicollinearity is present. In this example, we do not have multicollinearity.

2.7.4 Stata Syntax and Output for Multiple Linear Regression

The Stata syntax follows:

```
regress agedeath dx hyperten hypercho diabetes bmi , beta
```

STATA OUTPUT

Source	SS	df	MS	Number of obs =	2,031
				F(5, 2025)	= 35.33
Model	18078.464	5	3615.693	Prob > F	= 0.000
Residual	207241.859	2,025	102.342	R-squared	= 0.080
				Adj R-squared	= 0.078
Total	225320.323	2,030	110.995	Root MSE	= 10.116

Comments: The dependent variable is AGEDEATH with predictors: DIABETES, DX, HYPERCHO, BMI, and HYPERTEN. The variation explained by the predictors is 8%. BMI, DX, and hypertension are significant predictors. The five predictors jointly affect the age at death. The analysis of variance p-value is <0.0001, which indicates that one or more covariates significantly affect the outcome.

AGEDEATH	Coef	Std Err	t	P > t	Beta
DX	0.718	0.086	8.390	0.000	0.180
HYPERTEN	3.892	0.483	8.060	0.000	0.184
HYPERCHO	0.006	0.474	0.010	0.991	0.000
DIABETES	-1.010	0.807	-1.250	0.211	-0.028
BMI	-0.304	0.052	-5.890	0.000	-0.129
_ CONS	86.330	1.341	64.370	0.000	–

Comments: Regression parameter estimates' impact of the covariate on the outcome shows significance for BMI, DX, and hypertension. Regression parameter estimates for the model p-values for impact of the covariate on the outcome show significance for BMI, DX, and hypertension. Diabetes and hypercholesterolemia are not significant.

2.8 Statistical Tests for Binary Outcomes

Modeling binary outcomes is similar to modeling continuous outcomes in that we want to model the mean parameter of the distribution with certain assumptions. We begin with one sample.

TEST OF ONE SAMPLE PROPORTION

In this case, however, the mean of the binary outcome is the proportion or the probability. In the group of patients, we have 1,681 AD patients and 350 nondemented (normal) individuals. Of patients diagnosed with AD, 140 (8.33%) have active or recent diagnosis of diabetes. Of the normal patients, 47 (13.43%) patients have been diagnosed with diabetes. Thus the proportion of patients with diabetes in the AD group is $\dfrac{140}{1{,}681} = 0.0833$, and the proportion of patients with diabetes in the normal group is $\dfrac{47}{350} = 0.134$.

We use a one-sample test of proportions as a statistical test for binary data with no predictors, to test hypotheses about population proportions. For this statistical test, the null hypothesis is $H_0\colon p = p_0$, where p_0 is the hypothesized value. The alternative hypothesis is selected as one of the following:

$$H_a: p \neq p_0$$
$$H_a: p > p_0$$
$$H_a: p < p_0.$$

The test statistic z is computed as

$$z = \frac{\hat{p} - p_0}{p_0(1 - p_0)/\sqrt{n}}$$

and is compared to the value z_α^*. Beginners sometimes ask why the test statistic follows a Z-distribution and not a t-distribution. The answer lies in the distribution. When we use the analysis for continuous data and the observations are assumed to be normally distributed, we do not know the variance, as the variance is not related to the mean in the normal data. When you deal with binary data, however, the variance is known once the mean is established.

Problem: We believe that 10% of AD patients are diabetic. In our sample of observations, the proportion of diabetic AD patients is 0.083, or 8.33%. How do the data support or dispute the claim? The hypotheses for the one-sample test of proportions is

$$H_0: p_{\text{diabetes,AD}} = 0.10$$
$$H_a: p_{\text{diabetes,AD}} < 0.10.$$

Solution: From the test of proportions, we obtain a test statistic value of 111.62, and the one-sided p-value is <0.0001. This suggests that the proportion of AD patients with diabetes is statistically significantly less than 10%. Remember, we are never asking these questions about the sample that we have, but rather about the population. There are times when we are interested in comparing the parameters from two or more populations, however. We compare proportions across two groups using the two-sample test of proportions. One uses a chi-square test for comparing proportions. But that is only applicable when the researcher is interested in two-tailed tests. In other words, the research hypothesis is about identifying a difference and not necessarily about which population has the smaller or larger proportion.

The SAS syntax follows:

```
PROC FREQ DATA=CHAP2;
TABLES DIABETES/BINOMIAL(p=0.1);
WHERE DX = 1;
RUN;
```

SAS OUTPUT

The FREQ Procedure

DIABETES	Frequency	Percent	Cumulative Frequency	Cumulative Percent
0	1541	91.67	1541	91.67
1	140	8.33	1681	100.00

Binomial Proportion

DIABETES = 0

Proportion	0.917
ASE	0.007
95% Lower Conf Limit	0.904
95% Upper Conf Limit	0.930
Exact Conf Limits	
95% Lower Conf Limit	0.903
95% Upper Conf Limit	0.930

Test of H0: Proportion = 0.1

ASE under H0	0.007
Z	111.618
One-sided Pr > Z	< .0001
Two-sided Pr > |Z|	< .0001

TEST FOR COMPARING PROPORTIONS FOR TWO GROUPS

We compare the proportion of patients with diabetes between the AD and normal groups. We are interested in testing whether the proportion of patients with diabetes in the AD group is lower than the proportion of patients with diabetes in the normal group. The hypotheses are as follows.

$$H_0: p_{\text{diabetes,AD}} = p_{\text{diabetes},N}$$
$$H_a: p_{\text{diabetes,AD}} < p_{\text{diabetes},N}$$

We perform this test with the help of statistical software (SAS, R, SPSS, and Stata) and find that, on average, the proportion of patients with diabetes in the AD group is statistically significantly lower than the proportion of patients with diabetes and a nondemented diagnosis (p-value $= 0.003$).

2.8.1 SAS Syntax and Output for Comparing Proportions for Two Groups

The SAS syntax follows:

```
PROC FREQ DATA=DTA;
     TABLES DX*DIABETES/ CHISQ;
RUN;
```

SAS OUTPUT

		Table of DX by DIABETES		
DX			DIABETES	
Frequency				
Percent				
Row Pct				
Col Pct		0	1	Total
	1	1541	140	1681
		75.87	6.89	82.77
		91.67	8.33	
		83.57	74.87	

DX			DIABETES	
	8	303	47	350
		14.92	2.31	17.23
		86.57	13.43	
		16.43	25.13	
Total		1844	187	2031
		90.79	9.21	100.00

Comments: Each cell gives the observed count, the percentage, the row percentage, and the column percentage. There are 2,031 patients.

Statistics for Table of DX by DIABETES

Statistic	DF	Value	Prob
Chi-Square	1	9.014	0.003
Likelihood Ratio Chi-Square	1	8.224	0.004
Continuity Adj. Chi-Square	1	8.414	0.004
Mantel-Haenszel Chi-Square	1	9.010	0.003
Phi Coefficient		0.067	
Contingency Coefficient		0.067	
Cramer's V		0.067	

Comments: The p-value for the test of independence is between $p = 0.003$ and $p = 0.004$, depending on which test statistic one uses. There is a significant difference between diagnosis and diabetes.

Fisher's Exact Test	
Cell (1,1) Frequency (F)	1541
Left-sided Pr <= F	0.999
Right-sided Pr >= F	0.003
Table Probability (P)	0.001
Two-sided Pr <= P	0.004

Sample Size = 2031

Comments: The Fisher's exact test, which is best for small cell values, has a *p*-value of 0.001. There is a significant difference between proportion of diabetics across diagnosis.

2.8.2 R Syntax and Output for Comparing Proportions for Two Groups

The R syntax follows:

```
¹prop.test(x = c(nrow(AD_dta[AD_dta$DIABETES==1,]),
      nrow(normal_dta[normal_dta$DIABETES==1,])),
n = c(nrow(AD_dta),
      nrow(normal_dta)), alternative = "two.sided",correct =
TRUE)
```

¹prop.test performs test of proportions. The value x = specifies the number of successes (the count of the event of interest), n = specifies the total number of trials, alternative is used to specify the alternative hypothesis being tested, and correct = TRUE implements a Yates continuity correction. In this case, we are comparing the proportion of individuals with diabetes between the AD and normal groups.

R OUTPUT

```
##
##  2-sample test for equality of proportions with continuity
##  correction
##
## data:  c(nrow(AD_dta[AD_dta$DIABETES == 1, ]),
nrow(normal_dta[normal_dta$DIABETES ==  out of c(nrow(AD_dta),
nrow(normal_dta))    1, ])) out of c(nrow(AD_dta), nrow(normal_dta))
## X-squared = 8.4142, df = 1, p-value = 0.003723
## alternative hypothesis: two.sided
## 95 percent confidence interval:
```

```
##   -0.09081232 -0.01119159
## sample estimates:
##     prop 1       prop 2
## 0.08328376 0.13428571
```

Comments: The p-value for the test of independence is $p = 0.003$ based on the chi-square test statistic. There is a significant difference proportion of diabetics based on diagnosis.

2.8.3 SPSS Syntax and Output for Comparing Proportions for Two Groups

The SPSS syntax follows:

```
GET
    SAS DATA=C:\User\Documents\Data\ch2data.sas7bdat'.
DATASET NAME DataSet1 WINDOW=FRONT.
CROSSTABS
    /TABLES=DIABETES BY DX
    /FORMAT=AVALUE TABLES
    /STATISTICS=CHISQ PHI
    /CELLS=COUNT
    /COUNT ROUND CELL
    /METHOD=EXACT TIMER(5).
```

SPSS OUTPUT

Case Processing Summary

	Cases					
	Valid		Missing		Total	
	N	Percent	N	Percent	N	Percent
DIABETES * DX	2031	100.0%	0	0.0%	2031	100.0%

DIABETES * DX Cross tabulation

Count

			DX	
		1	8	Total
DIABETES	0	1541	303	1844
	1	140	47	187
Total		1681	350	2031

Comments: Each cell gives the observed count. There are 2,031 patients.

Chi-Square Tests

	Value	df	Asymptotic Significance (2-sided)	Exact Sig. (2-sided)	Exact Sig. (1-sided)	Point Probability
Pearson Chi-Square	9.014[a]	1	.003	.003	.003	
Continuity Correction[b]	8.414	1	.004			
Likelihood Ratio	8.223	1	.004	.004	.003	
Fisher's Exact Test				.004	.003	
Linear-by-Linear Association	9.010[c]	1	.003	.003	.003	.001
N of Valid Cases	2031					

a. 0 cells (0.0%) have expected count less than 5. The minimum expected count is 32.23.
b. Computed only for a 2×2 table
c. The standardized statistic is 3.002.

Comments: The p-value for the test of independence is between $p = 0.003$ and $p = 0.004$, depending on which test statistic one uses. There is a significant difference between diagnosis and diabetes.

Symmetric Measures

		Value	Approximate Significance	Exact Significance
Nominal by Nominal	Phi	.067	.003	.003
	Cramer's V	.067	.003	.003
N of Valid Cases		2031		

Comments: These are measures of association. The approximate p and the exact p tell that there is an association. They are 0.003.

2.8.4 Stata Syntax and Output for Comparing Proportions for Two Groups

The Stata syntax follows:

```
tabulate dx_ad diabetes,    cell   chi2   exact   expected
lrchi2  rowsort
```

STATA OUTPUT

```
+--------------------+
Key
---------------------
frequency
expected frequency
cell percentage
+--------------------+
          DIABETES
AD        0            1          Total

1         1,541        140        1,681
          1,526.2      154.8      1,681.0
             75.87       6.89        82.77

0           303         47          350
            317.8       32.2        350.0
             14.92       2.31        17.23
```

```
Total           1,844            187             2,031
                1,844.0          187.0           2,031.0
                  90.79            9.21             100.00
```

Comments: Each cell gives the observed count, the percentage, the row percentage, and the column percentage. There are 2,031 patients.

```
Pearson chi2(1)             =   9.014      Pr  =   0.003
likelihood-ratio chi2(1)    =   8.224      Pr  =   0.004
Fisher's exact              =                       0.004
1-sided Fisher's exact      =                       0.003
```

Comments: The p-value for the test of independence is between $p = 0.003$ and $p = 0.004$, depending on which test statistic one uses. There is a significant difference between diagnosis and diabetes.

2.9 Statistical Tests for Categorical Outcomes

We now introduce statistical tests and models for categorical data. By categorical data, we are referring to the response variable consisting of a finite set of manageable categories, and not on some infinite quantitative scale. We review the chi-square test of independence, which is used to identify associations between the factors consisting of two or more categories and the categorical response. For example, we may be interested in investigating whether there is an association between race (several categories) and diagnosis (AD vs. normal) in our cohort. The test of independence, which is a chi-square test, addresses how the response and group factors are related by comparing the expected and observed values in each category.

Problem: We ask a question about the association between diagnosis (AD vs. normal) and gender. Questions about two variables at a time should be cautioned, as variables usually exist in a system. Bivariate analysis is good to use as a starting point in a system of variables. It should not necessarily be the end to it all.

Table 2.4 Diagnosis by Gender

	Gender		
Diagnosis	Male	Female	Total
AD	928	753	1,681
	45.69%	37.08%	82.77%
Normal	139	211	350
	6.84%	10.39%	17.23%
Total	1,067	964	2,031
	52.54%	47.46%	

Solution: The association between diagnosis (normal or AD) and gender will answer the question. We had no prior knowledge of the distribution of males and females; thus we are looking at the test of independence rather than the test of homogeneity. A contingency table of the results is given (table 2.4). The table is a 2 × 2 because there are two rows and two columns.

The chi-square test statistic is $\chi^2 = 27.88$, and the p-value is <0.0001. The small p-value (less than $\alpha = 0.05$) suggests that one cannot support the null hypothesis because there is such a low probability of its existence even though we gave it such a great chance to exist. In statistical language, we reject the null hypothesis and conclude that there is an association between diagnosis and gender. It appears based on our dataset that men are more likely to have AD.

2.9.1 SAS Syntax and Output for a Chi-Square Test

The SAS syntax follows:

```
¹PROC FREQ DATA=CHAP2;
²TABLES SEX*DX / CHISQ;
RUN;
```

¹PROC FREQ is used for testing proportions and performing chi-square tests.
²The TABLES statement creates a 2 × 2 contingency table. The CHISQ option performs the chi-square test of independence.

SAS OUTPUT

Table of SEX by DX			
SEX(SEX)	DX		
Frequency Percent Row Pct Col Pct	1	8	Total
1	928 45.69 86.97 55.21	139 6.84 13.03 39.71	1067 52.54
2	753 37.08 78.11 44.79	211 10.39 21.89 60.29	964 47.46
Total	1681 82.77	350 17.23	2031 100.00

Comments: The contingency table provides the frequency the overall percentage, the row percentage, and the column percentage. For example, in cell (1,1), there is a count of 928 with an overall percentage of 928/2,031, a row percentage of 86.97%, or 928/1,067, and a column percentage of 55.21%, or 928/1,681.

Statistics for Table of SEX by DX			
Statistic	DF	Value	Prob
Chi-Square	1	27.878	<.0001
Likelihood Ratio Chi-Square	1	27.943	<.0001
Continuity Adj. Chi-Square	1	27.260	<.0001
Mantel-Haenszel Chi-Square	1	27.864	<.0001
Phi Coefficient		0.117	
Contingency Coefficient		0.116	
Cramer's V		0.117	

Comments: There is a significant association between gender and diagnosis, $p < 0.0001$.

Fisher's Exact Test	
Cell (1,1) Frequency (F)	928
Left-Sided Pr <= F	1.0000
Right-Sided Pr >= F	<.0001
Table Probability (P)	<.0001
Two-Sided Pr <= P	<.0001

Comments: There is a significant relationship between gender and diagnosis, $p < .0001$. Fisher's exact test gave a value of $p < .0001$. The test is best for small cell frequencies.

2.9.2 R Syntax and Output for a Chi-Square Test

The R syntax follows:

```
¹tbl <- table(chap2$SEX, chap2$DX)
²chisq.test(tbl)
```

[1]The table() function creates a contingency table.
[2]The function chisq.test() performs the chi-square test of independence.

R OUTPUT

```
chisq.test(tbl)
##
##   Pearson's Chi-squared test with Yates' continuity correction
##
## data:   tbl
## X-squared = 27.26, df = 1, p-value = 1.778e-07
```

Comments: There is a significant relationship between gender and group, as the p-value for the chi-square test is $p = 1.778e\text{-}07$.

2.9.3 SPSS Syntax and Output for a Chi-Square Test

The SPSS syntax follows:

```
CROSSTABS
  /TABLES=SEX BY DX
  /FORMAT=AVALUE TABLES
  /STATISTICS=CHISQ CC PHI LAMBDA
  /CELLS=COUNT EXPECTED ROW SRESID
  /COUNT ROUND CELL
  /METHOD=EXACT TIMER(5).
```

SPSS OUTPUT

Cross tabulation of SEX * DX

			DX		Total
			1	8	
SEX	1	Count	928	139	1067
		Expected Count	883.1	183.9	1067.0
		% within SEX	87.0%	13.0%	100.0%
		Standardized Residual	1.5	-3.3	
	2	Count	753	211	964
		Expected Count	797.9	166.1	964.0
		% within SEX	78.1%	21.9%	100.0%
		Standardized Residual	-1.6	3.5	
Total		Count	1681	350	2031
		Expected Count	1681.0	350.0	2031.0
		% within SEX	82.8%	17.2%	100.0%

Comments: The contingency table provides the frequency the overall percentage, the row percentage, and the column percentage. For example, in cell (1,1), there is a count of 928 with an overall percentage of 928/2,031, a row percentage of 86.97%, or 928/1,067, and a column percentage of 55.21%, or 928/1,681.

Chi-Square Tests

	Value	df	Asymptotic Significance (2-sided)	Exact Sig. (2-sided)	Exact Sig. (1-sided)	Point Probability
Pearson Chi-Square	27.878[a]	1	.000	.000	.000	
Continuity Correction[b]	27.260	1	.000			
Likelihood Ratio	27.943	1	.000	.000	.000	
Fisher's Exact Test				.000	.000	
Linear-by-Linear Association	27.864[c]	1	.000	.000	.000	.000
N of Valid Cases	2031					

a. 0 cells (0.0%) have expected count less than 5. The minimum expected count is 166.13.
b. Computed only for a 2×2 table
c. The standardized statistic is 5.279.

Comments: There is a significant relationship between gender and diagnosis (chi-square $p < .0001$; likelihood ratio chi-square $p < .0001$). Fisher's exact test (a test best for small cell frequencies) gave a value of $p < .0001$.

2.9.4 Stata Syntax and Output for a Chi-Square Test

The Stata syntax follows:

```
tabulate sex dx, cchi2 chi2 exact lrchi2
```

STATA OUTPUT

	DX		
SEX	1	8	Total
1	928	139	1,067
	2.3	11.0	13.2
2	753	211	964
	2.5	12.1	14.6
Total	1,681	350	2,031
	4.8	23.1	27.9

```
Pearson chi2(1)             =   27.878              Pr =  0.000

likelihood-ratio chi2(1)    =   27.943              Pr =  0.000

Fisher's exact              =                             0.000

  1-sided Fisher's exact    =                             0.000
```

Comments: There is a significant relationship between gender and diagnosis (chi-square $p < 0.0001$; likelihood ratio chi-square $p < 0.0001$).
Fisher's exact test gave a value of $p < 0.0001$.

2.10 Logistic Regression Models

To model binary data, we present a set of binary models known as logistic regression models. These models identify the relationship between a set of multivariable predictors and the mean of a binary response variable on a special nonlinear scale. It interprets in the form
of odds. We define this type of model as

$$
\log\left(\frac{p}{1-p}\right) = \beta_0 + \beta_1 X_1 + \beta_2 X_2 + \beta_3 X_3 + \beta_4 X_4 + \beta_5 X_5,
$$

where p is the probability of the event occurring, $\dfrac{p}{1-p}$ is the odds of
the event occurring, and $\log\left(\dfrac{p}{1-p}\right)$ is the log odds of the event. The
binary outcome is assumed to follow a Bernoulli trial. These trials are
assumed independent, so the sum of Bernoulli trials is a binomial.
Hence we will often refer to the set of data as having a binomial distribution. As such, we know the mean (np) is the number of trials
times (n) probability (p). Its variance is $np(1-p)$. This is indication that
the variance is related to the mean, which means that as we make
statements about the mean, we are influencing the variance. This is
unlike linear regression models where the variance and the mean have
no relationship, and we assume that the variance stays constant as we
move from one subpopulation to the next. Similar to linear regression, however, X represents the covariates of interest, and β represents
the regression coefficients relating the covariates to the log odds. This

is easily converted to the odds scale or to the probability scale. Both scales lend to meaningful and easily understood interpretations.

Problem: Are diagnosis (DX), BMI, systolic blood pressure (BPSYS), diastolic blood pressure (BPDIAS), and heart rate (HRATE) associated with the probability of diabetes?

Solution: Our example models the probability of diabetes (DB) as it pertains to diagnosis (DX), BMI, systolic blood pressure (BPSYS), diastolic blood pressure (BPDIAS), and heart rate (HR). Any of the four statistical programs yield the fitted model:

$$\log\left(\frac{\hat{p}_{DB}}{1-\hat{p}_{DB}}\right) = -5.73 - 0.34\text{DX} + 0.12\text{BMI} + 0.02\text{BPSYS}$$
$$- 0.05\text{BPDIAS} + 0.02\text{HR}.$$

We find that BMI, blood pressure measurements, and heart rate are statistically significant predictors of a diabetes diagnosis, although the diagnosis of AD is not statistically significantly associated with the probability of developing diabetes. It is possible that other factors are associated with diabetes, but they were not included in this model. The coefficient for DX, the diagnosis, is -0.34, with a p-value of 0.0686. Recall that a normal diagnosis ($=0$) is the reference category, as compared to a diagnosis of AD ($=1$). Since the p-value is greater than 0.05, we know that diagnosis does not have a significant impact on the probability of diabetes. For the sake of interpretation, however, the odds ratio is $e^{-0.34} = 0.71$. Thus AD patients are 0.71 times more likely to have diabetes compared to normal patients. This interpretation is confusing; instead, we are interested in saying that normal patients are $\frac{1}{0.71} = 1.40$ times more likely to have diabetes than AD patients. Thus this would indicate that normal patients are more likely to have diabetes than AD patients are. Recall, however, that diagnosis was not statistically significant in the analysis, so we cannot draw this conclusion. We may consider the variable BMI, which was found to be statistically significantly associated with diabetes ($p < 0.0001$). The parameter estimate for BMI was 0.1228, and thus the odds ratio is $e^{0.1228} = 1.13$. This indicates that for every one-point increase in BMI, the patient is 1.13 times more likely to be diabetic. We obtained these results using any of four statistical software programs, SAS, R, SPSS, and Stata.

2.10.1 SAS Syntax and Output for Logistic Regression Models

The SAS syntax follows:

```
[1]PROC LOGISTIC DATA=CHAP2 DESCENDING;
CLASS DX(REF="8");
MODEL DIABETES = DX BMI BPSYS BPDIAS HRATE;
RUN;
[2]PROC GENMOD DATA=CHAP2 DESCENDING;
CLASS DX(REF="8");
MODEL DIABETES = DX BMI BPSYS BPDIAS HRATE/dist = BIN LINK = LOGIT;
QUIT;
```

[1]PROC LOGISTIC fits logistic regression models. By default, it gives probability that the outcome = 0. The DESCENDING option is used to model the probability that the outcome = 1.
[2]PROC GENMOD is an alternate procedure that fits generalized linear models, of which logistic regression is a member. The distribution for logistic regression is binomial (DIST = BIN), and the link function is the logit link (LINK = LOGIT). We return to this in chapter 3.

SAS OUTPUT

The LOGISTIC Procedure

Model Information	
Data Set	WORK.CHAP2
Response Variable	DIABETES
Number of Response Levels	2
Model	binary logit
Optimization Technique	Fisher's scoring

Comments: There is no closed form to solve obtain regression estimates. We rely on the Fisher's scoring algorithm as our optimization technique to obtain parameter estimates.

Ordered Value	Response Profile DIABETES	Total Frequency
1	1	187
2	0	1844

Probability modeled is DIABETES=1.

Model Convergence Status

Convergence criterion (GCONV=1E-8) satisfied.

Comments: We are modeling the probability of diabetes at present. We are doing $\log \dfrac{\text{Prob (diabetic)}}{\text{Prob (not diabetic)}}$, not $\log \dfrac{\text{Prob (not diabetic)}}{\text{Prob (diabetic)}}$. If we did, then the coefficient signs are reversed. The model converges, which is important to know.

Test	Testing Global Null Hypothesis: BETA=0 Chi-Square	DF	Pr > ChiSq
Likelihood Ratio	94.904	5	<.0001
Score	99.598	5	<.0001
Wald	89.597	5	<.0001

Comments: BMI, systolic blood pressure (BPSYS), diastolic blood pressure (BPDIAS), and heart rate (HRATE) have significant effects on diabetes in our dataset. The five covariates in the model together are significant ($p < .0001$).

```
                    Analysis of Maximum Likelihood Estimates
 Parameter   DF   Estimate   Standard Error   Wald Chi-Square   Pr > ChiSq
 Intercept    1    -5.905         0.846            48.710          <.0001
 DX           1    -0.171         0.094             3.318          0.069
 BMI          1     0.123         0.016            57.754          <.0001
 BPSYS        1     0.017         0.004            14.099          0.000
 BPDIAS       1    -0.049         0.009            29.658          <.0001
 HRATE        1     0.025         0.007            13.312          0.000
```

Comments: The fitted logistic model is:

$$\log\left(\frac{\hat{p}_{DB}}{1-\hat{p}_{DB}}\right) = -5.91 - 0.17\text{DX} + 0.12\text{BMI} + 0.02\text{BPSYS}$$
$$- 0.05\text{BPDIAS} + 0.03\text{HR}.$$

```
                              Odds Ratio Estimates
              Effect     Point Estimate     95% Wald Confidence Limits
 DX          1 vs 8          0.711               0.492          1.026
 BMI                         1.131               1.095          1.167
 BPSYS                       1.017               1.008          1.026
 BPDIAS                      0.952               0.936          0.969
 HRATE                       1.025               1.012          1.039
```

Comments: If a variable has odds ratio greater than 1, then it tells about a change in that covariate that will result in the input. For example, BMI (1.131) says that for every extra unit in BMI, a patient is 1.131 times more likely to be diabetic. This is similar for the other continuous co-variates, BPSYS and HRATE. For BPDIAS (less than 1), however, we are saying that one more unit in BPDIAS results in a patient who is 0.952 times likely to be diabetic. Therefore they are 1/0.952 times more likely to be nondiabetic. As for the binary factor DX, we are saying that someone in group DX = 1 is 0.711 times more likely to be diabetic, meaning that they are 1/0.711 times more likely to be nondiabetic.

The GENMOD Procedure

Model Information	
Data Set	WORK.CHAP2
Distribution	Binomial
Link Function	Logit
Dependent Variable	DIABETES

Comments: In chapter 3, we address generalized linear models and their three components. There, we will learn about the random component (distribution), link function, and systematic component.

PROC GENMOD Is Modeling the Probability That DIABETES='1'.

Algorithm converged.

Analysis of Maximum Likelihood Parameter Estimates

Parameter		DF	Estimate[d]	Standard Error	Wald Confidence 95% Limits		Wald Chi-Square	Pr > ChiSq
Intercept		1	-5.734	0.857	-7.415	-4.054	44.740	<.0001
DX	1	1	-0.342	0.188	-0.709	0.026	3.320	0.069
DX	8	0	0.000	0.000	0.000	0.000	.	.
BMI		1	0.123	0.016	0.091	0.154	57.750	<.0001
BPSYS		1	0.017	0.005	0.008	0.026	14.100	0.000
BPDIAS		1	-0.049	0.009	-0.066	-0.031	29.670	<.0001
HRATE		1	0.025	0.007	0.012	0.038	13.310	0.000
Scale		0	1.0000	0.0000	1.0000	1.0000		

Comments: BMI, systolic blood pressure (BPSYS), diastolic blood pressure (BPDIAS), and heart rate (HRATE) have significant effects on diabetes in our dataset.

2.10.2 R Syntax and Output for Logistic Regression Models

The R syntax follows:

```
chap2$DX <- as.factor(chap2$DX)
chap2<- within(chap2, DX <- relevel(DX, ref = "8"))
```

```
¹reg<-glm(DIABETES~DX+BMI+BPSYS+BPDIAS+HRATE,family=binomial
(link="logit"),data= chap2)
summary(reg)
```

[1]The function glm() fits logistic regression models. The distribution and link function are family=binomial(link="logit").

R OUTPUT

```
summary(reg)
##
## Call:
## glm(formula = DIABETES ~ DX + BMI + BPSYS + BPDIAS + HRATE,
family = binomial(link = "logit"),
##      data = chap2)
##
## Deviance Residuals:
##     Min       1Q    Median        3Q       Max
## -1.4983  -0.4678  -0.3629  -0.2818    2.7625
##
## Coefficients:
##               Estimate  Std. Error  z value  Pr(>|z|)
## (Intercept) -5.734441    0.857273   -6.689  2.24e-11 ***
## DX1         -0.341685    0.187600   -1.821  0.068553 .
## BMI          0.122754    0.016153    7.599  2.97e-14 ***
## BPSYS        0.016754    0.004461    3.756  0.000173 ***
## BPDIAS      -0.048787    0.008956   -5.447  5.12e-08 ***
## HRATE        0.024777    0.006791    3.649  0.000264 ***
## ---
## Signif. codes:  0 '***' 0.001 '**' 0.01 '*' 0.05 '.' 0.1 ' ' 1
##
## (Dispersion parameter for binomial family taken to be 1)
##
##     Null deviance: 1248.3  on 2030  degrees of freedom
```

```
## Residual deviance: 1153.4  on 2025  degrees of freedom
## AIC: 1165.4
##
## Number of Fisher Scoring iterations: 5
```

Comments: BMI, systolic blood pressure (BPSYS), diastolic blood pressure (BPDIAS), and heart rate (HRATE) have significant effects on diabetes in our dataset.

2.10.3 SPSS Syntax and Output for Logistic Regression Models

The SPSS syntax follows:

```
FREQUENCIES VARIABLES=DIABETES
  /NTILES=4
  /PERCENTILES=25.0 75.0
  /STATISTICS=STDDEV VARIANCE RANGE MINIMUM MAXIMUM MEAN MEDIAN
MODE SUM SKEWNESS SESKEW KURTOSIS
      SEKURT
  /ORDER=ANALYSIS.
LOGISTIC REGRESSION VARIABLES DIABETES
  /METHOD=ENTER DX BMI BPSYS BPDIAS HRATE
  /CONTRAST (DX)=Indicator
  /CLASSPLOT
  /PRINT=GOODFIT CI(95)
  /CRITERIA=PIN(0.05) POUT(0.10) ITERATE(20) CUT(0.5).
```

SPSS OUTPUT

Omnibus Tests of Model Coefficients

		Chi-square	df	Sig.
Step 1	Step	94.904	5	.000
	Block	94.904	5	.000
	Model	94.904	5	.000

Comments: BMI, systolic blood pressure (BPSYS), diastolic blood pressure (BPDIAS), and heart rate (HRATE) have significant effects on diabetes in our dataset.

Hosmer and Lemeshow Test

Step	Chi-square	df	Sig.
1	6.421	8	.600

Comments: The Hosmer and Lemeshow test tells if the model is a good fit. In this case, the test has value 6.412, with p-value 0.600. This tells that the model is a good fit.

Variables in the Equation

	B	S.E.	Wald	df	Sig.	Exp(B)	95% C.I. for EXP(B) Lower	Upper
Step 1ª DX(1)	-.342	.188	3.317	1	.069	.711	.492	1.026
BMI	.123	.016	57.749	1	.000	1.131	1.095	1.167
BPSYS	.017	.004	14.104	1	.000	1.017	1.008	1.026
BPDIAS	-.049	.009	29.669	1	.000	.952	.936	.969
HRATE	.025	.007	13.313	1	.000	1.025	1.012	1.039
Constant	-5.734	.857	44.743	1	.000	.003		

a. Variable(s) entered on step 1: DX, BMI, BPSYS, BPDIAS, HRATE.

Comments: The output reports the logistic regression parameter estimates (B) and standard errors (S.E.), the Wald chi-square statistic, degrees of freedom (df), p-value (Sig.), estimate of the odds (Exp(B)), and the 95% confidence interval for the odds. BMI, systolic blood pressure (BPSYS), diastolic blood pressure (BPDIAS), and heart rate (HRATE) have significant effects on diabetes in our dataset. If a variable has an odds ratio greater than 1, then it tells about a change in that covariate will result in the input. For example, the odds for BMI (1.131) indicate that for every extra unit in BMI, a patient is 1.131 times more likely to be diabetic. This is similar for the other continuous covariates, BPSYS and HRATE. For BPIAS (less than 1), however, we are saying that a person with one more unit in BPDIA is 0.952 times likely to be diabetic. Therefore that person is 1/0.952 times more likely to be nondiabetic. As for the binary factor DX, we are saying that someone in group DX = 1 is 0.711 times more likely to have diabetes.

2.10.4 Stata Syntax and Output for Logistic Regression Models

The Stata syntax follows:

```
logistic diabetes bmi bpsys bpdias hrate dx, coef
```

STATA OUTPUT

Logistic regression				No. of obs	= 2,031
				LR chi2(5)	= 94.90
				Prob > chi2	= 0.000
Log likelihood = -576.690				Pseudo R2	= 0.076

Diabetes.	Coef.	Std. Err.	z	P>z	[95% Conf. Interval]
BMI	0.123	0.016	7.600	0.000	[0.091, 0.154]
BPSYS	0.017	0.004	3.760	0.000	[0.008, 0.025]
BPDIAS	-0.049	0.009	-5.450	0.000	[-0.066, -0.031]
HRATE	0.025	0.007	3.650	0.000	[0.011, 0.038]
DX	0.049	0.027	1.820	0.069	[-0.004, 0.101]
_CONS	-6.125	0.847	-7.230	0.000	[-7.785, -4.465]

Comments: BMI, systolic blood pressure (BPSYS), diastolic blood pressure (BPDIAS), and heart rate (HRATE) have significant effects on diabetes in our dataset. The type of diagnosis has no impact.

2.11 Summary and Discussions

This chapter provides a brief overview of introductory statistical applications for modeling the mean of normally distributed responses and for the mean of Bernoulli responses. These models include addressing questions strictly about the mean with the use of multivariable (covariates or factors) to help explain differences in the responses. This cadre of models depends on the response and the predictors used. Some key ideas for readers to take away as they contemplate on the appropriate model to explore are:

1. Identify the response variable and the covariates and or factors.
2. Examine the assumptions and evaluate how well they are satisfied.
3. Statistical modeling is not an exact science, but the more the assumptions are satisfied, the better the fit of the model.

2.12 Exercises

Using the data subset for chapter 2 (http://www.public.asu.edu/~jeffreyw /), answer the following questions.

1. Are there differences in ages of patients with and without diabetes?
2. How do age, gender, and BMI relate to diabetes? By adding these other variables, how does it change the relationship, and what type of statistical models may one use and why?
3. Using one of the statistical programs, construct a 2 × 2 contingency table demonstrating the proportion of cases with diabetes as it compares to hypertension. Is there a statistical difference?
4. How are the data spread for the variable age at death? Does this suggest fitting different models to explain the age at death?

Chapter 3

Generalized Linear Models

3.1 Motivating Example

In dementia research, the data often consist of many different variables. Some variables may have a known effect on the onset of Alzheimer's disease (AD), while the impact of the other variables remains unknown. This chapter introduces generalized linear models (GLMs), which are used to address the challenges of identifying covariate associations. We introduce linear models and general linear models, and demonstrate how these are a subset of GLMs. We provide a number of examples as we distinguish the uses of these models. In particular, we examine how covariates typically measured in dementia research, including demographics as well as cardiovascular risk factors such as body mass index (BMI) and years of smoking, are used to predict cognitive scores and clinical diagnoses.

In order to demonstrate applications of generalized linear models, we evaluate a subset of data obtained from National Alzheimer's Coordinating Center (NACC). We have information on the baseline visits of 761 patients visiting Alzheimer's Disease Center (ADC) 4967 between October 2005 and April 2014. The information collected at the baseline visit includes demographic information as well as physical and clinical assessments. A subset of the data evaluated in this chapter is shown in table 3.1.

3.2 Introduction to Generalized Linear Models

Generalized linear models (GLMs) are an extension of linear models and general linear models. We refer to these models as marginal models, as our interest is primarily in the mean of the distribution of the outcomes. When the outcome is binary, the mean is called a proportion.

Table 3.1 Subset of Data

ADC	ID	CDRSUM	DX_AD	AGE	BMI	SEX	NIHR	DIABETES
4967	1705	4.5	1	78	28.7	1	1	0
4967	1927	0.5	1	83	29.3	1	2	1
4967	5856	5	1	87	29.5	1	1	0
4967	7646	3	0	60	34.4	1	2	1
4967	7824	1.5	0	64	25.2	2	1	0
4967	7866	7	1	78	19.6	2	1	0
4967	8553	5	0	73	26.6	1	1	0
4967	8802	0	0	67	52.1	2	1	0
4967	8956	4.5	1	68	26.9	1	1	0
4967	9747	0	0	75	20.1	2	1	0

For example, GLMs may be used to investigate whether BMI and years of smoking are different in people with a clinical diagnosis of AD compared to persons without AD. Because AD diagnosis is binary, we use the covariates BMI and years of smoking to understand the proportion of subjects with AD.

Linear models are a subset of general linear models, while general linear models are a subset of generalized linear models (fig. 3.1). General linear models are a specialized case of generalized linear models. We discuss the latter in chapters 4 and 5. We outline generalized linear models on the basis of three components.

3.2.1 Linear Models

A linear model is used to identify the impact of continuous covariates on the mean of a normally distributed response variable. For example, one may use a linear model to understand the impact of age (continuous variable) on the mean of blood pressure measurements (normally distributed population of outcomes). Linear models consist of the outcome or mean of the response (left-hand side) and the systematic part, a linear combination of a set of covariates and factors (right-hand side), which are connected by an identity link function. The outcome, or the variable of interest, is also referred to as the predicted variable, response variable, target variable, or the so-called Y variable. These models are referred to as linear models, as an identity

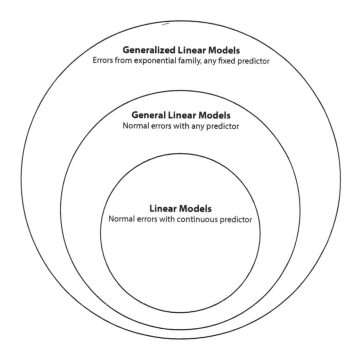

Figure 3.1 Relationship between linear models, general linear models, and generalized linear models.

link function is used to relate the mean parameter of the normal distribution and the covariates. The general form of a linear model is presented for each subject i as

$$\text{response}_i = \text{systematic part}_i + \text{error}_i.$$

The systematic or explanation part is a linear combination of covariates such that

$$\text{systematic part} = \sum_{j=1}^{p} \beta_j * X_j$$

for p covariates of interest, where β_j is the parameter indicating the impact of the covariate X_j on outcome Y. The term ϵ_i is used to represent the random error that is left unexplained after the selected covariates are taken into account. Although the errors are nonmeasurable, we assume the errors follow a normal distribution. Thus the general form of the linear model for a unit i or subject i,

$$Y_i = \beta_0 + \beta_1 X_{1i} + \beta_2 X_{2i} + \cdots \beta_p X_{pi} + \epsilon_i,$$

for the response Y, with p covariates $X_{1i}, \ldots, X_{pi}$, parameters $\beta_0, \ldots, \beta_p$, and error term ϵ_i. For the example of predicting blood pressure (outcome variable, on the left-hand side) based on age (covariate, on the right-hand side), the response would be the blood pressure measurement, and the systematic part would be a function of the patient's age such that:

$$BP_i = \beta_0 + \beta_1 * age_i + \epsilon_i.$$

The parameter β_0 is the intercept term (which denotes the predicted blood pressure (BP) when *age* is zero, which may be nonsensical), and the parameter β_1 denotes the impact of the single covariate *age* on blood pressure.

Additionally, the term *linear model* usually refers to the conventional linear regression model with a continuous response/outcome variable (left-hand side) and continuous covariates (right-hand side). It relies on the assumption that each outcome comes from a normal distribution. If the outcomes are not normally distributed, we can use a Box-Cox transformation (Box and Cox 1964) to make the response variable normally distributed. For example, in dementia research, our interest may be to predict the age of dementia onset. Most persons are diagnosed with dementia after age 65, and the risk increases as one ages; thus there are few individuals diagnosed with dementia at an early age, and many more later in life. These data are often negatively skewed and therefore not normally distributed. In order to fit a linear model on these data, we would need to transform the age of dementia onset to become approximately normally distributed. But this transformation makes the interpretation of the predictor variable more challenging.

3.2.2 General Linear Models

The term *general linear model* usually refers to conventional linear regression models with a continuous response variable (such as blood pressure) similar to the linear model, but it can include both continuous and categorical predictors (such as age and diabetes status). This allows one to incorporate predictors such as indicators for obesity status, gender, and race along with continuous predictors. General linear models include the analysis of variance (ANOVA), analysis of covariance (ANCOVA), regression analysis, factor analysis, cluster analysis, and discriminant function analysis, among others. The outcomes are assumed to originate from a normally distributed subpopulation.

3.2.3 Generalized Linear Models

The term *generalized linear model* (GLM) refers to a larger class of models, including general linear models and linear models (McCullagh and Nelder 1989; Dobson and Barnett 2008). Generalized linear models (GLMs) allow one to model the relationship between a response, which is not limited to the normal distribution, and one or more continuous and categorical predictors. In GLMs, the outcome variable has a distribution belonging to the exponential family. This allows one to model continuous, count, binary, and categorical outcomes. Generalized linear models allow one to address questions such as: How are cardiovascular risk factors (including BMI and number of years smoking), age, and gender related to whether a subject will be diagnosed with AD? In a general sense, our goal in fitting GLMs is to "explain" as much of the variability in the outcome as possible. We consider questions such as: How much variability do BMI, years smoking, age, and gender account for in AD diagnoses? If an outcome variable always had the same result, then there would be nothing to model. Our desire is to explain the difference in outcomes with predictors.

There are three components in a generalized linear model:

1. The *random component* refers to the distribution of the responses (left-hand side). It describes the unmeasurable effects in our model. These unmeasurable effects include the "pure randomness" that represents unexpected circumstances as well as additional predictors and effects that are not included in the model (such as patients from different centers or clinics, or patient attributes that were not collected during the study). Unlike linear models, the distribution does not have to be normal. For example, the binomial distribution implies the outcome is binary, and our interest is the probability of an event occurring. In fact, as previously mentioned, the random component of GLMs can follow any distribution from a family of distributions referred to as the exponential family of distributions.

2. The *systematic component* refers to the portion of the variation in the outcomes that is explained by the predictors (right-hand side). Statistically, it is specified as the linear combination of the predictors, denoted by the matrix $X = (X_1, \ldots, X_p)$ in the model, with the regression parameter β, to give $\beta_0 + \beta_1 X_1 + \cdots + \beta_p X_p$. The impact of each predictor is determined by the magnitude and direction of the corresponding parameter estimate.

3. The *link function* connects the systematic and random components. We have noted that the random component addresses the left-hand side of the model through the distribution of the outcomes. In addition, we note that the systematic component makes up the right-hand side of the model and consists of the predictors and the regression parameters $\beta_0, \ldots, \beta_p$. The link function joins the two components, thereby forming the model. The user determines the link function, although there are common link functions (canonical link) typically selected on the basis of the distribution of the random component.

In summary, a GLM consists of

$$f(\text{random component}) = \text{systematic component},$$

where the function $f(\cdot)$ represents the link function. The systematic component is a linear combination of the parameters and the predictors.

We assume a function of the mean is equal to some linear combination of the covariates. For example, when evaluating the mean of the Mini-Mental State Examination (MMSE) score or the probability of an AD diagnosis, the systematic component may be a combination of age, gender and select cardiovascular risk factors.

GLMs are a broad class of models that include linear regression, ANOVA, Poisson regression, and log-linear models, among others. A summary of GLMs is reproduced in table 3.2 (Agresti 1990). The table displays various types of GLMs, the specification of the random and systematic components, and common link functions used for these GLMs. For example, table 3.2 (row 4) shows the components of a regression model. The random component assumes a binomial distribution, the systematic component contains covariates or factors, and there is a logit link.

The fitting of statistical models is a process with the following steps:

1. *Identify the objective of the study*: What do you want to say about the outcomes?

Table 3.2 Generalized Linear Models and Components

Model	Random	Link	Systematic
Linear regression	Normal	Identity	Continuous
ANOVA	Normal	Identity	Categorical
ANCOVA	Normal	Identity	Both*
Logistic regression	Binomial	Logit	Both*
Loglinear	Poisson	Log	Categorical
Poisson regression	Poisson	Log	Both*
Multinomial response	Multinomial	Generalized logit	Both*

*Indicates continuous and categorical predictors.

2. *Model selection*: Identify the appropriate type of model for the question being investigated. There is no such thing as "the" model; rather, we say "a" model, as it is possible to consider multiple models with varying covariates.
3. *Model structure*: Determine the type of relation between the covariates and outcome.
4. *Model assumptions*: Check assumptions about the outcome and form of the data.
5. *Model fit*: Check how well the data support the relation between the predictors and outcomes.
6. *Parameter estimates and interpretation*: Identify the impact of the covariates, and interpret the effect on the outcome.

3.2.4 Assumptions When Fitting GLMs

In statistical modeling, we make certain assumptions to fit models to data. In GLMs, the assumptions are:

1. Unlike linear models, the outcomes of GLMs do not have to come from a normal distribution. We assume that it comes from a distribution that belongs to the exponential family of distributions.
2. The mechanism that gives rise to an outcome is not related to the mechanism that gives rise to other outcomes. In fact, we say that the outcomes $Y_1, \ldots, Y_n$ are independently distributed. Thus the errors are independent.
3. GLMs do not assume a linear relationship between the mean of outcome variable and the predictors, but it does assume linear relationship between a function of the mean of the distribution (specified using the link function) and the predictors. Because we are interested in a function of the mean, we often refer to these as marginal or population-averaged models.

When we fit linear models, we assume that the variance of the outcomes at any given predictor value (referred to as a subpopulation) is the same at any other predictor value. In an evaluation of the relationship between age (predictor) and blood pressure (outcome), we assume the variance of blood pressure at any age is the same. We refer to this assumption as the homogeneity of variance. We do not require this assumption when we fit GLMs, however. In many cases, this is not an issue, as for many distributions in the exponential family the variance is related to the mean.

3.2.5 Issues Affecting the Systematic Component of a GLM

It is seldom the case that the predictors in the model are uncorrelated, so it is important to understand the correlation structure among the predictors. For example, consider a patient that is obese, has elevated blood pressure, elevated fasting plasma glucose, high serum triglycerides, and/or low high-density lipoprotein (HDL) levels. In addition, if a person has at least three of these five medical conditions, he or she is considered to have metabolic syndrome and has an increased risk of type 2 diabetes and cardiovascular disease. These factors are all associated, but what if one wants to evaluate the contribution of each specific variable to a dementia diagnosis?

When two or more predictors in a model may be strongly predictive of a third predictor, a situation known as multicollinearity exists. Multicollinearity refers to the correlation between the covariates. A useful statistic for detecting multicollinearity is the variance inflation factor (VIF). If there is moderate correlation, inferences from the GLM will not be seriously affected. With significant correlation, however, we must take some precautions. The high correlation means that the information provided by the covariates is duplicated and can result in parameter estimates that lead to an incorrect conclusion. Such a model is unstable, which should be avoided. Thus it is important to look out for cases of high correlation using the variance inflation factor or some other appropriate means. A common statistical rule of thumb is that a VIF greater than 10 indicates significant multicollinearity. When two predictors are perfectly correlated, they are said to be aliased, and the GLM will not have a unique solution. When they are nearly perfectly correlated, the model may give results, but the extreme correlation will result in a highly unstable model. The fitting procedure may fail to converge, and even if the model run is successful, the estimated coefficients will be useless. Such problems are avoided by identifying and properly handling correlations among predictors. But if we fitted a statistical model for prediction rather than to understand the impact of each individual predictor, multicollinearity is not a problem.

3.2.6 Examples of Generalized Linear Models

Generalized linear models are used in many clinical studies. Consider the following analysis by Irimata et al. (2018). In the study, patients with various dementia subtypes, including AD, dementia with Lewy bodies (DLB), frontotemporal dementia (FTD), or vascular dementia (VaD) were evaluated throughout the course of the study to identify the impact of cardiovascular risk factors on cognitive change. A simplified model of the relationship between the cardiovascular risk factors and MMSE, a measure of cognitive functioning, is:

$$
\begin{aligned}
\text{MMSE} = {} & \beta_0 + \beta_1 * \text{BMI} + \beta_2 * \text{years smoking} + \beta_3 * \text{atrial fibrillation} \\
& + \beta_4 * \text{diabetes} + \beta_5 * \text{hypertension} \\
& + \beta_6 * \text{hypercholesterolemia} + \epsilon_i.
\end{aligned}
$$

This is an example of multiple linear regression.

Multiple linear regression models represent the relationship between the mean of a continuous response variable and a set of covariates. For example, we may be interested in how BMI and the number of years since the dementia diagnosis affect MMSE. We consider a GLM with an identity link and normal errors, given the scale of MMSE and that MMSE is normally distributed for each subpopulation.

1. Random component: $Y =$ MMSE is a continuous response or outcome variable that follows a normal distribution.
2. Systematic component: A linear combination of covariates that are continuous or categorical. In our example,

$$= \beta_0 + \beta_1 \text{age} + \cdots + \beta_p \text{BMI}$$

is linear in the parameters.

3. Link component: Identity link, which models the mean directly.

Model:

$$\text{mean (MMSE)} = E(\text{MMSE}) = \beta_0 + \beta_1 \text{age} + \cdots + \beta_p \text{BMI}.$$

Logistic regression models represent how a binary response variable Y depends on a set of p predictors, $X_1, \ldots, X_p$. For example, the outcome may be the presence or absence of a condition or diagnosis, such as the presence or absence of AD. The occurrence of the event is usually measured as 1, and the nonoccurrence of an event is measured as 0. Suppose we are interested in knowing whether MMSE and BMI as continuous covariates have a differential effect on AD diagnosis versus no AD diagnosis. Then our GLM has binomial error (whether or not the subject had an AD diagnosis) and a logistic link $\text{logit}(p_{\text{AD}})$. The model addresses the logit (the log odds of an event occurring) as a function of covariates. In other words, we do not look for linearity on the probability scale, but rather on the logit scale.

1. Random component: The distribution of Y is binomial, where p_{AD} is the probability of an AD diagnosis.
2. Systematic component: The covariates are age and BMI, both continuous, and thus the systematic component is $\beta_0 + \beta_1 \text{MMSE} + \beta_2 \text{BMI}$, which is linear in the parameters.
3. Link function: In logistic regression, the link function is the logit link, which is the log of the odds. The odds are the ratio of two probabilities, event versus nonevent. While binary data are commonly analyzed using logistic regression (with the logit link), they can also be modeled with other types of models such as the probit, log-log, and complimentary log-log (which implement different link functions) (table 3.2).

Our model is:

$$\log\left(\frac{p_{AD}}{p_{no\,AD}}\right) = \beta_0 + \beta_1 BMI + \cdots + \beta_p MMSE$$

Log-linear models are used to model the expected cell counts as a function of levels of categorical variables. For example, one may want to study whether a certain frequency of persons (the response has a Poisson error) with or without an AD diagnosis is associated with se- lect cardiovascular factors, such as diabetes (categorized as recent/ active or remote/inactive/absent) and hypercholesterolemia (catego- rized in three categories as recent/active, remote/inactive, or absent). One may use a log-linear model:

1. Random component: The number of patients in a certain cat- egory (the count) is our response variable, which is Poisson.
2. Systematic component: The covariates are discrete variables used in cross-classification $(2 \times 2 \times 2 \times 2 \times 3)$ and are linear in the parameters.
3. Link function: Our outcome variable is frequency of persons with and without AD. We model on the logarithmic scale; thus we have a log link.

The log-linear model is equivalent to a Poisson regression model when all explanatory variables are categorical.
Our model:

$$\log\,(\text{cell count}) = \beta_0 + \beta_1 AD + \beta_2 \text{diabetes} + \beta_3 HC_1 + \beta_4 HC_2,$$

where AD and diabetes are binary variables, and hypercholesterol- emia is a categorical variable with three categories denoted by indi- cator variables HC_1 and HC_2. The three values of hypercholesterol- emia (categorical) used two indicator variables to produce equivalent binary format as:

$HC_1 = 1$ and $HC_2 = 0$ for recent/active, $HC_1 = 0$ and $HC_2 = 1$
for remote/inactive, and $HC_1 = 0$ and $HC_2 = 0$ for absent.

Generalized linear models do the same things that linear models do and more.

1. We do not need to transform the outcome Y to have a normal distribution, as we can switch scales through the link function. We once relied on the Box-Cox transformation to obtain normality. In dementia research, GLMs are advantageous because we often evaluate outcomes that are not necessarily normally distributed.
2. Selecting the link function is separate from the choice of the random component. Thus we have more flexibility in modeling.
3. If the link produces additive effects, we do not need constant variance.
4. Generalized linear models are fit using maximum likelihood estimation, in the same way that linear models are fit. As is well known, maximum likelihood estimates have great properties.
5. All the inference methods and the model checking include chi-square tests such as the Wald and likelihood ratio tests. Similar to linear models, we can still apply statistical diagnostics.
6. Linear models have a linear predictor and an identity link. Generalized linear models have linear predictor on several scales.
7. Responses are independent. This is still true for generalized linear models.

3.3 Fitting Continuous Generalized Linear Models

We now describe how to fit GLMs with a continuous response using SAS, R, SPSS, and Stata. We evaluate the Clinical Dementia Rating Scale Sum of Boxes (CDR-SUM), which is a measure of cognitive ability and daily functioning (O'Bryant et al. 2008). The CDR-SUM is an overall dementia rating that assesses memory, orientation, judgment and problem solving, community affairs, home and hobbies, and personal care (Hughes et al. 1982). Each category is rated on a scale of

0 to 3 for a total CDR-SUM score ranging between 0 and 18. Higher scores indicate severe dementia and cognitive impairment. For the binary case, we evaluate the probability of a patient having a clinical diagnosis of AD. For both examples, we evaluate the data at baseline for 761 patients from the nonidentifiable ADC 4967. The first visit for each patient occurred between October 2005 and April 2014.

Problem: Do diagnosis, age, BMI, diabetes, hypertension, and hypercholesterolemia affect the CDR-SUM score?

Solution: We evaluate the predictors diagnosis (AD, DLB, FTD, VaD or normal), age, BMI, diabetes (DIABETES), hypertension (HYPERTEN), and hypercholesterolemia (HYPERCHO) on CDR-SUM:

$$\widehat{CDR} = -0.74 + 4.36(\text{Diagnosis} = AD) + 3.85(\text{Diagnosis} = DLB)$$
$$+ 5.21(\text{Diagnosis} = FTD) + 2.55(\text{Diagnosis} = VaD)$$
$$+ 0.03\,AGE - 0.02\,BMI + 0.17\,DIABETES$$
$$+ 0.02\,HYPERTEN - 0.49\,HYPERCHO.$$

The regression parameter estimates, standard errors, and p-values are reported in table 3.3. From our analysis, we found that diagnosis, age, and hypercholesterolemia are significant predictors of a patient's CDR-SUM score in our cohort. We fit these data using SAS, R, SPSS, and Stata.

Table 3.3 Estimates, Standard Errors, and p-Values

	Estimate	Std Err	p-Value
Intercept	−0.739	0.879	0.401
Diagnosis = AD	4.359	0.235	<0.0001
Diagnosis = DLB	3.848	0.787	<0.0001
Diagnosis = FTD	5.212	0.518	<0.0001
Diagnosis = VaD	2.546	1.008	0.012
AGE	0.025	0.009	0.006
BMI	−0.022	0.018	0.236
DIABETES	0.168	0.286	0.557
HYPERTEN	0.020	0.185	0.914
HYPERCHO	−0.487	0.182	0.007

3.3.1 SAS Code and Output

The SAS syntax follows:

```
¹PROC GENMOD DATA = CHAP3;

²CLASS DIAGNOSIS(REF="Normal");

³MODEL CDRSUM = DIAGNOSIS AGE BMI DIABETES HYPERTEN HYPERCHO;

RUN;
```

[1]PROC GENMOD fits generalized linear models.
[2]The variable DIAGNOSIS is specified as categorical. The reference category is "Normal."
[3]The model statement has no options, so by default we have linear regression.

SAS OUTPUT

Model Information		
Data Set	WORK.DTA	
Distribution	Normal	
Link Function	Identity	
Dependent Variable	CDRSUM	CDRSUM

Comments: The Model Information table indicates that the random component is normally distributed with an identity link, and the dependent variable is CDR-SUM. It summarizes the dataset being evaluated; the assumed error distribution (random component), the link function, and the dependent variable (outcome).

Class Level Information		
Class	Levels	Values
Diagnosis	5	AD DLB FTD VaD Normal

Comments: The class variable Diagnosis is categorical with five levels. The Class Level Information table lists all of the categorical variables in the dataset (specified by the CLASS statement in the SAS code) as well as the possible values for each variable.

Criteria for Assessing Goodness of Fit

Criterion	DF	Value	Value/DF
Deviance	751	4373.733	5.824
Scaled Deviance	751	761.000	1.013
Pearson Chi-Square	751	4373.733	5.824
Scaled Pearson X2	751	761.000	1.013
Log Likelihood		-1745.207	
Full Log Likelihood		-1745.207	
AIC (smaller is better)		3512.415	
AICC (smaller is better)		3512.767	
BIC (smaller is better)		3563.396	

Comments: A set of goodness-of-fit statistics reveals that the model is a good fit. The scaled deviance and scaled Pearson X2 are close to one when the fit is good. For criteria such as the Akaike's information criterion (AIC), Akaike's information criterion with a correction for small sample sizes (AICC), and the Bayesian information criterion (BIC), the values can be compared between models where smaller values indicate a better fit.

Algorithm converged.

Comments: This statement is important, as there are times when the model does not converge, so the results, if given, are useless.

Analysis of Maximum Likelihood Parameter Estimates

Parameter	Estimate	Standard Error	Wald 95% Confidence Limits		Pr > ChiSq
Intercept	-0.739	0.879	-2.463	0.985	0.401
Diagnosis AD	4.359	0.235	3.899	4.820	<.0001
Diagnosis DLB	3.848	0.787	2.306	5.390	<.0001
Diagnosis FTD	5.212	0.518	4.196	6.227	<.0001
Diagnosis VaD	2.546	1.008	0.570	4.522	0.012
Diagnosis Normal	0.000	0.000	0.000	0.000	.
Age	0.025	0.009	0.007	0.043	0.006
BMI	-0.022	0.018	-0.058	0.014	0.236
Diabetes	0.168	0.286	-0.393	0.729	0.557
Hypertension	0.020	0.185	-0.343	0.383	0.914
Hypercholesterolemia	-0.487	0.182	-0.843	-0.131	0.007
Scale	2.397	0.062	2.280	2.521	

Comments: Age, diagnosis, and hypercholesterolemia are also significant in their explanation of the differences in CDR-SUM. The maximum likelihood parameter estimates are reported in the Estimate column. These are the estimated regression coefficients. The confidence intervals for each parameter estimate are also reported in the output. The p-values for testing the significance of each covariate are reported in this column. The p-values (Pr > Chisq) tell us what is significant. Generally, a significance level of 0.05 is used such that the covariates with p-values less than 0.05 are considered significant. AD, DLB, FTD, and VaD are significantly different from normal in explaining CDR-SUM.

3.3.2 R Code and Output

The R syntax follows:

```
1dta$Diagnosis <- as.factor(dta$Diagnosis)
2dta <- within(dta, Diagnosis <- relevel(Diagnosis, ref = "Normal"))
```

```
³reg <- glm(CDRSUM~Diagnosis+AGE+BMI+DIABETES+HYPERTEN+HYPERCHO,
data=dta)
⁴summary(reg)
```

[1]The as.factor() function declares the factor variables.

[2]This statement is used to set the comparison category of diagnosis to "Normal."

[3]The glm() function is the generalized linear models function.

[4]The summary statement summarizes the model output, including the parameter estimates and *p*-values, which is saved in REG.

R OUTPUT

```
summary(reg)
##
## Call:
## glm(formula = CDRSUM ~ Diagnosis + AGE + BMI + DIABETES + HYPERTEN +
## HYPERCHO, data = dta)
##
## Deviance Residuals:
##     Min      1Q   Median       3Q      Max
## -5.3113  -1.4522  -0.0967   0.9548   8.7425
##
## Coefficients:
##                 Estimate Std. Error t value Pr(>|t|)
## (Intercept)    -0.738915   0.885221  -0.835  0.40414
## DiagnosisAD     4.359284   0.236458  18.436  < 2e-16 ***
## DiagnosisDLB    3.847654   0.791933   4.859 1.44e-06 ***
## DiagnosisFTD    5.211638   0.521409   9.995  < 2e-16 ***
## DiagnosisVaD    2.546024   1.014913   2.509  0.01233 *
## AGE             0.025179   0.009293   2.710  0.00689 **
## BMI            -0.021779   0.018484  -1.178  0.23906
## DIABETES        0.168174   0.288074   0.584  0.55954
## HYPERTEN        0.019957   0.186517   0.107  0.91482
## HYPERCHO       -0.486997   0.182852  -2.663  0.00790 **
## ---
```

```
## Signif. codes:  0 '***' 0.001 '**' 0.01 '*' 0.05 '.' 0.1 ' ' 1
##
## (Dispersion parameter for gaussian family taken to be 5.823879)
##
##     Null deviance: 6848.7  on 760  degrees of freedom
## Residual deviance: 4373.7  on 751  degrees of freedom
## AIC: 3512.4
##
## Number of Fisher Scoring iterations: 2
```

Comments: The maximum likelihood parameter estimates are reported in the Estimate column. These are the estimated regression coefficients. The confidence intervals for each parameter estimate are also reported in the output. The p-values for testing the significance of each covariate are reported. The p-values tell us what is significant. The covariates with less than 0.05 are considered significant. AD, DLB, FTD, and VaD are significantly different from normal in explaining CDR-SUM. Age, diagnosis, and hypercholesterolemia are also significant in their explanation of the differences in CDR-SUM.

3.3.3 SPSS Code and Output

The SPSS syntax follows:

```
* Generalized Linear Models.
GENLIN CDRSUM BY Diagnosis (ORDER=ASCENDING) WITH AGE BMI
DIABETES HYPERTEN HYPERCHO
  /MODEL Diagnosis AGE BMI DIABETES HYPERTEN HYPERCHO
INTERCEPT=YES
 DISTRIBUTION=NORMAL LINK=IDENTITY
  /CRITERIA SCALE=MLE COVB=MODEL PCONVERGE=1E-006(ABSOLUTE)
SINGULAR=1E-012 ANALYSISTYPE=3(WALD)
    CILEVEL=95 CITYPE=WALD LIKELIHOOD=FULL
  /EMMEANS TABLES=Diagnosis SCALE=ORIGINAL
  /MISSING CLASSMISSING=EXCLUDE
  /PRINT CPS DESCRIPTIVES MODELINFO FIT SUMMARY SOLUTION.
```

SPSS OUTPUT

Model Information

Dependent Variable	CDRSUM
Probability Distribution	Normal
Link Function	Identity

Comments: The Model Information table summarizes the specified model. In this case, the assumed error distribution for the random component is normal, the link function is the identity link, and the dependent variable evaluated is CDR-SUM.

Omnibus Test

Likelihood Ratio Chi-Square	df	Sig
342.991	9	.000

Comments: The dependent variable, CDR-SUM, and the model containing the covariates Diagnosis, AGE, BMI, DIABETES, HYPERTEN, and HYPERCHO are compared against the intercept-only model.

Parameter Estimates

Parameter	B	Std. Error	95% Wald Confidence Interval		Hypothesis Test		
			Lower	Upper	Wald Chi-Square	df	Sig.
(Intercept)	-.739	.8794	-2.462	.985	.706	1	.401
[Diagnosis=AD]	4.359	.2349	3.899	4.820	344.403	1	.000
[Diagnosis=DLB]	3.848	.7867	2.306	5.390	23.920	1	.000
[Diagnosis=FTD]	5.212	.5180	4.196	6.227	101.236	1	.000
[Diagnosis=VaD]	2.546	1.0082	.570	4.522	6.377	1	.012
[Diagnosis=Normal]	0[a]	.	.	.	.	.	.
AGE	.025	.0092	.007	.043	7.440	1	.006
BMI	-.022	.0184	-.058	.014	1.407	1	.236
DIABETES	.168	.2862	-.393	.729	.345	1	.557

Parameter	B	Std. Error	95% Wald Confidence Interval		Hypothesis Test		
			Lower	Upper	Wald Chi-Square	df	Sig.
HYPERTEN	.020	.1853	-.343	.383	.012	1	.914
HYPERCHO	-.487	.1816	-.843	-.131	7.188	1	.007
(Scale)	5.747[b]	.2946	5.198	6.355			

Dependent Variable: CDRSUM
Model: (Intercept), Diagnosis, AGE, BMI, DIABETES, HYPERTEN, HYPERCHO
a. Set to zero because this parameter is redundant.
b. Maximum likelihood estimate.

Comments: Age, diagnosis, and hypercholesterolemia are also significant in their explanation of the differences in CDR-SUM. The maximum likelihood parameter estimates are reported in the B column. These are the estimated regression coefficients. The confidence intervals for each parameter estimate are also reported (Lower, Upper) in the output. The p-values for testing the significance of each covariate are reported in this column. The p-values (Sig) tell us what is significant. The covariates with p-values less than $\alpha = 0.05$ are considered significant. FTD and Normal are significantly different from VaD in explaining CDR-SUM. The scale parameter is 5.747.

3.3.4 Stata Syntax and Output

The Stata syntax and output follow:

```
glm cdrsum contr_ad contr_dlb contr_ftd contr_vad age bmi
diabetes hyperten hypercho, family(gaussian) link(identity)
```

STATA OUTPUT

```
Iteration 0:  log likelihood=-1887.658
Generalized linear models            No. of obs      =      761
Optimization  :  ML                  Residual df     =      751
                                     Scale parameter =    8.468
Deviance      =      6359.778  (1/df) Deviance       =    8.468
```

```
Pearson          =      6359.778    (1/df) Pearson    =    8.468

Variance function:    V(u) = 1        [Gaussian]

Link function         g(u) = u        [Identity]

                                         AIC      =   4.994

Log likelihood  =  -1887.658            BIC      =   1377.168
```

Comments: The maximum likelihood (ML) optimization technique is used to evaluate this linear model. The scaled parameter is 8.468, which suggests that there are factors that need to be addressed. This is the linear regression with the identity link.

CDRSUM	Coef.	Std. Err.	z	P>z	[95% Conf. Interval]	
CONTR_AD	0.461	1.036	0.440	0.656	-1.570	2.491
CONTR_DLB	1.503	0.649	2.310	0.021	0.230	2.775
CONTR_FTD	3.172	2.920	1.090	0.277	-2.552	8.895
CONTR_VAD	2.133	0.795	2.680	0.007	0.576	3.691
AGE	0.054	0.011	5.010	0.000	0.033	0.075
BMI	-0.047	0.022	-2.150	0.031	-0.091	-0.004
DIABETES	0.544	0.346	1.570	0.117	-0.135	1.223
HYPERTEN	0.116	0.226	0.510	0.608	-0.328	0.560
HYPERCHO	-0.405	0.221	-1.830	0.067	-0.838	0.028
_CONS	1.189	1.063	1.120	0.263	-0.893	3.272

Comments: Age and diagnosis are significant in their explanation of the differences in CDR-SUM. The maximum likelihood parameter estimates are reported in the Coefficient column. These are the estimated regression coefficients. The confidence intervals for each parameter estimate are also reported in the output. The p-values for testing the significance of each covariate are reported in this column. The p-values $(P > |z|)$ tell us what is significant at a certain level of significance. The covariates with p-values less than 0.05 are considered significant. DLB and VaD are significantly different from normal in explaining CDR-SUM. The 95% confidence interval is also helpful. If the interval contains a zero, then the predictor is not significant. The interval gives a range of possible values.

3.4 Fitting Binary Generalized Linear Models

In binary data, we cannot use linear models, as we do not have a continuous response. Instead, we use logistic regression with a logit link $\log\left(\dfrac{p}{1-p}\right)$, where p is the probability of the event of interest, such as the probability of an AD diagnosis. For covariates of interest $(X_1, \ldots, X_p)$, we express the logistic regression model as

$$\log\left(\frac{p}{1-p}\right) = \beta_0 + \beta_1 X_1 + \cdots + \beta_p X_p,$$

which are written in the nonlinear form $P = \dfrac{e^{\beta_0 + \beta_1 X_1 + \cdots + \beta_p X\_{p_2}}}{1 + e^{\beta_0 + \beta_1 X_1 + \cdots + \beta\_{p_2} X_p}}$. To use this model, the data must satisfy the following conditions.

1. The occurrence of an event for a patient (such as an AD diagnosis) is not affected by any other patient's outcome.
2. The probability of the event remains the same.
3. The number of patients selected is known before we collect the information.

Problem: Do gender, age, CDR-SUM and race (denoted by NIHR) have an impact on whether one has AD?

Solution: We evaluate the probability of a patient being diagnosed with AD. The response, AD diagnosis, is binary, indicating whether the patient had an AD diagnosis ($0 = $ no AD diagnosis, $1 = $ AD diagnosis). The three conditions above are satisfied, so we fit a logistic regression model. We obtain the following coefficient estimates (table 3.4).

We can express the parameter estimates in the logistic model form:

$$\log\left(\frac{\hat{p}_{AD}}{\hat{p}_{\overline{AD}}}\right) = -5.99 + 0.03\text{female} + 0.1\text{age} + 0.72\text{CDR}$$

$$+ 0.28(\text{race} = 2) + 0.40(\text{race} = 5) + 1.38(\text{race} = 6),$$

Table 3.4 Estimates, Standard Errors, and *p*-Values

Parameter	Estimate	Std Err	*p*-Value
Intercept	−5.989	0.963	<0.001
SEX = 2 (Female)	0.0306	0.221	0.890
AGE	0.074	0.013	<0.001
CDRSUM	0.716	0.062	<0.001
NIHR = 2	0.280	0.403	0.487
NIHR = 5	0.404	1.302	0.757
NIHR = 6	1.384	1.297	0.286

where age and CDR-SUM score are significant predictors of an AD diagnosis. Race and gender showed no significant impact in our cohort. We show how these results are obtained through SAS, R, SPSS, and Stata.

3.4.1 SAS Code and Output

The SAS syntax follows:

```
PROC GENMOD DATA = DTA DESCENDING;
2CLASS DX_AD SEX(REF="1") NIHR(REF="1");
3MODEL DX_AD = SEX AGE CDRSUM NIHR / DIST=BIN LINK=logit TYPE3;
run;
```

[2]Used to identify categorical variables and select the reference categories.
[3]The model statement specifies the outcome and predictors, as well as the distribution of the random component (BIN) and the link function (logit).

SAS OUTPUT

Model Information	
Data Set	WORK.DTA
Distribution	Binomial
Link Function	Logit
Dependent Variable	DX_AD

Comments: The Model Information table identifies the dataset being evaluated, the assumed error distribution (random component is binomial), the link function (logit) and the dependent variable (DX of Alzheimer's or not).

Class Level Information		
Class	Levels	Values
DX_AD	2	1 0
SEX	2	2 1
NIHR	4	2 5 6 1

Comments: The responses have two levels, gender has two levels, and race (NIHR) has four levels.

Response Profile		
Ordered Value	DX_AD	Total Frequency
1	1	579
2	0	182

Comments: The response DX_AD = 1 is an Alzheimer's disease diagnosis that occurred 579 times in the data. We are modeling the probability that DX_AD = 1 through the logit function.

PROC GENMOD Is Modeling the Probability That DX_AD='1'

Criteria for Assessing Goodness of Fit			
Criterion	DF	Value	Value/DF
Log Likelihood		-267.554	
Full Log Likelihood		-267.554	
AIC (smaller is better)		549.108	
AICC (smaller is better)		549.257	
BIC (smaller is better)		581.551	

Comments: These are goodness-of-fit measures to help identify or compare one model with another. The smaller the value, the better the model.

Algorithm converged.

Comments: Not all models converge. Such a note means the model ran and the results are accepted.

Parameter		Estimate	Standard Error	Wald 95% Confidence Limits		Wald Chi-Square	Pr > ChiSq
Intercept		-5.989	0.963	-7.876	-4.103	38.72	<.001
SEX	2	0.0306	0.221	-0.402	0.464	0.02	0.890
AGE		0.074	0.013	0.049	0.099	32.93	<.001
CDRSUM		0.716	0.062	0.595	0.837	134.22	<.001
NIHR	2	0.280	0.403	-0.509	1.069	0.48	0.487
NIHR	5	0.404	1.302	-2.149	2.956	0.10	0.757
NIHR	6	1.384	1.297	-1.158	3.926	1.14	0.286
NIHR	1	0.000	0.000	0.000	0.000	.	.
Scale		1.000	0.000	1.000	1.000		

Comments: The maximum likelihood parameter estimates are reported in the Estimate column. These are the estimated regression coefficients. The confidence intervals for each parameter estimate are also reported in the output. The p-values (Pr > ChiSq) for testing the significance of each covariate are reported. Age and CDR-SUM are significant ($p < 0.001$) predictors in identifying the differences between in the two diagnosed groups.

LR Statistics for Type 3 Analysis			
Source	DF	Chi-Square	Pr > ChiSq
SEX	1	0.02	0.889
AGE	1	39.13	<.0001
CDRSUM	1	238.87	<.0001
NIHR	3	1.77	0.623

Comments: Likelihood ratio statistics for sex, age, CDR-SUM, and NIHR are computed.

3.4.2 R Code and Output

The R syntax follows:

```
dta$SEX <- as.factor(dta$SEX)
dta <- within(dta, SEX <- relevel(SEX, ref = "1"))
dta$NIHR <- as.factor(dta$NIHR)
dta <- within(dta, NIHR <- relevel(NIHR, ref = "1"))
¹reg2<-glm(DX_AD~SEX+AGE+CDRSUM+NIHR,family=binomial(link="logit
"),data=dta)
summary(reg2)
```

[1]For the logistic regression a member of GLMs, the glm() function has family as binomial, and the link is logit.

R OUTPUT

```
summary(reg2)
##
## Call:
## glm(formula = DX_AD ~ SEX + AGE + CDRSUM + NIHR, family = binomial(link =
"logit"),
##      data = dta)
##
## Deviance Residuals:
##     Min       1Q    Median       3Q       Max
## -4.2535   0.0221   0.2399   0.5540   2.5838
##
## Coefficients:
##               Estimate Std. Error z value Pr(>|z|)
## (Intercept) -5.98927    0.96252   -6.222 4.89e-10 ***
## SEX2         0.03063    0.22093    0.139    0.890
## AGE          0.07380    0.01286    5.739 9.54e-09 ***
## CDRSUM       0.71550    0.06176   11.585  < 2e-16 ***
## NIHR2        0.27991    0.40255    0.695    0.487
```

```
## NIHR5         0.40372    1.30219    0.310     0.757
## NIHR6         1.38405    1.29680    1.067     0.286
## ---
## Signif. codes: 0  '***' 0.001 '**' 0.01 '*' 0.05 '.' 0.1 ' ' 1
##
## (Dispersion parameter for binomial family taken to be 1)
##
##     Null deviance: 837.27  on 760  degrees of freedom
## Residual deviance: 535.11  on 754  degrees of freedom
## AIC: 549.11
##
## Number of Fisher Scoring iterations: 6
```

Comments: The maximum likelihood parameter estimates are reported in the Estimate column. These are the estimated regression coefficients. The confidence intervals for each parameter estimate are also reported in the output. The p-values (`Signif. codes`) for testing the significance of each covariate are reported in this column. Age and CDR-SUM are significant ($p < 0.001$) predictors in identifying the differences between the two groups

3.4.3 SPSS Syntax and Output

The SPSS syntax follows:

```
* Generalized Linear Models.
GENLIN DX_AD (REFERENCE=LAST) BY SEX NIHR (ORDER=ASCENDING)
WITH AGE CDRSUM
   /MODEL SEX AGE CDRSUM NIHR INTERCEPT=YES
  DISTRIBUTION=BINOMIAL LINK=LOGIT
   /CRITERIA METHOD=FISHER(1) SCALE=1 COVB=MODEL
MAXITERATIONS=100 MAXSTEPHALVING=5
     PCONVERGE=1E-006(ABSOLUTE) SINGULAR=1E-012
ANALYSISTYPE=3(WALD) CILEVEL=95 CITYPE=WALD
     LIKELIHOOD=FULL
   /EMMEANS TABLES=SEX SCALE=ORIGINAL
```

```
/EMMEANS TABLES=NIHR SCALE=ORIGINAL
/MISSING CLASSMISSING=EXCLUDE
/PRINT CPS DESCRIPTIVES MODELINFO FIT SUMMARY SOLUTION.
```

SPSS OUTPUT

Generalized Linear Models

Model Information

Dependent Variable	DX_AD
Probability Distribution	Binomial
Link Function	Logit

Comments: The Model Information table provides a summary of the dataset being evaluated. The assumed error distribution (random component) is binomial, the link function is logit, and the binary dependent variable is DX, whether Alzheimer's or not.

Omnibus Test

Likelihood Ratio Chi-Square	df	Sig.
302.157	6	.000

Dependent Variable: DX_AD
Model: (Intercept), SEX, AGE, CDRSUM, NIHR
a. Compares the fitted model against the intercept-only model.

Comments: This is a test for all coefficients equal to zero.

Parameter Estimates

Parameter	B	Std. Error	95% Wald Confidence Interval		Hypothesis Test		
			Lower	Upper	Wald Chi-Square	df	Sig.
(Intercept)	7.053	.584	5.909	8.198	145.872	1	.000
[NIHR=6]	-.035	.896	-1.791	1.722	.001	1	.969
[NIHR=5]	-.236	1.097	-2.383	1.912	.046	1	.830
[NIHR=2]	-.173	.291	-.744	.398	.353	1	.552
[NIHR=1]	0[a]	.	.	.	.	.	.

| Parameter | B | Std. Error | 95% Wald Confidence Interval | | Hypothesis Test | | |
			Lower	Upper	Wald Chi-Square	df	Sig.
[SEX=2]	.334	.162	.016	.651	4.238	1	.040
[SEX=1]	0[a]	.	.	.	.	.	.
CDRSUM	-.488	.027	-.541	-.435	326.994	1	.000
AGE	-.040	.008	-.056	-.025	25.459	1	.000
(Scale)	4.772[b]	.245	4.316	5.276			

Dependent Variable: DX
Model: (Intercept), NIHR, SEX, CDRSUM, AGE
a. Set to zero because this parameter is redundant.
b. Maximum likelihood estimate.

Comments: The maximum likelihood parameter estimates are reported in the Estimate column. These are the estimated regression coefficients. The confidence intervals for each parameter estimate are also reported in the output. The p-values (Pr > ChiSq) for testing the significance of each covariate are reported. Age and CDR-SUM are significant ($p < .001$) predictors in identifying the differences between in the two diagnosed groups.

3.4.4 Stata Syntax and Output

The Stata syntax and output follow:

```
. glm dx_ad age cdrsum i.nihr i.sex, family(binomial 1) link(logit)
```

STATA OUTPUT

```
Iteration 0:   log likelihood = -299.61799

Iteration 1:   log likelihood = -268.25816

Iteration 2:   log likelihood = -267.55446

Iteration 3:   log likelihood = -267.55416

Iteration 4:   log likelihood = -267.55416
```

Comments: The iteration shows that convergence was obtained after four iterations.

```
Generalized linear  models                    No. of obs  =  761
Optimization:       ML                        Residual df =  754
              Scale parameter     =   1
Deviance     =        535.108        (1/df) Deviance  =   .7097
Pearson      =      10134.015        (1/df) Pearson   = 13.440
```

Comments: The scale deviance is less than 1.

```
Variance function:  V(u) = u*(1-u)        [Bernoulli]
Link function:      g(u) = ln(u/(1-u))    [Logit]
           AIC              =  .722
Log likelihood             = -267.554  BIC =   -4467.405
```

Comments: The Bernoulli is an independent trial at each outcome. The variance is related to the mean.

DX_AD	Coef.	Std. Err.	z	P>z	[95% Conf.	Interval]
AGE	0.074	0.013	5.740	0.000	0.049	0.099
CDRSUM	0.715	0.062	11.590	0.000	0.594	0.837
NIHR						
2	0.280	0.403	0.700	0.487	-0.509	1.069
5	0.404	1.302	0.310	0.757	-2.149	2.956
6	1.384	1.297	1.070	0.286	-1.158	3.926
SEX	0.031	0.221	0.140	0.890	-0.402	0.464
_CONS	-5.989	0.963	-6.220	0.000	-7.876	-4.103

Comments: The dependent variable is DX_AD modeled by sex, age, CDR-SUM, and NIHR. The maximum likelihood parameter estimates are reported for each covariate. These are the estimated regression coefficients. The confidence intervals for each parameter estimate are also reported in the output. The p-values ($Pr > |z|$) for testing the significance of each covariate are reported in this column. Age and CDR-SUM are significant ($p < 0.001$) predictors in identifying the differences between the two groups.

3.5 Summary and Discussion

It was originally believed that in order to model data or to understand the mean response, the response random variable had to be normally distributed. Initially, in the case when it was not normally distributed, we transformed the outcome to change the scale to be normally distributed. For example, the age of diagnosis for AD is typically over 65. Hence, we would need to transform the data if we wanted to use linear models to model the age of diagnosis. With the advent of the GLMs, however, we are able model the mean directly and not transform the data to be normal or approximately normal. The GLM allows us to model the mean for distributions belonging to the exponential family. The observations are independent. In evaluating our dementia data, GLMs allow us to model CRD-SUM, MMSE, the probability of AD, the probability of diabetes, and the number of patients with a certain disease. Such models rely on independent observations and obtain the regression coefficients based on the maximum likelihood approach, which has many nice properties.

3.6 Exercises

Consider NACC data collected from a certain center. We examine data from ADC 4967 (http://www.public.asu.edu/~jeffreyw/). The information includes the patient's identification number, sex (1 = male, 2 = female), MMSE (a measure of cognition) and age as predictors of the outcome of interest, and AD diagnosis (1 = diagnosed with AD, 0 = no AD diagnosis) model. Do the following:

1. What is the link function?
2. Write out the model.
3. Do age, gender, and MMSE have differential effects on AD?
4. Are males more likely to be diagnosed with AD than females?
5. Do you find the MMSE to be significant in the model?
6. Based on the data, who do you think is most likely to be diagnosed AD?

Chapter 4

Hierarchical Regression Models for Continuous Responses

4.1 Motivating Example

Longitudinal studies are used to collect and analyze information on patients over time, resulting in multiple observations per patient. These studies usually evaluate changes in the relationship between variables as time progresses. For example, a researcher may wish to assess the relationship between cognitive ability—measured by the Mini-Mental State Examination (MMSE) and Clinical Dementia Rating Scale Sum of Boxes (CDR-SUM) scores—and cardiovascular risk factors, such as diabetes mellitus, hypertension, hypercholesterolemia, smoking, and body mass index (BMI) on subjects diagnosed with Alzheimer's disease (AD) or dementia with Lewy bodies (DLB) (Bergland et al. 2017). Another example includes evaluating how a patient's cognition changes over time after receiving a particular drug.

In chapter 3, we evaluated the CDR-SUM score (Hughes et al. 1982; O'Bryant et al. 2008), a measure of cognitive ability and daily functioning. We consider the baseline visit, a single time-point, for each patient in Alzheimer's Disease Center (ADC) 4967 to identify associations between the CDR-SUM and cardiovascular risk factors. This type of study, which evaluates one time-point per subject, is called a cross-sectional study. The analysis revealed a number of associations but did not answer questions about the relationship between cardiovascular risk factors and cognition over time. In addition, the analysis did not evaluate associations within particular ADCs or patients. To address these questions, we rely on hierarchical models or nested models. We discuss such models in this chapter.

In our study of longitudinal data, we fit hierarchical regression models to a continuous response from a subset of NACC data. We

Table 4.1 Subset of Data

ADC	ID	MOFROMINDEX	AGE	BMI	DIABETES	HYPERTEN	HYPERCHO	CDRSUM
4967	1705	0	78	28.7	0	1	1	4.5
4967	1705	12	79	27.5	0	1	1	4.5
4967	1705	23	80	27.1	0	1	1	5.5
4967	1927	0	83	29.3	1	0	1	0.5
4967	1927	13	84	28.7	1	0	1	0.5
4967	5856	0	87	29.5	0	1	1	5
4967	5856	12	88	29.2	0	1	1	8
4967	5856	23	89	25.7	0	1	1	8
4967	7646	0	60	34.4	1	1	1	3
4967	7646	9	61	35.8	1	1	1	2

evaluate the association between CDR-SUM and cardiovascular risk factors across several visits using various models. We concentrate on evaluating patients with a minimum of two visits. The data consist of 45,508 visits from 12,258 patients from 35 ADCs. All visits occur between June 2005 and March 2015. These patients have various dementia diagnoses, including AD (5,222 patients), DLB (189 patients), frontotemporal dementia (FTD) (600 patients), vascular dementia (VaD) (117 patients), and those lacking a dementia diagnosis (normal) (6,130 patients). A sample of the data analyzed in this chapter is shown in table 4.1.

4.2 Graphical Presentation of Hierarchical Continuous Data

Figure 4.1 shows a two-level hierarchical data structure, which represents longitudinal or clustered data. In longitudinal data, there are many patients in a study, and each patient has multiple measurements collected at different time-points, as is the case in the present example. In clustered data, the subjects are grouped into clusters by certain similarities, such as patients within ADCs. We approach the analysis in the same manner for both longitudinal and clustered data. To analyze the data in figure 4.1, we use a two-level analysis (as we have two-level data). We can evaluate additional levels if we have additional layers of information, such as a three-level analysis, if we have information on the ADC that each patient visits.

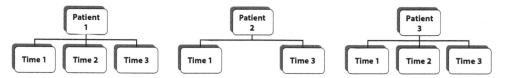

Figure 4.1 Diagram of a hierarchical structure.

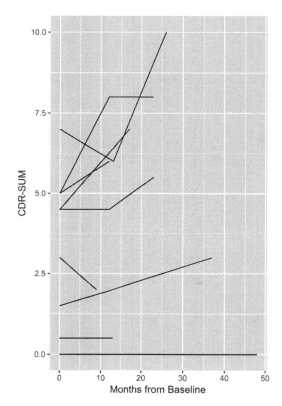

Figure 4.2 Plot of CDR-SUM by time from baseline (months).

To demonstrate the use of graphical methods for longitudinal data, we plot the data for the subset of patients shown in table 4.1. Figure 4.2 displays a line plot of the CDR-SUM over time for this group of 10 patients. The graphical display of the measurements over time shows that each patient has a different curve. This curve represents the change in time for each patient. This type of plot can be obtained using any of the four statistical programs, SAS, R, SPSS, and Stata.

The line plot shows that each of the 10 patients has a different change in CDR-SUM score during the course of the study after the baseline measurement. Note that two patients have a CDR-SUM score of zero for all time-points, which is why it appears there are only nine lines on the plot. While most patients seem to have an increase in the CDR-SUM score, indicating cognitive decline throughout the study, there are a few with decreasing scores. The nonparallel lines suggest that there are different factors affecting the responses over time. We want to identify such factors that lead to these changes.

4.2.1 SAS Syntax for Longitudinal Plots

```
¹SYMBOL1 VALUE = CIRCLE COLOR = BLACK INTERPOL = JOIN REPEAT = 10;
²PROC GPLOT DATA=dta4967_10subj;
³PLOT CDRSUM*MOFROMINDEX = ID / NOLEGEND;
RUN;
```

[1]Defines plot settings: circular, black symbols that are joined by a line.
[2]PROC GPLOT plots in SAS. The datafile is named dta4967_10subj.
[3]This plots CDRSUM on the y-axis, MOFROMINDEX on the x-axis, and identifies each line by the patient ID.

4.2.2 R Syntax for Longitudinal Plots

```
¹library(ggplot2)
²p <- ggplot(data = dta4967_10subj, aes(x = MOFROMINDEX,
y = CDRSUM, group = ID)) + xlab("Months from Baseline")
+ ylab("CDR-SUM")
³p + geom_line()
```

[1]The library ggplot2 is used for producing graphs and charts.
[2]This creates a plot for 10 subjects from ADC 4967, with time (months) on the x-axis and the CDR-SUM scores on the y-axis. The points are grouped by ID.

[3]The option geom_line() plots a line graph. The option geom_point() plots points for each value.

4.2.3 SPSS Syntax for Longitudinal Plots

To produce a "multiple" line plot, showing CDR-SUM differences across months for various patients, in SPSS using the pull-down menu, click on Graphs → Chart Builder → Line. Click on the graph next to Multiple, and drag it into the chart preview area. Put the dependent variable (CDRSUM) into the "Y axis?" box. Put "months" into the "X axis?" box. Into "Set color:", select the independent variable (IV) for which you want separate lines on the graph (in this case, patient ID).

4.2.4 Stata Syntax for Longitudinal Plots

```
encode varname, gen(varname1)
scatter mean varname1, xlabel(, valuelabel) || rcap upper lower
varname1 || line upper mean lower varname1
```

4.3 Marginal Models for Correlated Data

In chapter 3, we presented generalized linear models (GLMs), in which the responses were assumed independent, as there was only one outcome per patient. In this chapter, however, we analyze clustered and longitudinal data that have more than one outcome per person (or sampling unit). As the data contain multiple measurements obtained on the same individuals, we cannot expect the observations to be independent. In longitudinal data, measurements obtained on the same individual at different time points are more similar than measurements obtained on different individuals. We require more complex models to properly account for the correlation. We focus on marginal models in this section (Liang and Zeger 1986; Zeger and Liang 1986) and discuss a subject-specific model using random effects in the next section (Stroup 2012).

The dataset introduced in section 4.1 contains information on 12,258 patients. Each patient has between 2 and 10 visits in the study.

Table 4.2 Frequency of Total Number of Visits in Longitudinal Data

Visits	2	3	4	5	6	7	8	9	10
Frequency	4,356	2,780	1,818	1,188	750	569	466	277	54
	35.5%	22.7%	14.8%	9.7%	6.1%	4.6%	3.8%	2.3%	0.4%

The breakdown of the total number of visits for each patient in our subset is shown in table 4.2.

Marginal models are population-averaged models, which are used to model the mean through an adjustment to the random component. In hierarchical data, we often use generalized estimating equations (GEEs) (Liang and Zeger 1986; Zeger and Liang 1986) to fit a model that accounts for correlation. The GEE specifies a working correlation structure, which accounts for the repeated measures, or clustering in the data. The working correlation structures include independent (IN), compound symmetry (CS), autoregressive (AR), and unstructured (UN). In each of these structures, the off-diagonal values in the matrix indicate the correlation between the measurements at different time-points (in repeated measures data) or the correlation between the subjects within a cluster (in clustered data). We present these correlation structures using the example of three repeated measurements on patients, which produces a 3×3 correlation matrix. While we focus on the interpretation of the correlation structure for longitudinal data, these are also applicable to clustered data with three subjects or units within the cluster.

The independent (IN) working correlation structure is of the form

$$\Sigma = \begin{bmatrix} 1 & 0 & 0 \\ 0 & 1 & 0 \\ 0 & 0 & 1 \end{bmatrix},$$

which has ones on the diagonal and zeros in the off diagonal. The independent working correlation structure assumes independence between the measurements at each time-point for a patient. In this case, one is assuming that the observation at one time-point is independent of an observation at another time-point. For example, the CDR-SUM score for patient with ID 1705 at the baseline visit is independent of the CDR-SUM score for the same patient (ID 1705) at the second visit. In practice, this structure should not be used when any level of correlation is assumed to exist between the repeated measurements.

The compound symmetry (CS), or exchangeability, working correlation structure is of the form

$$\Sigma = \begin{bmatrix} 1 & \rho & \rho \\ \rho & 1 & \rho \\ \rho & \rho & 1 \end{bmatrix},$$

which assumes that all time-points are associated by the common correlation parameter ρ. Thus we assume that the relationship is the same between measurements on the same patient at all time-points. For example, we assume that the CDR-SUM score for patient 1705 at baseline is correlated to the CDR-SUM score at the second visit by ρ, and the baseline CDR-SUM score is correlated to the CDR-SUM score at the third visit by ρ. This is usually a stringent condition.

The autoregressive order 1 (AR(1)) working correlation structure is of the form

$$\Sigma = \begin{bmatrix} 1 & \rho & \rho^2 \\ \rho & 1 & \rho \\ \rho^2 & \rho & 1 \end{bmatrix}.$$

If we implement an autoregressive correlation structure, we assume that the correlation between time-points decreases as the time-points are further apart. To utilize this correlation structure for our data, we assume that CDR-SUM evaluations between visits further apart are less correlated. For instance, the baseline CDR-SUM score for patient

1705 is weakly correlated with the CDR-SUM score at the third visit, as compared to the correlation between the CDR-SUM scores at baseline and second visit.

The unstructured (UN) working correlation structure is of the form

$$\Sigma = \begin{bmatrix} 1 & \rho_{12} & \rho_{13} \\ \rho_{21} & 1 & \rho_{23} \\ \rho_{31} & \rho_{32} & 1 \end{bmatrix}.$$

This correlation matrix assumes that there are unique correlations between every time-point. While the unstructured correlation structure (UN) is flexible, it requires the most parameters to be estimated and can lead to convergence issues in cases where there are many time-points. In our example evaluating CDR-SUM score, this indicates that the correlation of scores within a patient varies between every single score at various time-points.

Statistically, GEE works as follows. Prior to considering correlated observations, we use a set of equations to obtain the estimates of our regression parameters β_I based on independent observations by solving

$$\sum_{i=1}^{n} X_i'(Y_i - X_i\beta_I) = 0.$$

When we have correlated data, however, we use the working correlation matrix to obtain estimates of the regression parameters β_C. Thus we solve the system of equations

$$\sum_{i=1}^{n} X_i' \Sigma_i^{-1} (Y_i - X_i\beta_C) = 0$$

by specifying a working covariance structure Σ, which is readily available in statistical software packages, including SAS, R, SPSS, and Stata. The GEE method produces consistent estimates even if the working correlation structure is misspecified (specified incorrectly) (Pepe and Anderson 1994).

Problem: Do age, BMI, diabetes, hypertension, and hypercholesterolemia have an impact on CDR-SUM while accounting for the random effect due to patients?

Solution: We assess the associations between CDR-SUM and cardiovascular risk factors while accounting for the correlation structure between visits for each patient. We consider the variables time since baseline measured in months (MOFROMINDEX), age, BMI, diabetes, hypertension (HYPERTEN), and hypercholesterolemia (HYPERCHO). Patients are identified through their ID. We apply GEE and account for the correlation through a working correlation matrix. We consider four correlation structures, IN, CS, AR, and UN. Although we know that measurements on the same patient over time should be correlated, we include the independent working correlation structure for comparison. The four correlation structures are compared by evaluating the Quasilikelihood under the Independence model Criterion (QIC) proposed by Pan (2001) for each model (lower is better). Based on the model fit results, we report the GEE model fit for the AR(1) correlation structure (table 4.3).

Table 4.4 summarizes the significant predictors in each analysis for various working correlation structures across the four software programs.

In our example, the results remain fairly consistent between these four working correlation structures. In general, the results indicate that time since the baseline visit, age, BMI, and hypertension are significantly associated with the CDR-SUM score. Regardless of which analysis or software was used, hypercholesterolemia was not identified

Table 4.3 Parameter Estimates for the GEE Model

Parameter	Estimate	Std Err	p-Value
Intercept	−1.049	0.333	0.002
MOFROMINDEX	0.027	0.001	<0.0001
AGE	0.063	0.004	<0.0001
BMI	−0.031	0.006	<0.0001
DIABETES	0.157	0.081	0.052
HYPERTEN	−0.172	0.044	<0.0001
HYPERCHO	−0.067	0.035	0.059

Table 4.4 Significant Predictors by Working Correlation Matrix for Statistical Programs

	Independent	AR(1)	Compound Symmetry	Unstructured
SAS	Time	Time	Time	Did not converge
	Age	Age	Age	
	BMI	BMI	BMI	
	Diabetes	Hypertension	Diabetes	
	Hypertension		Hypertension	
R	Time	Time	Time	Time
	Age	Age	Age	Age
	BMI	BMI	BMI	BMI
	Diabetes	Diabetes	Diabetes	Diabetes
	Hypertension	Hypertension	Hypertension	Hypertension
SPSS	Time	Time	Time	Time
	Age	Age	Age	Age
	BMI	BMI	BMI	BMI
	Diabetes	Diabetes	Diabetes	Diabetes
	Hypertension	Hypertension	Hypertension	Hypertension
Stata	Time	Time	Time	Did not converge
	Age	Age	Age	
	BMI	BMI	BMI	
	Diabetes	Hypertension	Diabetes	
	Hypertension		Hypertension	

as a statistically significant predictor. Although the parameter estimates are consistent, it is important to pay close attention to the standard errors. In the case of correlated data, the standard errors will be smaller if we incorrectly assumed an independent correlation structure. We use SAS, R, SPSS, and Stata to compute these estimates.

4.3.1 SAS Syntax and Output for GEE

Independent Working Correlation Matrix

The SAS syntax follows:

```
¹PROC GENMOD DATA = LONGITUDINAL;
²CLASS VISITNUM ID;
³MODEL CDRSUM = MOFROMINDEX AGE BMI DIABETES HYPERTEN HYPERCHO;
⁴REPEATED SUBJECT= ID / WITHIN=VISITNUM TYPE=IND CORRW;
RUN;
```

[1]PROC GENMOD for fitting GLMs and GEEs.

[2]The CLASS statement identifies categorical variables and sets the reference category. For GEE, the variable listed in the WITHIN= option (4) is listed in the CLASS statement.

[3]The model statement defines the outcome = predictors.

[4]The REPEATED statement is used to specify the source of correlation in the data. SUBJECT= identifies the variable on which there are repeated measurements. In this case, each subject (identified by ID) has multiple measurements. The WITHIN= statement identifies the variable that denotes the various measurements on the SUBJECT= variable. In this case, the multiple measurements per subject are identified by the visit number (VISITNUM). TYPE= specifies the working correlation structure, where IND is independent

SAS OUTPUT

The GENMOD Procedure		
Model Information		
Dataset	WORK.LONGITUDINAL	
Distribution	Normal	
Link Function	Identity	
Dependent Variable	CDRSUM	CDRSUM

Comments: The random component is assumed to be normally distribution, and an identify link function is used. The response variable is CDRSUM.

Algorithm converged.

Comments: The output indicates that the model converged. Convergence refers to the convergence status of estimating procedure. It is important to check convergence, as not all models converge. In order to interpret the model output, the model must converge, or the results may not be reliable.

GEE Model Information	
Correlation Structure	Independent
Within-Subject Effect	VISITNUM (10 levels)
Subject Effect	ID (12258 levels)
Number of Clusters	12258
Correlation Matrix Dimension	10
Maximum Cluster Size	10
Minimum Cluster Size	2

Comments: The working correlation matrix is independent, with a dimension of 10. There are 12,258 clusters (subjects). The GEE model information summarizes the specified correlation structure, the subject, and the within-subject effect (which the correlation structure is defined for). The maximum cluster size determines the size of the working correlation structure.

	Col1	Col2	Col3	Col4	Col5	Col6	Col7	Col8	Col9	Col10
				Working Correlation Matrix						
Row1	1.0000	0.0000	0.0000	0.0000	0.0000	0.0000	0.0000	0.0000	0.0000	0.0000
Row2	0.0000	1.0000	0.0000	0.0000	0.0000	0.0000	0.0000	0.0000	0.0000	0.0000
Row3	0.0000	0.0000	1.0000	0.0000	0.0000	0.0000	0.0000	0.0000	0.0000	0.0000
Row4	0.0000	0.0000	0.0000	1.0000	0.0000	0.0000	0.0000	0.0000	0.0000	0.0000
Row5	0.0000	0.0000	0.0000	0.0000	1.0000	0.0000	0.0000	0.0000	0.0000	0.0000
Row6	0.0000	0.0000	0.0000	0.0000	0.0000	1.0000	0.0000	0.0000	0.0000	0.0000
Row7	0.0000	0.0000	0.0000	0.0000	0.0000	0.0000	1.0000	0.0000	0.0000	0.0000
Row8	0.0000	0.0000	0.0000	0.0000	0.0000	0.0000	0.0000	1.0000	0.0000	0.0000
Row9	0.0000	0.0000	0.0000	0.0000	0.0000	0.0000	0.0000	0.0000	1.0000	0.0000
Row10	0.0000	0.0000	0.0000	0.0000	0.0000	0.0000	0.0000	0.0000	0.0000	1.0000

Comments: The working correlation matrix, which is the estimated correlation structure used in GEE, is displayed. In the independent case, this is an identity matrix. But in other correlation structures, the matrix will contain the estimated correlation parameters.

GEE Fit Criteria	
QIC	45542.513
QICu	45515.000

Comments: The QIC statistic is used to compare the model fit. Lower QIC values indicate a better model fit.

Analysis of GEE Parameter Estimates

Empirical Standard Error Estimates

Parameter	Estimate	Standard Error	95% Confidence Limits		Z	Pr > |Z|
Intercept	0.113	0.359	-0.591	0.817	0.310	0.753
MOFROMINDEX	-0.017	0.001	-0.019	-0.015	-17.050	<.0001
AGE	0.058	0.004	0.051	0.066	14.730	<.0001
BMI	-0.043	0.007	-0.057	-0.029	-5.980	<.0001
DIABETES	0.484	0.124	0.241	0.727	3.910	<.0001
HYPERTEN	-0.305	0.075	-0.452	-0.158	-4.070	<.0001
HYPERCHO	0.029	0.070	-0.108	0.167	0.420	0.675

Comments: The Analysis of GEE Parameter Estimates table contains the parameter estimates, standard errors, confidence intervals (limits), and the p-values (Pr > \|Z\|) for the association of each covariate on the outcome. Time since baseline (MOFROMINDEX), age, BMI, diabetes, and hypertension (HYPERTEN) are significant drivers of CDR-SUM. Hypercholesterolemia (HYPERCHO) is not a significant covariate.

Autoregressive Working Correlation Matrix
The SAS syntax follows:

```
PROC GENMOD DATA = LONGITUDINAL;
   CLASS VISITNUM ID;
   MODEL CDRSUM = MOFROMINDEX AGE BMI DIABETES HYPERTEN
HYPERCHO;
¹REPEATED SUBJECT= ID / WITHIN=VISITNUM TYPE=AR CORRW;
RUN;
```

[1]The working correlation matrix is specified as autoregressive structure, TYPE=AR.

SAS OUTPUT

	Col1	Col2	Col3	Col4	Col5	Col6	Col7	Col8	Col9	Col10
Row1	1.000	0.882	0.777	0.685	0.604	0.532	0.469	0.414	0.365	0.322
Row2	0.882	1.000	0.882	0.777	0.685	0.604	0.532	0.469	0.414	0.365
Row3	0.777	0.882	1.000	0.882	0.777	0.685	0.604	0.532	0.469	0.414
Row4	0.685	0.777	0.882	1.000	0.882	0.777	0.685	0.604	0.532	0.469
Row5	0.604	0.685	0.777	0.882	1.000	0.882	0.777	0.685	0.604	0.532
Row6	0.532	0.604	0.685	0.777	0.882	1.000	0.882	0.777	0.685	0.604
Row7	0.469	0.532	0.604	0.685	0.777	0.882	1.000	0.882	0.777	0.685
Row8	0.414	0.469	0.532	0.604	0.685	0.777	0.882	1.000	0.882	0.777
Row9	0.365	0.414	0.469	0.532	0.604	0.685	0.777	0.882	1.000	0.882
Row10	0.322	0.365	0.414	0.469	0.532	0.604	0.685	0.777	0.882	1.000

Working Correlation Matrix

Comments: This is the estimated working correlation with an autoregressive structure (AR). The correlation parameter is estimated as $\hat{\rho} = 0.8816$.

Analysis of GEE Parameter Estimates
Empirical Standard Error Estimates

Parameter	Estimate	Standard Error	95% Confidence Limits		Z	Pr > |Z|
Intercept	−1.049	0.333	−1.701	−0.397	−3.150	0.002
MOFROMINDEX	0.027	0.001	0.025	0.029	31.180	<.0001
AGE	0.063	0.004	0.055	0.070	15.790	<.0001
BMI	−0.031	0.006	−0.042	−0.020	−5.420	<.0001
DIABETES	0.157	0.081	−0.001	0.315	1.940	0.052
HYPERTEN	−0.172	0.044	−0.258	−0.086	−3.920	<.0001
HYPERCHO	−0.067	0.035	−0.136	0.003	−1.890	0.059

Comments: The parameter estimates, standard errors, 95% confidence interval (95% Confidence Limits), test statistics (Z), and the *p*-values

$(\Pr > |Z|)$ for the association of each covariate on the outcome are reported in this table. Time since baseline (MOFROMINDEX), age, BMI, and hypertension (HYPERTEN) are significant drivers of CDR-SUM. Diabetes and hypercholesterolemia (HYPERCHO) are not found to be statistically significant.

Compound Symmetry Working Correlation Matrix
The SAS syntax follows:

```
PROC GENMOD DATA = LONGITUDINAL;
CLASS VISITNUM ID;
MODEL CDRSUM = MOFROMINDEX AGE BMI DIABETES HYPERTEN HYPERCHO;
¹REPEATED SUBJECT= ID / WITHIN=VISITNUM TYPE=CS CORRW;
RUN;
```

[1] The working correlation matrix is specified as compound symmetry by TYPE=CS.

SAS OUTPUT

	Col1	Col2	Col3	Col4	Col5	Col6	Col7	Col8	Col9	Col10
					Working Correlation Matrix					
Row1	1.000	0.799	0.799	0.799	0.799	0.799	0.799	0.799	0.799	0.799
Row2	0.799	1.000	0.799	0.799	0.799	0.799	0.799	0.799	0.799	0.799
Row3	0.799	0.799	1.000	0.799	0.799	0.799	0.799	0.799	0.799	0.799
Row4	0.799	0.799	0.799	1.000	0.799	0.799	0.799	0.799	0.799	0.799
Row5	0.799	0.799	0.799	0.799	1.000	0.799	0.799	0.799	0.799	0.799
Row6	0.799	0.799	0.799	0.799	0.799	1.000	0.799	0.799	0.799	0.799
Row7	0.799	0.799	0.799	0.799	0.799	0.799	1.000	0.799	0.799	0.799
Row8	0.799	0.799	0.799	0.799	0.799	0.799	0.799	1.000	0.799	0.799
Row9	0.799	0.799	0.799	0.799	0.799	0.799	0.799	0.799	1.000	0.799
Row10	0.799	0.799	0.799	0.799	0.799	0.799	0.799	0.799	0.799	1.0000

Exchangeable Working Correlation	
Correlation	0.799

Comments: This is the estimated working correlation with a compound symmetry (CS) structure. The correlation parameter is estimated as $\hat{\rho} = 0.799$.

Analysis of GEE Parameter Estimates

Empirical Standard Error Estimates

Parameter	Estimate	Standard Error	95% Confidence Limits		Z	Pr > |Z|
Intercept	-1.151	0.345	-1.828	-0.475	-3.330	0.001
MOFROMINDEX	0.017	0.001	0.016	0.018	23.620	<.0001
AGE	0.064	0.004	0.057	0.072	16.270	<.0001
BMI	-0.021	0.007	-0.034	-0.008	-3.220	0.001
DIABETES	0.228	0.093	0.046	0.409	2.460	0.014
HYPERTEN	-0.245	0.050	-0.343	-0.147	-4.910	<.0001
HYPERCHO	-0.065	0.045	-0.154	0.024	-1.420	0.154

Comments: The parameter estimates, standard errors, 95% confidence interval (95% Confidence Limits), test statistics (Z), and the *p*-values (Pr > |Z|) for the association of each covariate on the outcome are reported in this table. Time since baseline (MOFROMINDEX), age, BMI, diabetes, and hypertension (HYPERTEN) are significant drivers of CDR-SUM. Hypercholesterolemia (HYPERCHO) is not a significant predictor.

Unstructured Working Correlation Matrix

The SAS syntax follows:

```
PROC GENMOD DATA = LONGITUDINAL;
CLASS VISITNUM ID;
MODEL CDRSUM = MOFROMINDEX AGE BMI DIABETES  HYPERTEN  HYPERCHO ;
¹REPEATED SUBJECT= ID / WITHIN=VISITNUM TYPE=UN CORRW;
run;
```

[1]The working correlation matrix is specified unstructured correlation TYPE=UN.

SAS OUTPUT

	Col1	Col2	Col3	Col4	Col5	Col6	Col7	Col8	Col9	Col10
				Working Correlation Matrix						
Row1	1.000	0.687	0.627	0.561	0.555	0.585	0.602	0.639	0.668	0.734
Row2	0.687	1.000	0.829	0.708	0.649	0.670	0.676	0.702	0.739	0.797
Row3	0.627	0.829	1.000	0.890	0.784	0.777	0.765	0.769	0.817	0.831
Row4	0.561	0.708	0.890	1.000	0.898	0.857	0.831	0.821	0.871	0.909
Row5	0.555	0.649	0.784	0.898	1.000	0.939	0.924	0.884	0.927	0.939
Row6	0.585	0.670	0.777	0.857	0.939	1.000	0.939	0.939	0.939	0.939
Row7	0.602	0.676	0.765	0.831	0.924	0.939	1.000	0.939	0.939	0.939
Row8	0.639	0.702	0.769	0.821	0.884	0.939	0.939	1.000	0.939	0.939
Row9	0.668	0.739	0.817	0.871	0.927	0.939	0.939	0.939	1.000	0.939
Row10	0.734	0.797	0.831	0.909	0.939	0.939	0.939	0.939	0.939	1.000

Comments: The estimated working correlation matrix with an unstructured (UN) correlation structure is shown. Each off-diagonal correlation term is estimated.

Parameter	Estimate	Standard Error	95% Confidence Limits		Z	Pr > |Z|
		Analysis of GEE Parameter Estimates				
		Empirical Standard Error Estimates				
Intercept	2.060	2.323	−2.494	6.614	0.890	0.375
MOFROMINDEX	0.006	0.004	−0.002	0.015	1.460	0.145
AGE	0.017	0.033	−0.048	0.082	0.520	0.605
BMI	−0.004	0.014	−0.032	0.025	−0.260	0.798
DIABETES	0.107	0.158	−0.203	0.417	0.680	0.499
HYPERTEN	−0.064	0.088	−0.237	0.108	−0.730	0.464
HYPERCHO	−0.081	0.081	−0.239	0.078	−1.000	0.318

Comments: The parameter estimates, standard errors, 95% confidence interval (95% Confidence Limits), test statistics (Z), and the p-values (Pr > $|Z|$) are reported as usual. In this case, however, the log displays a warning message:

Note: No convergence of GEE parameter estimates after 50 iterations.

Warning: Iteration limit exceeded.

This warning indicates that the model did not converge, and thus the model results are not reliable.

4.3.2 R Syntax and Output for GEE

Independent Working Correlation Matrix
The R syntax follows:

```
¹library(gee)
#Order data using subject ID
²orderID <- order(as.integer(dta$ID))
dta <- dta[orderID,]
#Independent working correlation structure
³gee_ind_out <- gee(CDRSUM ~ MOFROMINDEX + AGE + BMT + DIABETES
+ HYPERTEN  + HYPERCHO ,
                    data = dta, id = ID, family = gaussian,
                    corstr = "independence")
⁴summary(gee_ind_out)
```

[1]The gee library contains the gee() function used to fit GEE models.
[2]To use gee() in R, the data are sorted in order of the variable with repeated measurements. In this case, we order the subject IDs (ID). The order() function obtains the order of the ID numbers, and then the following statement orders the data in terms of this order.
[3]The gee() function fits a model using GEE for the Outcome ~ Predictors (separated by + signs). The data = option specifies the data frame that the data are stored in, id = specifies the identifier for the variable on which there are repeated measurements, family = specifies the distribution of the outcome, and corstr = is used to specify the working correlation structure. Options for corstr = include "independence," "AR-M," "exchangeable," and "unstructured." For "AR-M,"

the order must also be specified by adding the option Mv=, which has a default value of 1 (order 1).

[4]The summary statement prints a summary of the GEE model fit, including parameter estimates, standard errors, and the z-values.

R OUTPUT

```
summary(gee_ind_out)
##
##   GEE:  GENERALIZED LINEAR MODELS FOR DEPENDENT DATA
##   gee S-function, version 4.13 modified 98/01/27 (1998)
##
## Model:
##  Link:                     Identity
##  Variance to Mean Relation: Gaussian
##  Correlation Structure:    Independent
##
## Call:
## gee(formula = CDRSUM ~ MOFROMINDEX + AGE + BMI + DIABETES  +
##     HYPERTEN + HYPERCHO , id = ID, data = dta, family = gaussian,
##     corstr = "independence")
##
## Summary of Residuals:
##       Min        1Q     Median        3Q       Max
## -5.149723 -2.712966 -1.927100  1.606512 17.228722
##
##
## Coefficients:
##                  Estimate     Naive S.E.      Naive z  Robust S.E.      Robust z
## (Intercept)    0.11287389  0.2009064854    0.5618230  0.359090026     0.3143331
## MOFROMINDEX   -0.01677928  0.0007950972  -21.1034377  0.000984228   -17.0481674
## AGE            0.05821298  0.0021229352   27.4209861  0.003952054    14.7298015
## BMI           -0.04297255  0.0041494785  -10.3561319  0.007183714    -5.9819405
## DIABETES       0.48401483  0.0661759709    7.3140571  0.123836135     3.9085105
## HYPERTEN      -0.30507177  0.0436936482   -6.9820623  0.074901949    -4.0729484
## HYPERCHO       0.02941989  0.0418072039    0.7037038  0.070150458     0.4193827
```

```
##
## Estimated Scale Parameter:   17.86296
## Number of Iterations:  1
##
## Working Correlation
##         [,1] [,2] [,3] [,4] [,5] [,6] [,7] [,8] [,9] [,10]
## [1,]      1    0    0    0    0    0    0    0    0     0
## [2,]      0    1    0    0    0    0    0    0    0     0
## [3,]      0    0    1    0    0    0    0    0    0     0
## [4,]      0    0    0    1    0    0    0    0    0     0
## [5,]      0    0    0    0    1    0    0    0    0     0
## [6,]      0    0    0    0    0    1    0    0    0     0
## [7,]      0    0    0    0    0    0    1    0    0     0
## [8,]      0    0    0    0    0    0    0    1    0     0
## [9,]      0    0    0    0    0    0    0    0    1     0
## [10,]     0    0    0    0    0    0    0    0    0     1
```

Comments: The parameter estimates, standard errors, and z-values for the association of each covariate on the outcome are listed. Time since baseline (MOFROMINDEX), age, BMI, diabetes, and hypertension (HYPERTEN) are found to be statistically significant predictors of CDR-SUM. Hypercholesterolemia (HYPERCHO) is not found to affect CDR-SUM, however. The identity working correlation matrix is for the independent case.

Autoregressive Working Correlation Matrix
The R syntax follows:

```
#Autoregressive working correlation structure
¹gee_ar_out <- gee(CDRSUM ~ MOFROMINDEX + AGE + BMI + DIABETES
+ HYPERTEN  + HYPERCHO ,
                  data = dta, id = ID, family = gaussian,
                  corstr = "AR-M", Mv=1)
summary(gee_ar_out)
```

[1]GEE is performed for the Outcome ~ Predictors, with an autoregressive working correlation structure. This is specified using the option corstr = "AR-M," where the order of the autocorrelation is specified by Mv=1 (which is the default value).

R OUTPUT

```
summary(gee_ar_out)
##
##  GEE:  GENERALIZED LINEAR MODELS FOR DEPENDENT DATA
##  gee S-function, version 4.13 modified 98/01/27 (1998)
##
## Model:
## Link:                      Identity
## Variance to Mean Relation: Gaussian
## Correlation Structure:     AR-M , M = 1
##
## Call:
## gee(formula = CDRSUM ~ MOFROMINDEX + AGE + BMI + DIABETIC
##     HYPERTEN + HYPERCHO , id = ID, data = dta, family = gaussian,
##     corstr = "AR-M", Mv = 1)
##
## Summary of Residuals:
##       Min        1Q    Median        3Q       Max
## -7.254701 -3.502216 -2.342302  1.423265 17.435510
##
##
## Coefficients:
##                 Estimate    Naive S.E.    Naive z Robust S.E.  Robust z
## (Intercept)  -1.02054311 0.3162895649 -3.226610 0.332345465 -3.070730
## MOFROMINDEX   0.02645105 0.0007702436 34.341144 0.000865850 30.549222
## AGE           0.06259704 0.0037136790 16.855803 0.003963894 15.791806
## BMI          -0.03189050 0.0053793605 -5.928307 0.005727937 -5.567537
## DIABETES      0.16737025 0.0811259852  2.063091 0.081080385  2.064251
## HYPERTEN     -0.17466972 0.0444972457 -3.925405 0.043984233 -3.971190
## HYPERCHO     -0.06636031 0.0393542003 -1.686232 0.035644333 -1.861735
```

```
##
## Estimated Scale Parameter:  19.48162
## Number of Iterations:  4
##
## Working Correlation
##              [,1]       [,2]       [,3]       [,4]       [,5]       [,6]
## [1,]  1.0000000  0.8745837  0.7648966  0.6689660  0.5850668  0.5116898
## [2,]  0.8745837  1.0000000  0.8745837  0.7648966  0.6689660  0.5850668
## [3,]  0.7648966  0.8745837  1.0000000  0.8745837  0.7648966  0.6689660
## [4,]  0.6689660  0.7648966  0.8745837  1.0000000  0.8745837  0.7648966
## [5,]  0.5850668  0.6689660  0.7648966  0.8745837  1.0000000  0.8745837
## [6,]  0.5116898  0.5850668  0.6689660  0.7648966  0.8745837  1.0000000
## [7,]  0.4475156  0.5116898  0.5850668  0.6689660  0.7648966  0.8745837
## [8,]  0.3913898  0.4475156  0.5116898  0.5850668  0.6689660  0.7648966
## [9,]  0.3423031  0.3913898  0.4475156  0.5116898  0.5850668  0.6689660
## [10,] 0.2993727  0.3423031  0.3913898  0.4475156  0.5116898  0.5850668
##              [,7]       [,8]       [,9]      [,10]
## [1,]  0.4475156  0.3913898  0.3423031  0.2993727
## [2,]  0.5116898  0.4475156  0.3913898  0.3423031
## [3,]  0.5850668  0.5116898  0.4475156  0.3913898
## [4,]  0.6689660  0.5850668  0.5116898  0.4475156
## [5,]  0.7648966  0.6689660  0.5850668  0.5116898
## [6,]  0.8745837  0.7648966  0.6689660  0.5850668
## [7,]  1.0000000  0.8745837  0.7648966  0.6689660
## [8,]  0.8745837  1.0000000  0.8745837  0.7648966
## [9,]  0.7648966  0.8745837  1.0000000  0.8745837
## [10,] 0.6689660  0.7648966  0.8745837  1.0000000
```

Comments: Time since baseline (MOFROMINDEX), age, BMI, diabetes, and hypertension (HYPERTEN) are found to be statistically significant, while hypercholesterolemia (HYPERCHO) is not a statistically significant predictor of CDR-SUM. The correlation coefficient is $\hat{\rho} = 0.8746$.

Compound Symmetry Working Correlation Matrix
The R syntax follows:

```
#Compound symmetry working correlation structure
¹gee_cs_out <- gee(CDRSUM ~ MOFROMINDEX + AGE + BMI + DIABETES
+ HYPERTEN  + HYPERCHO ,
                    data = dta, id = ID, family = gaussian,
                    corstr = "exchangeable")
summary(gee_cs_out)
```

[1]GEE is performed with an exchangeable or compound symmetry correlation matrix.

R OUTPUT

```
summary(gee_cs_out)
##
##   GEE:  GENERALIZED LINEAR MODELS FOR DEPENDENT DATA
##   gee S-function, version 4.13 modified 98/01/27 (1998)
##
## Model:
##  Link:                     Identity
##  Variance to Mean Relation: Gaussian
##  Correlation Structure:    Exchangeable
##
## Call:
## gee(formula = CDRSUM ~ MOFROMINDEX + AGE + BMI + DIABETES  +
##     HYPERTEN  + HYPERCHO , id = ID, data = dta, family = gaussian,
##     corstr = "exchangeable")
##
## Summary of Residuals:
##      Min         1Q     Median        3Q        Max
## -6.487472 -3.480193 -2.492375   1.331599 17.331306
##
##
```

```
## Coefficients:
##               Estimate   Naive S.E.   Naive z  Robust S.E.   Robust z
## (Intercept) -1.15126918 0.3173340919 -3.627940 0.3452278018 -3.334810
## MOFROMINDEX  0.01697162 0.0005383944 31.522657 0.0007185778 23.618348
## AGE          0.06431055 0.0036991198 17.385367 0.0039521029 16.272490
## BMI         -0.02118905 0.0055002904 -3.852351 0.0065717254 -3.224275
## DIABETES     0.22781139 0.0809374983  2.814658 0.0926606276  2.458557
## HYPERTEN    -0.24534997 0.0453134168 -5.414511 0.0500117825 -4.905843
## HYPERCHO    -0.06460076 0.0408313155 -1.582138 0.0453551234 -1.424332
##
## Estimated Scale Parameter:  19.01802
## Number of Iterations:  5
##
## Working Correlation
##            [,1]      [,2]      [,3]      [,4]      [,5]      [,6]
##  [1,] 1.0000000 0.7987651 0.7987651 0.7987651 0.7987651 0.7987651
##  [2,] 0.7987651 1.0000000 0.7987651 0.7987651 0.7987651 0.7987651
##  [3,] 0.7987651 0.7987651 1.0000000 0.7987651 0.7987651 0.7987651
##  [4,] 0.7987651 0.7987651 0.7987651 1.0000000 0.7987651 0.7987651
##  [5,] 0.7987651 0.7987651 0.7987651 0.7987651 1.0000000 0.7987651
##  [6,] 0.7987651 0.7987651 0.7987651 0.7987651 0.7987651 1.0000000
##  [7,] 0.7987651 0.7987651 0.7987651 0.7987651 0.7987651 0.7987651
##  [8,] 0.7987651 0.7987651 0.7987651 0.7987651 0.7987651 0.7987651
##  [9,] 0.7987651 0.7987651 0.7987651 0.7987651 0.7987651 0.7987651
## [10,] 0.7987651 0.7987651 0.7987651 0.7987651 0.7987651 0.7987651
##            [,7]      [,8]      [,9]     [,10]
##  [1,] 0.7987651 0.7987651 0.7987651 0.7987651
##  [2,] 0.7987651 0.7987651 0.7987651 0.7987651
##  [3,] 0.7987651 0.7987651 0.7987651 0.7987651
##  [4,] 0.7987651 0.7987651 0.7987651 0.7987651
##  [5,] 0.7987651 0.7987651 0.7987651 0.7987651
##  [6,] 0.7987651 0.7987651 0.7987651 0.7987651
##  [7,] 1.0000000 0.7987651 0.7987651 0.7987651
```

```
## [8,]  0.7987651 1.0000000 0.7987651 0.7987651
## [9,]  0.7987651 0.7987651 1.0000000 0.7987651
## [10,] 0.7987651 0.7987651 0.7987651 1.0000000
```

Comments: The GEE model output suggests that time since baseline (MOFROMINDEX), age, BMI, diabetes, and hypertension (HYPERTEN) significantly drive the CDR-SUM score, while hypercholesterolemia (HYPERCHO) does not have a significant impact. The working correlation structure is also displayed, which has an estimated correlation coefficient of $\hat{\rho} = 0.799$.

Unstructured Working Correlation Matrix
The R syntax follows:

```
#Unstructured working correlation structure
¹gee_un_out <- gee(CDRSUM ~ MOFROMINDEX + AGE + BMI + DIABETES
+ HYPERTEN  + HYPERCHO ,
                    data = dta, id = ID, family = gaussian,
                    corstr = "unstructured")
summary(gee_un_out)
```

[1]GEE is performed with an unstructured (UN) working correlation structure in which every correlation coefficient is individually estimated.

R OUTPUT

```
summary(gee_un_out)
##
## GEE:  GENERALIZED LINEAR MODELS FOR DEPENDENT DATA
## gee S-function, version 4.13 modified 98/01/27 (1998)
##
## Model:
## Link:                    Identity
```

```
##   Variance to Mean Relation: Gaussian
##   Correlation Structure:      Unstructured
##
## Call:
## gee(formula = CDRSUM ~ MOFROMINDEX + AGE + BMI + DIABETES   +
##      HYPERTEN  + HYPERCHO , id = ID, data = dta, family = gaussian,
##      corstr = "unstructured")
##
## Summary of Residuals:
##       Min          1Q     Median          3Q         Max
## -4.974257 -2.841571 -2.123366   1.653614 17.389692
##
##
## Coefficients:
##                   Estimate    Naive S.E.     Naive z  Robust S.E.     Robust z
## (Intercept) -0.376108378 0.2703138742 -1.3913765 0.3604315221 -1.0434947
## MOFROMINDEX -0.003055424 0.0008296047 -3.6829877 0.0008618203 -3.5453142
## AGE          0.059942182 0.0029296261 20.4606933 0.0040928628 14.6455390
## BMI         -0.039746726 0.0053855444 -7.3802616 0.0068190557 -5.8287728
## DIABETES     0.428246427 0.0842404634  5.0836191 0.1131633279  3.7843216
## HYPERTEN    -0.294565171 0.0528827339 -5.5701578 0.0637548737 -4.6202769
## HYPERCHO     0.029144952 0.0492985267  0.5911932 0.0568864571  0.5123355
##
## Estimated Scale Parameter:  17.99501
## Number of Iterations:  4
##
## Working Correlation
##               [,1]         [,2]         [,3]         [,4]         [,5]
## [1,] 1.000000000 0.678873085 0.384927249 0.208157146 0.122757018
## [2,] 0.678873085 1.000000000 0.522619000 0.270195424 0.145854384
## [3,] 0.384927249 0.522619000 1.000000000 0.349601396 0.181738008
## [4,] 0.208157146 0.270195424 0.349601396 1.000000000 0.211655829
## [5,] 0.122757018 0.145854384 0.181738008 0.211655829 1.000000000
```

```
## [6,]  0.076813939 0.088254500 0.104425122 0.115692695 0.135440835
## [7,]  0.046814134 0.052061231 0.059457906 0.064141099 0.072198359
## [8,]  0.027280597 0.029256393 0.031588020 0.032853465 0.034852625
## [9,]  0.011323590 0.012296268 0.013541958 0.014062581 0.014647378
## [10,] 0.001633555 0.001703739 0.001655199 0.001795384 0.001819689
##               [,6]        [,7]        [,8]        [,9]       [,10]
## [1,]  0.07681394 0.046814134 0.027280597 0.011323590 0.001633555
## [2,]  0.08825450 0.052061231 0.029256393 0.012296268 0.001703739
## [3,]  0.10442512 0.059457906 0.031588020 0.013541958 0.001655199
## [4,]  0.11569270 0.064141099 0.032853465 0.014062581 0.001795384
## [5,]  0.13544084 0.072198359 0.034852625 0.014647378 0.001819689
## [6,]  1.00000000 0.079466599 0.036797614 0.015274803 0.001918100
## [7,]  0.07946660 1.000000000 0.037925071 0.015845863 0.002022627
## [8,]  0.03679761 0.037925071 1.000000000 0.016664457 0.001999136
## [9,]  0.01527480 0.015845863 0.016664457 1.000000000 0.002056503
## [10,] 0.00191810 0.002022627 0.001999136 0.002056503 1.000000000
```

Comments: The output displays the estimates, standard errors, and z-values for each covariate in the analysis. The results suggest that all predictors except hypercholesterolemia (HYPERCHO) are statistically significant predictors of CDR-SUM.

4.3.3 SPSS Syntax and Output for GEE

Independent Working Correlation Matrix
The SPSS syntax follows:

```
* Generalized Estimating Equations.
GENLIN CDRSUM WITH AGE BMI MOFROMINDEX DIABETES HYPERTEN HYPERCHO
  /MODEL AGE BMI MOFROMINDEX DIABETES HYPERTEN HYPERCHO INTERCEPT=YES
  DISTRIBUTION=NORMAL LINK=IDENTITY
  /CRITERIA SCALE=MLE PCONVERGE=1E-006(ABSOLUTE) SINGULAR=1E-012
ANALYSISTYPE=3(WALD) CILEVEL=95
    LIKELIHOOD=FULL
```

```
/REPEATED SUBJECT=MOFROMINDEX*BMI*AGE*DIABETES*HYPERTEN*HYPERCHO SORT=YES
  CORRTYPE=INDEPENDENT ADJUSTCORR=YES COVB=ROBUST
/MISSING CLASSMISSING=EXCLUDE
/PRINT DESCRIPTIVES MODELINFO FIT SUMMARY SOLUTION WORKINGCORR.
```

SPSS OUTPUT

Model Information		
Dependent Variable		CDRSUM
Probability Distribution		Normal
Link Function		Identity
Subject Effect	1	MOFROMINDEX
	2	BMI
	3	AGE
	4	DIABETES
	5	HYPERTEN
	6	HYPERCHO
Working Correlation Matrix Structure		Independent

Comments: This model uses an identity link function and assumes a normal distribution for the random component. The response variable is CDRSUM.

Parameter Estimates							
			95% Wald Confidence Interval		Hypothesis Test		
Parameter	B	Std. Error	Lower	Upper	Wald Chi-Square	df	Sig.
(Intercept)	.113	.3591	−.591	.817	.099	1	.753
HYPERCHO	.029	.0702	−.108	.167	.176	1	.675
HYPERTEN	−.305	.0749	−.452	−.158	16.589	1	.000
DIABETES	.484	.1238	.241	.727	15.276	1	.000
MOFROMINDEX	−.017	.0010	−.019	−.015	290.640	1	.000
BMI	−.043	.0072	−.057	−.029	35.784	1	.000

| Parameter | B | Std. Error | 95% Wald Confidence Interval | | Hypothesis Test | | |
			Lower	Upper	Wald Chi-Square	df	Sig.
AGE	.058	.0040	.050	.066	216.967	1	.000
(Scale)	17.863						

Dependent Variable: CDRSUM
Model: (Intercept), HYPERCHO, HYPERTEN, DIABETES, MOFROMINDEX, BMI, AGE

Comments: The parameter estimates, standard errors, confidence intervals, and the *p*-values (Sig.) for the association of each covariate on the outcome are reported. Age, BMI, time since baseline (MOFROMINDEX), diabetes, and hypertension are all significant drivers of CDR-SUM. Hypercholesterolemia is not found to be a significant covariate.

Working Correlation Matrix

| Measurement | Measurement | | | | | | |
	1	2	3	4	5	6	7
1	1.000	.000	.000	.000	.000	.000	.000
2	.000	1.000	.000	.000	.000	.000	.000
3	.000	.000	1.000	.000	.000	.000	.000
4	.000	.000	.000	1.000	.000	.000	.000
5	.000	.000	.000	.000	1.000	.000	.000
6	.000	.000	.000	.000	.000	1.000	.000
7	.000	.000	.000	.000	.000	.000	1.000

Comments: The estimated working correlation matrix is given. In the independent case, this is an identity matrix. In other correlation structures, however, the matrix will contain the estimated correlation parameters. The working correlation matrix is of dimension 10, as the most repeated measurements any subject has is 10. The maximum cluster size determines the size of the working correlation structure.

Autoregressive Working Correlation Matrix

The SPSS syntax follows:

```
GENLIN CDRSUM WITH AGE BMI MOFROMINDEX DIABETES HYPERTEN
HYPERCHO
  /MODEL AGE BMI MOFROMINDEX DIABETES HYPERTEN HYPERCHO
INTERCEPT=YES
  DISTRIBUTION=NORMAL LINK=IDENTITY
  /CRITERIA SCALE=MLE PCONVERGE=1E-006(ABSOLUTE)
SINGULAR=1E-012 ANALYSISTYPE=3(WALD) CILEVEL=95
    LIKELIHOOD=FULL
  /REPEATED SUBJECT=MOFROMINDEX*BMI*AGE*DIABETES*HYPERTEN*HYPER
CHO SORT=YES
    CORRTYPE=AR(1) ADJUSTCORR=YES COVB=ROBUST MAXITERATIONS=100
PCONVERGE=1e-006(ABSOLUTE) UPDATECORR=1
  /MISSING CLASSMISSING=EXCLUDE
  /PRINT DESCRIPTIVES MODELINFO FIT SUMMARY SOLUTION
WORKINGCORR.
```

SPSS OUTPUT

Parameter Estimates

| Parameter | B | Std. Error | 95% Wald Confidence Interval | | Hypothesis Test | | |
			Lower	Upper	Wald Chi-Square	df	Sig.
(Intercept)	-1.049	0.333	-1.701	-.397	9.954	1	.002
HYPERCHO	-.067	0.035	-.136	.002	3.573	1	.059
HYPERTEN	-.172	0.044	-.258	-.086	15.359	1	.000
DIABETES	.157	0.081	-.001	.315	3.778	1	.052
MOFROMINDEX	.027	0.001	.025	.029	972.503	1	.000
BMI	-.031	0.006	-.042	-.020	29.405	1	.000
AGE	.063	0.004	.055	.070	249.398	1	.000
(Scale)	19.532						

Dependent Variable: CDRSUM
Model: (Intercept), HYPERCHO, HYPERTEN, DIABETES, MOFROMINDEX, BMI, AGE

Comments: The results suggest that all covariates except hypercholesterolemia have a statistically significant impact on CDR-SUM.

Compound Symmetry Working Correlation Matrix
The SPSS syntax follows:

```
* Generalized Estimating Equations.
GENLIN CDRSUM WITH AGE BMI MOFROMINDEX DIABETES HYPERTEN
HYPERCHO
  /MODEL AGE BMI MOFROMINDEX DIABETES HYPERTEN HYPERCHO
INTERCEPT=YES
   DISTRIBUTION=NORMAL LINK=IDENTITY
   /CRITERIA SCALE=MLE PCONVERGE=1E-006(ABSOLUTE)
SINGULAR=1E-012 ANALYSISTYPE=3(WALD) CILEVEL=95
      LIKELIHOOD=FULL
   /REPEATED SUBJECT=MOFROMINDEX*BMI*AGE*DIABETES*HYPERTEN*HYPER
CHO SORT=YES
      CORRTYPE=EXCHANGEABLE ADJUSTCORR=YES COVB=ROBUST
MAXITERATIONS=100 PCONVERGE=1e-006(ABSOLUTE)
      UPDATECORR=1
   /MISSING CLASSMISSING=EXCLUDE
   /PRINT DESCRIPTIVES MODELINFO FIT SUMMARY SOLUTION
WORKINGCORR.
```

SPSS OUTPUT

Parameter Estimates

| Parameter | B | Std. Error | 95% Wald Confidence Inter. | | Hypothesis Test | | |
			Lower	Upper	Wald Chi-Square	df	Sig.
(Intercept)	-1.151	.345	-1.828	-.475	11.121	1	.001
HYPERCHO	-.065	.045	-.153	.024	2.029	1	.154
HYPERTEN	-.245	.050	-.343	-.147	24.067	1	.000
DIABETES	.228	.093	.046	.409	6.044	1	.014

| Parameter | B | Std. Error | 95% Wald Confidence Inter. | | Hypothesis Test | | |
			Lower	Upper	Wald Chi-Square	df	Sig.
MOFROMINDEX	.017	.001	.016	.018	557.828	1	.000
BMI	-.021	.007	-.034	-.008	10.396	1	.001
AGE	.064	.004	.057	.072	264.794	1	.000
(Scale)	19.018						

Dependent Variable: CDRSUM
Model: (Intercept), HYPERCHO, HYPERTEN, DIABETES, MOFROMINDEX, BMI, AGE

Comments: The results show the parameter estimates, standard, errors, confidence intervals, and p-values (Sig.). We find that hypercholesterolemia is not a significant covariate ($p = .154$), while all other covariates are found to have a significant impact on CDR-SUM.

Working Correlation Matrix

| Measurement | Measurement | | | | | | | | | |
	1	2	3	4	5	6	7	8	9	10
1	1.000	.799	.799	.799	.799	.799	.799	.799	.799	.799
2	.799	1.000	.799	.799	.799	.799	.799	.799	.799	.799
3	.799	.799	1.000	.799	.799	.799	.799	.799	.799	.799
4	.799	.799	.799	1.000	.799	.799	.799	.799	.799	.799
5	.799	.799	.799	.799	1.000	.799	.799	.799	.799	.799
6	.799	.799	.799	.799	.799	1.000	.799	.799	.799	.799
7	.799	.799	.799	.799	.799	.799	1.000	.799	.799	.799
8	.799	.799	.799	.799	.799	.799	.799	1.000	.799	.799
9	.799	.799	.799	.799	.799	.799	.799	.799	1.000	.799
10	.799	.799	.799	.799	.799	.799	.799	.799	.799	1.000

Dependent Variable: CDRSUM
Model: (Intercept), HYPERCHO, HYPERTEN, DIABETES, MOFROMINDEX, BMI, AGE

Comments: The working correlation matrix with a compound symmetry correlation structure is shown. The estimated correlation parameter is $\hat{\rho} = 0.799$.

Unstructured Working Correlation Matrix

The SPSS syntax follows:

```
* Generalized Estimating Equations.
GENLIN CDRSUM WITH AGE BMI MOFROMINDEX DIABETES HYPERTEN HYPERCHO
   /MODEL AGE BMI MOFROMINDEX DIABETES HYPERTEN HYPERCHO
INTERCEPT=YES
 DISTRIBUTION=NORMAL LINK=IDENTITY
   /CRITERIA SCALE=MLE PCONVERGE=1E-006(ABSOLUTE)
SINGULAR=1E-012 ANALYSISTYPE=3(WALD) CILEVEL=95
     LIKELIHOOD=FULL
   /REPEATED SUBJECT=MOFROMINDEX*BMI*AGE*DIABETES
*HYPERTEN*HYPERCHO  SORT=YES
     CORRTYPE=UNSTRUCTURED ADJUSTCORR=YES COVB=ROBUST
MAXITERATIONS=100 PCONVERGE=1e-006(ABSOLUTE)
     UPDATECORR=1
   /MISSING CLASSMISSING=EXCLUDE
   /PRINT DESCRIPTIVES MODELINFO FIT SUMMARY SOLUTION
WORKINGCORR.
```

SPSS OUTPUT

Parameter Estimates

Parameter	B	Std. Error	95% Wald Confidence Interval		Hypothesis Test		
			Lower	Upper	Wald Chi-Square	df	Sig.
(Intercept)	−.385	.323	−1.018	.248	1.421	1	.233
HYPERCHO	−.074	.038	−.149	.000	3.800	1	.051
HYPERTEN	−.171	.045	−.259	−.083	14.597	1	.000
DIABETES	.241	.089	.067	.416	7.339	1	.007
MOFROMINDEX	.013	.001	.011	.015	216.940	1	.000
BMI	−.035	.006	−.046	−.024	38.154	1	.000
AGE	.060	.004	.052	.067	245.855	1	.000
(Scale)	18.827						

Dependent Variable: CDRSUM
Model: (Intercept), HYPERCHO, HYPERTEN, DIABETES, MOFROMINDEX, BMI, AGE

Comments: The parameter estimates, standard errors, confidence intervals, and the *p*-values for the association of each covariate on the outcome are reported. Age, BMI, time since baseline (MOFROMINDEX), diabetes, and hypertension are all significant drivers of CDRSUM. Hypercholesterolemia ($p = 0.051$) is not found to be a significant covariate.

Working Correlation Matrix

Measurement	Measurement									
	1	2	3	4	5	6	7	8	9	10
1	1.000	.673	.613	.547	.540	.570	.587	.625	.655	.719
2	.673	1.000	.812	.692	.634	.656	.663	.692	.729	.788
3	.613	.812	1.000	.873	.769	.764	.754	.762	.811	.828
4	.547	.692	.873	1.000	.883	.844	.822	.817	.867	.911
5	.540	.634	.769	.883	1.000	.922	.917	.882	.922	.922
6	.570	.656	.764	.844	.922	1.000	.922	.922	.922	.922
7	.587	.663	.754	.822	.917	.922	1.000	.922	.922	.922
8	.625	.692	.762	.817	.882	.922	.922	1.000	.922	.922
9	.655	.729	.811	.867	.922	.922	.922	.922	1.000	.922
10	.719	.788	.828	.911	.922	.922	.922	.922	.922	1.000

Dependent Variable: CDRSUM
Model: (Intercept), HYPERCHO, HYPERTEN, DIABETES, MOFROMINDEX, BMI, AGE
a. Ridge value was added to the working correlation matrix to make it positive definite.

Comments: The working correlation matrix is unstructured (UN). The relationship between any two observations on the same person is the same.

4.3.4 Stata Syntax and Output for GEE

Independent Working Correlation Matrix
The Stata syntax follows:

```
xtgee cdrsum mofromindex bmi age hyperten hypercho diabetes,
family(gaussian) link(identity) corr(independent)
```

STATA OUTPUT

```
GEE population-averaged model          Number of obs      = 45508
Group variable:          cdrsum        Number of groups   = 12258
Link:                    identity  Obs per group:
Family:                  Gaussian                   min = 2
Correlation:             independent                avg = 3.7
                                                    max = 10
```

Comments: The GEE models have link identity, and the working correlation matrix is independent. There are 45,508 observations, with 12,258 subjects. The distribution of CDRSUM at any point is normal.

```
Scale parameter:         17.860        Prob > chi2    =    0.000
Pearson chi2(761):    812782.62        Deviance       =812782.62
Dispersion (Pearson):    17.860        Dispersion     =   17.860
```

Comments: There is a scale parameter on the variance of 17.860. The correlation in the observations results in a scaling of the variance.

CDRSUM	Coef.	Std. Err.	z	P>z	[95% Conf. Interval]	
BMI	-0.043	0.004	-10.360	0.000	-0.051	-0.035
MOFROMINDEX	-0.017	0.001	-21.110	0.000	-0.018	-0.015
AGE	0.058	0.002	27.420	0.000	0.054	0.062
DIABETES	0.484	0.066	7.310	0.000	0.354	0.614
HYPERTEN	-0.305	0.044	-6.980	0.000	-0.391	-0.219
HYPERCHO	0.029	0.042	0.700	0.482	-0.053	0.111
_CONS	0.113	0.201	0.560	0.574	-0.281	0.507

Comments: The output contains the parameter estimates, standard errors, z-values, p-values, and confidence intervals for the association of each covariate on CDR-SUM. Age, BMI, time since baseline (MOFROMINDEX), diabetes, and hypertension are identified as significant drivers of the outcome.

Autoregressive Working Correlation Matrix

The Stata syntax follows:

```
xtgee cdrsum mofromindex bmi age hyperten hypercho  diabetes,
family(gaussian) link(identity) corr(ar 1)
```

STATA OUTPUT

```
GEE population-averaged model         Number of obs    =  45508

Group variable:           cdrsum      Number of groups =  12258

Link:                     identity  Obs per group:

Family:                   Gaussian                  min =  2

Correlation:              independent               avg =  3.7

                                                    max =  10
```

Comments: The GEE models have link identity, and the working correlation matrix is independent (IN). There are 45,508 observations, within 12,258 subjects. The distribution of CDRSUM at any point is normal.

```
Scale parameter:       19.529   Prob > chi2   =      0.000
```

Comments: There is a scale parameter on the variance of 19.529. The correlation in the observations results in a scaling of the variance.

CDRSUM	Coef.	Std. Err.	z	P>z	[95% Conf. Interval]	
BMI	−0.031	0.005	−5.850	0.000	−.042	−.021
MOFROMINDEX	0.027	0.001	35.710	0.000	.026	.029
AGE	0.063	0.004	16.790	0.000	.055	.070
DIABETES	0.157	0.080	1.960	0.050	−.000	.314
HYPERTEN	−0.172	0.044	−3.930	0.000	−.257	−.086
HYPERCHO	−0.067	0.039	−1.740	0.082	−.143	.009
_CONS	−1.049	0.316	−3.320	0.001	−1.669	−.429

Comments: The parameter estimates, standard errors, z-values, p-values, and confidence intervals for the association of each covariate on CDR-SUM are given. Age, BMI, time since baseline (MOFRO-MINDEX), and hypertension (HYPERTEN) are identified as significant drivers of the outcome. We find that age, BMI, MOFROMIN-DEX, and HYPERTEN are significant drivers of CDR-SUM. Diabetes and hypercholesterolemia (HYPERCHO) are not found to be statistically significantly associated with the outcome.

Compound Symmetry Working Correlation Matrix
The Stata syntax follows:

```
xtgee cdrsum mofromindex bmi age hyperten hypercho diabetes,
family(gaussian) link(identity) corr(exchangeable)
```

STATA OUTPUT

```
GEE population-averaged model          Number of obs     =  45508
Group variable:          cdrsum        Number of groups  =  12258
Link:                    identity      Obs per group:
Family:                  Gaussian                  min  =  2
Correlation:             independent               avg  =  3.7
                                                   max  =  10
```

Comments: The GEE models have link identity, and the working correlation matrix is independent (IN). There are 45,508 observations, in 12,258 subjects. The distribution CDRSUM at any point is normal.

```
Scale parameter:         19.015   Prob > chi2   =      0.000
```

Comments: There is a scale parameter on the variance of 19.015. The correlation in the observations results in a scaling of the variance.

CDRSUM	Coef.	Std. Err.	z	P>z	[95% Conf. Interval]	
BMI	-0.021	0.005	-3.850	0.000	-0.032	-0.010
MOFROMINDEX	0.017	0.001	31.530	0.000	0.016	0.018
AGE	0.064	0.004	17.390	0.000	0.057	0.072
DIABETES	0.228	0.081	2.810	0.005	0.069	0.386
HYPERTEN	-0.245	0.045	-5.420	0.000	-0.334	-0.157
HYPERCHO	-0.065	0.041	-1.580	0.114	-0.145	0.015
_CONS	-1.151	0.317	-3.630	0.000	-1.773	-0.530

Comments: The parameter estimates, standard errors, z-values, p-values, and confidence intervals for the association of each covariate on CDR-SUM are given. Age, BMI, time since baseline (MOFROMINDEX), diabetes, and hypertension (HYPERTEN) are identified as significant drivers of the outcome. The GEE results suggest that all predictors except hypercholesterolemia (HYPERCHO, $p = 0.114$) are statistically significant predictors of the CDR-SUM score.

Unstructured Working Correlation Matrix

The Stata syntax follows:

```
xtgee cdrsum mofromindex bmi age hyperten hypercho diabetes,
family(gaussian) link(identity) corr(unstructured)
```

STATA OUTPUT

```
GEE population-averaged model        Number of obs   = 45508
Group variable:         cdrsum       Number of groups = 12258
Link:                   identity Obs per group:
Family:                 Gaussian                   min = 2
Correlation:            independent                avg = 3.7
                                                   max = 10
```

Comments: The GEE model has link identity, and the working correlation matrix is independent. There are 45,508 observations from 12,258 patients. The distribution CDRSUM at any point is normal.

```
Scale parameter:        20.224  Prob > chi2  =       0.000
```

Comments: There is a scale parameter on the variance of 20.224. The correlation in the observations results in a scaling of the variance.

CDRSUM	Coef.	Std. Err.	z	P>z	[95% Conf. Interval]	
BMI	-0.039	0.006	-6.540	0.000	-0.050	-0.027
MOFROMINDEX	0.034	0.001	33.660	0.000	0.032	0.036
AGE	0.061	0.004	16.630	0.000	0.054	0.068
DIABETES	0.210	0.091	2.310	0.021	0.032	0.389
HYPERTEN	-0.132	0.052	-2.550	0.011	-0.232	-0.031
HYPERCHO	-0.137	0.047	-2.920	0.003	-0.229	-0.045
_CONS	-0.715	0.323	-2.220	0.027	-1.347	-0.083

```
convergence not achieved r(430);
```

Comments: For the unstructured (UN) working correlation matrix, Stata reported the model output. The model did not converge, however, and thus we cannot rely on these results.

4.4 Two-Level Random Effects Models

For hierarchical data, subject-specific approaches such as random effects models are used as an alternative to marginal models. These approaches, which may also be referred to as multilevel models, incorporate the nested sources of variability at each level. In this section, we focus on the analysis of two-level hierarchical data, although as we will show in the next section, the approach is also applicable to three-level or higher hierarchical data. The key to analyzing hierarchical data is the use of random effects at each level of nesting to account for correlation in the hierarchical structure. The random effects are added into the model to account for unobservable effects that are known to exist but are not measured. For example, in our data, we may assume that the patients account for some of the variation. Some patients may tend to have higher CDR-SUM scores, while others tend to have lower CDR-SUM scores. Random effects can be positive or negative, but overall we assume that the average effect is zero (Breslow and Clayton 1993). We wish to evaluate the overall effect of each patient as well as measure variation in their repeated visits as the observations.

Intraclass correlation describes the correlation between observations within each level of the hierarchy. Strong intraclass correlation indicates that observations within a cluster of the hierarchy are strongly related, while weak intraclass correlation indicates that the observations within a cluster are not strongly related. Stronger correlation within the clusters must be accounted for using methods such as mixed models.

The following section is included as a complete but brief discussion of mixed models. Those unfamiliar with matrices can skip this section and follow the computer code and outputs.

STATISTICAL MODEL

In statistical notation, we define a linear mixed model as having the form

$$y = X\beta + Z\gamma + \epsilon$$

(observation = fixed part + random part + unexplained part),

where X is a $n \times p$ data matrix for the fixed effects, Z is the $n \times q$ design matrix for the random effects, β is the $p \times 1$ q parameters, γ is the $q \times 1$ vector of random effects parameters, and ϵ is the $n \times 1$ vector of error terms. It is assumed that $\gamma \sim N(0, G)$ and $\epsilon \sim N(0, R)$ and so the expectation of the observations y is

$$E(Y) = X\beta,$$

which is the same as the fixed model, but the variance of the observations y is

$$\text{var}(Y) = ZGZ^T + R$$

(Breslow and Clayton 1993). This is analyzed using Henderson's mixed model equations

$$\begin{pmatrix} X^T R^{-1} X & X^T R^{-1} Z \\ Z^T R^{-1} X & Z^T R^{-1} Z + G^{-1} \end{pmatrix} \begin{pmatrix} \hat{\beta} \\ \hat{\gamma} \end{pmatrix} = \begin{pmatrix} X^T R^{-1} y \\ Z^T R^{-1} y \end{pmatrix},$$

where $\hat{\beta}$ is the best linear unbiased estimator of β, and $\hat{\gamma}$ is the best linear unbiased predictor of γ (Verbeke and Molenberghs 2000). Thus we can solve the system of equations to obtain

$$\hat{\beta} = \left(X^T V^{-1} X \right)^{-1} X^T V^{-1} y$$

and

$$\hat{\gamma} = G Z^T V^{-1} (y - X\hat{\beta}).$$

The random effect is used to account for the impact of particular groups. For patients nested within ADCs, for example, the random effect estimates the impact the particular center has on the outcome as compared to other centers. In longitudinal studies, we expect measurements from the same patient to be similar to one another, and the random effect can account for differences between patients.

Problem: Do times since the baseline visit, age, BMI, diabetes, hypertension, and hypercholesterolemia jointly affect CDR-SUM while adjusting for patient effects?

Solution: One uses random effects models to account for the patient-level effects. We analyzed the longitudinal dataset containing visits for 12,258 patients, each with multiple visits, which was introduced in section 4.1. We consider a two-level model where we fit a mixed model with a random intercept for the patient effect. This allows us to account for the individual effects of the patients on the variability in the CDR-SUM measurements. We consider the variables time since baseline measured in months (MOFROMINDEX), age, BMI, diabetes, hypertension (HYPERTEN), and hypercholesterolemia (HYPERCHO). Patients are identified through their ID. The mixed-model parameter estimates are reported in table 4.5.

In the two-level model with a random intercept at the patient level, we find that the covariance parameter estimate is statistically significant at the 95% significance level as $\dfrac{\hat{\sigma}}{\text{SE}(\hat{\sigma})} = \dfrac{17.2119}{0.2330} = 73.87 > 1.96$, where $\hat{\sigma}$ and $\text{SE}(\hat{\sigma})$ are the point estimate and the standard error. This indicates that the patient as a random effect is significant. Thus the measurements within each patient are significantly correlated and differ from measurements on other patients. From the evaluation of the covariates, we find that time (months) since baseline visit, age, diabetes, and hypertension are significantly associated with the CDR-SUM score. This is the same result we found using GEE. The results found after using the four statistical software programs are summarized in table 4.6.

Table 4.5 Parameter Estimates for the Two-Level Mixed Model

Parameter	Estimate	Std Err	p-Value
Intercept	−1.391	0.322	<0.0001
MOFROMINDEX	0.018	0.000	<0.0001
AGE	0.065	0.004	<.0001
BMI	−0.013	0.005	0.011
DIABETES	0.183	0.075	0.014
HYPERTEN	−0.236	0.041	<0.0001
HYPERCHO	−0.061	0.036	0.092

Table 4.6 Significant Predictors for Two-Level Mixed Models for Statistical Programs

SAS	R	SPSS	Stata
Time	Time	Time	Time
Age	Age	Age	Age
BMI	BMI	BMI	BMI
Diabetes	Diabetes	Diabetes	Diabetes
Hypertension	Hypertension	Hypertension	Hypertension

4.4.1 SAS Syntax and Output for Two-Level Mixed Models

The SAS syntax follows:

```
¹PROC GLIMMIX DATA=LONGITUDINAL NOCLPRINT;
²CLASS ID;
³MODEL CDRSUM = MOFROMINDEX AGE BMI DIABETES HYPERTEN HYPERCHO/
DIST=NORMAL DDFM=RESIDUAL S;
⁴RANDOM INTERCEPT /SUBJECT=ID;
RUN;
```

[1]PROC GLIMMIX fits generalized linear mixed models. NOCL-PRINT suppresses output.
[2]The CLASS statement identifies categorical variables.
[3]The MODEL statement defines the outcome = predictors. DIST= is distribution of the outcome; DDFM= is the residual degrees of freedom method. The option S prints the solutions for the fixed effects table.
[4]Defines a random effect. Times are nested within patients (SUBJECT).

SAS OUTPUT

The GLIMMIX Procedure

Model Information

Dataset	WORK.LONGITUDINAL
Response Variable	CDRSUM
Response Distribution	Gaussian
Link Function	Identity
Variance Function	Default
Variance Matrix Blocked By	ID
Estimation Technique	Restricted Maximum Likelihood
Degrees of Freedom Method	Residual

Comments: The Model Information table summarizes information about the model specification and fit. The random component is assumed to follow a normal (Gaussian) distribution. The link is an identity link function. The regression coefficients are obtained using restricted maximum likelihood estimation.

Class-Level Information		
Class	Levels	Values
ID	12258	not printed

Comments: The Class-Level Information table displays information about categorical variables (specified using the class statement in SAS). ID is specified as a categorical variable, which has 12,258 different values.

Dimensions	
G-side Cov. Parameters	1
R-side Cov. Parameters	1
Columns in X	7
Columns in Z per Subject	1
Subjects (Blocks in V)	12258
Max Obs per Subject	10

Comments: There is a random effect covariance matrix (G-side) and a fixed effect covariance effect (R-side) in this model. There are six covariates plus the constant, for a total of seven columns in X. There is one random effect in the model (columns in Z), which represents the random intercept for the patient. There are 12,258 clusters, representing the 12,258 patients, and each patient has up to 10 observations.

Convergence Criterion (GCONV=1E-8) Satisfied.

Comments: The model converged. This is good news, as these models do not always converge. Convergence depends on the structure of the data and the sample sizes at each level. Do not confuse convergence with the model fit.

Fit Statistics	
-2 Res Log Likelihood	213245.5
AIC (smaller is better)	213249.5
AICC (smaller is better)	213249.5
BIC (smaller is better)	213264.3
CAIC (smaller is better)	213266.3
HQIC (smaller is better)	213254.5
Generalized Chi-Square	126040.0
Gener. Chi-Square / DF	2.77

Comments: The Fit Statistics table reports fit statistics including the −2 residual log likelihood (−2 Res Log Likelihood), Akaike information criterion (AIC), Akaike information criterion with a correction for small sample sizes (AICC), Bayesian information criterion (BIC), consistent Akaike information criterion (CAIC), Hannan-Quinn information criterion (HQIC), generalized chi-square, and the ratio of the generalized chi-square divided to degrees of freedom (DF). The model is usually considered a good fit when the generalized chi-square/DF is close to one. In this case, the value is 2.77. Thus there is more variation to address in this model than what is explained by the covariates that were included.

Covariance Parameter Estimates			
Cov Parm	Subject	Estimate	Standard Error
Intercept	ID	17.212	0.233
Residual		2.770	0.022

Comments: The estimated covariance for the random effect (Estimate) and the estimated standard error for the covariance estimate (Std Err) are provided. The z-value for the random intercept is

17.2119/0.2330 = 73.87 > 1.96. The significance of the covariance terms is determined by evaluating whether Estimate/Std Err > 1.96. Because the ratio in this example is greater than 1.96, we support the use of the random effects in patients in the model. The covariance parameter estimates, standard errors for the random error (residual), and the random effects (in this example, the intercept term for subject) are provided in this table.

Solutions for Fixed Effects					
Effect	Estimate	Standard Error	DF	t Value	Pr > |t|
Intercept	-1.391	0.322	45501	-4.320	<.0001
MOFROMINDEX	0.018	0.000	45501	36.130	<.0001
AGE	0.065	0.004	45501	16.720	<.0001
BMI	-0.013	0.005	45501	-2.550	0.011
DIABETES	0.183	0.075	45501	2.450	0.014
HYPERTEN	-0.236	0.041	45501	-5.820	<.0001
HYPERCHO	-0.061	0.036	45501	-1.690	0.092

Comments: The Solutions for Fixed Effects table provides the parameter estimates, standard error, t-value, and p-value (Pr > |t|) for the association between each covariate and the outcome. All the predictors other than hypercholesterolemia ($p = 0.092$) are found to be significant predictors of CDR-SUM.

4.4.2 R Syntax and Output for Two-Level Mixed Models

The R syntax follows:

```
1library(lme4)
#Two level mixed model - analyze patient effect
2mm_1_out <- glmer(CDRSUM ~ MOFROMINDEX + AGE + BMI + DIABETES
+ HYPERTEN + HYPERCHO + (1 | ID), family = gaussian(), data = dta)
3summary(mm_1_out)
```

[1]The library lme4 contains the glmer() function to fit generalized linear mixed models.

[2]The glmer() function fits a mixed model for the Outcome ~ Predictors. The data= option specifies that the variables in the model come from the dataset dta. The option (1 | ID) adds a random intercept for the subject level (ID).

[3]The summary statement prints a summary of the model fit and parameter estimates.

R OUTPUT

```
summary(mm_1_out)
## Linear mixed model fit by REML ['lmerMod']
## Formula:
## CDRSUM ~ MOFROMINDEX + AGE + BMI + DIABETES  + HYPERTEN  +
##     HYPERCHO  + (1 | ID)
##     Data: dta
##
## REML criterion at convergence: 213245.5
##
## Scaled residuals:
##     Min      1Q  Median      3Q     Max
## -6.1925 -0.3461 -0.0587  0.2678  7.8090
##
## Random effects:
##  Groups   Name        Variance Std.Dev.
##  ID   (Intercept) 17.21    4.149
##  Residual             2.77    1.664
## Number of obs: 45508, groups:  ID, 12258
##
## Fixed effects:
##                 Estimate Std. Error t value
## (Intercept)  -1.3905318 0.3217535  -4.322
## MOFROMINDEX   0.0179087 0.0004957  36.129
```

```
## AGE             0.0645184   0.0038589   16.719
## BMI            -0.0131468   0.0051517   -2.552
## DIABETES        0.1827774   0.0745981    2.450
## HYPERTEN       -0.2360210   0.0405604   -5.819
## HYPERCHO       -0.0611023   0.0362496   -1.686
##
## Correlation of Fixed Effects:
##               (Intr)  MOFROM  AG  BM  DIABET  HYPERT
## MOFROMINDEX   0.528
## AGE          -0.895  -0.625
## BMI          -0.507  -0.009   0.098
## DIABETES      0.029  -0.025  -0.024  -0.059
## HYPERTEN      0.084  -0.024  -0.112  -0.084  -0.062
## HYPERCHO     -0.002  -0.032  -0.026  -0.044  -0.075  -0.153
```

Comments: The R output for glmer() includes the estimates of the random effects and the estimates of the fixed effects. In this case, the covariance for the subject random intercept is estimated as 17.21 (which is standard error $\sqrt{17.21} = 4.149$). For the fixed effects, the parameter estimates, standard errors, and t-values for the association between each covariate and the outcome are provided. We find that all the predictors other than hypercholesterolemia are significant after adjusting for patient and center effect.

4.4.3 SPSS Syntax and Output for Two-Level Mixed Models

The linear mixed-effects models (MIXED) procedure in SPSS enables you to fit linear mixed-effects models to data sampled from normal distributions (McCulloch and Searle 2000; Verbeke and Molenberghs 2000). Correlated data, such as repeated measurements, are common in the measurements of survey respondents or in clinical studies. The MIXED procedure fits correlated data and unequal variances, unlike the general linear model procedure GLM. The MIXED procedure allows patients to have an unequal number of measurements, as is the case in our example of CDR-SUM scores, since patients had a varying number of visits. MIXED is based on maximum likelihood (ML) and restricted maximum likelihood (REML) methods. The ML and REML yield asymptotically efficient estimators for balanced and unbalanced designs. The asymptotic normality of ML and REML estimators, furthermore, conveniently allows us to make inferences on the covariance parameters of the model.

The SPSS syntax follows:

```
GET FILE ="C:\User\Documents\Data\chap4.sav "
mixed cdrsum with MOFROMINDEX AGE BMI DIABETES HYPERTEN
HYPERCHO
 /fixed = MOFROMINDEX AGE BMI DIABETES HYPERTEN HYPERCHO
 /print = solution
 /random = intercept | subject(ID).
```

SPSS OUTPUT

Parameter	Estimate	Std. Error	t	Sig.	95% Confidence Interval	
					Lower Bound	Upper Bound
Intercept	-1.391	.322	-4.322	.000	-2.021	-.760
MOFROMINDEX	.018	.001	36.129	.000	.017	.019
AGE	.065	.004	16.719	.000	.057	.072
BMI	-.013	.005	-2.552	.011	-.023	-.003
DIABETES	.183	.075	2.450	.014	.037	.329
HYPERTEN	-.236	.041	-5.819	.000	-.316	-.157
HYPERCHO	-.061	.036	-1.686	.092	-.132	.010

Comments: The parameter estimates, standard error, t-value (t), and p-value (Sig.) for the association between each covariate and the outcome are given. The variable hypercholesterolemia is not significant ($p = 0.092$). All the other predictors are significant after adjusting for patient effect.

Estimates of Covariance Parameters

Parameter			Estimate	Std. Error
Residual			2.770	.022
Intercept [subject = ID]		Variance	17.212	.233

Comments: The random effect parameter for the subject level has a z-value of $17.212/.233 = 73.87$. This is significantly larger than the value of two. As such, we support the use of the random effects in patients in the model. The covariance parameter estimates and standard errors for the random error (residual) and the random effects (in this example, the intercept term for ID) are provided in this table. The significance of the covariance terms is determined by evaluating whether estimate/standard error > 1.96.

4.4.4 Stata Syntax and Output for Two-Level Mixed Models

The Stata syntax follows:

```
. mixed cdrsum mofromindex age diabetes        hyperten
hypercho        id:
```

STATA OUTPUT

```
Performing EM optimization:
Performing gradient-based optimization:
Iteration 0:    log likelihood = -106601.33
Iteration 1:    log likelihood = -106601.33
```

Comments: Stata uses an expectation-maximization (EM) algorithm to fit the model and obtain the estimates.

```
Computing standard errors:
Mixed-effects ML regression    Number of obs    =    45,508
Group variable: id             Number of groups =    12,258
```

```
                    Obs per group:

                              min   =           2

                              avg   =         3.7

                              max   =          10

                    Wald chi2(5)    =     3954.06
Log likelihood = -106601.33     Prob > chi2   =      0.0000
```

Comments: There are 12,258 clusters. They have between 2 and 10 observations. The Wald chi-square for testing the joint significance has a value of 3,954.06.

CDRSUM	Coef.	Std. Err.	z	P>z	[95% Conf. Interval]	
MOFROMINDEX	0.018	0.000	36.110	0.000	0.017	0.019
AGE	0.065	0.004	17.040	0.000	0.058	0.073
DIABETES	0.171	0.074	2.300	0.021	0.025	0.317
HYPERTEN	-0.245	0.040	-6.050	0.000	-0.324	-0.165
HYPERCHO	-0.065	0.036	-1.800	0.072	-0.136	0.006
_CONS	-1.807	0.278	-6.510	0.000	-2.351	-1.263

Comments: The parameter estimate (Coef.), standard error, t-value, and p-value ($P>z$) for the association between each covariate and the outcome are given. Hypercholesterolemia is found not to be significant ($p = 0.072$). All the other predictors are significant after adjusting for patient and center effect.

Random-Effects Parameters	Estimate	Std. Err.	[95% Conf. Interval]	
id: Identity				
var(_cons)	17.240	0.233	16.789	17.702
var(Residual)	2.768	0.022	2.727	2.811

Comments: The random effects parameter for the subject effect (var(_cons)) has a confidence interval (16.789, 17.702). This does not include zero. As such, we support the use of the random effects in patients in the model. The covariance parameter estimates and standard errors for the random error (residual) and the random effects (in this example, var(_cons)) are provided in this table. The significance of the covariance terms is determined by the exclusion of zero.

4.5 Three-Level Random Effects Models

Hierarchical data also arise with more than one level of clustering. In section 4.4, patients in the dataset have repeated measurements. In turn, however, the patients are nested within one of 35 ADCs. Thus we have a three-level hierarchical structure. An appropriate model must account for the correlation that exists between patients from the same ADC. In the two-level model, we had one random effect to address the ties within the patients. For the three-level model, we add a second random effect to address the patients nested within the center random effects. Thus in our three-level model we include two random effects, one for the patient level and one for the ADC level.

The random effects mixed model can also be extended analogously to account for hierarchical structures with more than three levels. Each additional level of nesting is accounted for with the inclusion of an additional random effect. Random slope terms are possible, depending on which level of the data they pertain to. The linear mixed model follows the same form provided in section 4.4, though the dimensions of Z and γ vary based on the number of random effects. The statistical properties of the estimators, as well as the corresponding assumptions, also remain the same. Practically, it is challenging to fit these higher-level models because it is difficult to obtain convergence in statistical software.

Problem: Do baseline visit, age, BMI, diabetes, hypertension, and hypercholesterolemia jointly affect CDR-SUM over time while adjusting for patient and center effects?

Solution: We utilize a three-level random effects model to address both levels of nesting in the data, with one random intercept term for the patient level and one random intercept term for the center-level effects. We consider as predictors time since baseline measured in months (MOFROMINDEX), age, BMI, diabetes, hypertension (HYPERTEN), and hypercholesterolemia (HYPERCHO). Each of the times measured on each patient is identified by ID, and the patients within the centers are identified through the center number (ADC). The parameter estimates are reported in table 4.7.

We find that the patient and center effects are both statistically significant for patient $\dfrac{15.5723}{0.2124} = 73.32 > 1.96$ and for ADC $\dfrac{1.6091}{0.4162} = 3.87 > 1.96$. This indicates that, in addition to the patients accounting for a significant amount of variation in CDR-SUM, the center effect explains variation in the outcome. Thus patients within the same center tend to be more similar than patients between different centers, and observations from the same patient tend to be more similar than observations from different patients. We also find that the same covariates and cardiovascular risk factors are statistically significant. The significance of the predictors, obtained using the four statistical software programs, is reported in table 4.8.

Table 4.7 Parameter Estimates for the Three-Level Mixed Model

Parameter	Estimate	Std Err	p-Value
Intercept	−1.265	0.389	0.001
MOFROMINDEX	0.018	0.000	<0.0001
AGE	0.063	0.004	<0.0001
BMI	−0.013	0.005	0.010
DIABETES	0.182	0.074	0.013
HYPERTEN	−0.228	0.040	<0.0001
HYPERCHO	−0.061	0.036	0.091

Table 4.8 Significant Predictors for Three-Level Mixed Models for Statistical Programs

SAS	R	SPSS	Stata
Time (months)	Time (months)	Did not converge	Time (months)
Age	Age		Age
BMI	BMI		BMI
Diabetes	Diabetes		Diabetes
Hypertension	Hypertension		Hypertension
			Hypercholesterolemia

4.5.1 SAS Syntax and Output for Three-Level Mixed Models

The SAS syntax follows:

```
PROC GLIMMIX DATA=LONGITUDINAL NOCLPRINT;
CLASS ADC ID;
MODEL CDRSUM = MOFROMINDEX AGE BMI DIABETES HYPERTEN HYPERCHO /
DIST=NORMAL DDFM=RESIDUAL S;
¹RANDOM INTERCEPT /SUBJECT=ID(ADC);
²RANDOM INTERCEPT/SUBJECT=ADC;
RUN;
```

¹Visits are nested within the patients.
²Patients are nested within ADCs.

SAS OUTPUT

Dimensions	
G-side Cov. Parameters	2
R-side Cov. Parameters	1
Columns in X	7
Columns in Z per Subject	762
Subjects (Blocks in V)	35
Max Obs per Subject	2955

Comments: The G-side covariance parameters account for the random effects, while the R-side covariance parameters account for the fixed effect (error term). There are two parameters for the random effects ($\sigma^2_{\text{patients}}$ and σ^2_{center}), as we assume that the patient $\sim N(0, \sigma^2_{\text{patients}})$ and center $\sim N(0, \sigma^2_{\text{center}})$.

Covariance Parameter Estimates			
Cov Parm	Subject	Estimate	Standard Error
Intercept	ID(ADC)	15.572	0.212
Intercept	ADC	1.609	0.416
Residual		2.771	0.0215

Comments: The patient random effect parameter for the subject level (ID) has a z-value of $15.5723/0.2124 = 73.32 > 1.96$. This is significantly larger than the value of two. As such, we support the use of the random effects in patients in the model. In addition, the covariance for the center random intercept has a z-value of $1.6091/0.4162 = 3.87$, which is also larger than the value of two. We support this center random effect in the model.

Solutions for Fixed Effects					
Effect	Estimate	Standard Error	DF	t Value	Pr > |t|
Intercept	−1.265	0.389	45501	3.25	0.001
MOFROMINDEX	0.018	0.000	45501	36.45	<.0001
AGE	0.063	0.004	45501	16.28	<.0001
BMI	−0.013	0.005	45501	−2.58	0.010
DIABETES	0.182	0.074	45501	2.47	0.013
HYPERTEN	−0.228	0.040	45501	−5.65	<.0001
HYPERCHO	−0.061	0.036	45501	−1.69	0.091

Comments: The Solutions for Fixed Effects table presents the parameter estimates; standard error, t-value, and p-value for the association between each covariate and the outcome are given. We find that hypercholesterolemia is not a significant predictor of CDR-SUM. All the other predictors are found to be statistically significant after adjusting for patient and center effect.

4.5.2 R Syntax and Output for Three-Level Mixed Models

The R syntax follows:

```
#Three level mixed model - analyze patient and center effects
¹mm_2_out <- glmer(CDRSUM ~ MOFROMINDEX + AGE + BMI + DIABETES +
HYPERTEN
                   + HYPERCHO + (1 | ID) + (1 | ADC),
                   family = gaussian(), data = dta)
summary(mm_2_out)
```

[1]Two random intercepts are specified in this mixed model and call for the subject level (ID) and the center level (ADC).

R OUTPUT

```
summary(mm_2_out)
## Linear mixed model fit by REML ['lmerMod']
## Formula:
## CDRSUM ~ MOFROMINDEX + AGE + BMI + DIABETES + HYPERTEN +
##      HYPERCHO + (1 |      ID) + (1 |      ADC)
##     Data: dta
##
## REML criterion at convergence: 212205.8
##
## Scaled residuals:
##      Min       1Q   Median       3Q      Max
## -6.1695  -0.3504  -0.0612   0.2666   7.8114
##
## Random effects:
##  Groups    Name         Variance  Std.Dev.
##      ID    (Intercept)  15.572    3.946
##     ADC    (Intercept)   1.609    1.268
##  Residual                2.771    1.665
## Number of obs: 45508, groups:  ID, 12258; ADC, 35
##
```

```
## Fixed effects:
##                 Estimate Std. Error t value
## (Intercept)    -1.265151   0.388958  -3.253
## MOFROMINDEX     0.018043   0.000495  36.454
##       AGE       0.062655   0.003849  16.276
##       BMI      -0.013088   0.005077  -2.578
## DIABETES        0.181998   0.073610   2.472
## HYPERTEN       -0.227570   0.040291  -5.648
## HYPERCHO       -0.061014   0.036039  -1.693
##
## Correlation of Fixed Effects:
##              (Intr) MOFROM AG BM DIABET HYPERT
## MOFROMINDEX   0.437
## AGE          -0.740 -0.624
## BMI          -0.416 -0.013  0.102
## DIABETES      0.019 -0.028 -0.018 -0.058
## HYPERTEN      0.061 -0.030 -0.100 -0.084 -0.060
## HYPERCHO     -0.004 -0.035 -0.022 -0.046 -0.076 -0.152
```

Comments: The estimate of the covariance for the subject-level random intercept is 15.572, while the estimate of the covariance for the center-level random effect is 1.609. We identify time since baseline (MOFROMINDEX), age, BMI, diabetes, and hypertension as significant predictors of CDR-SUM.

4.5.3 SPSS Syntax and Output for Three-Level Mixed Models

The SPSS syntax follows:

```
GET FILE = "C:\User\Documents\Data\chap4.sav"
mixed CDRSUM with MOFROMINDEX AGE BMI DIABETES HYPERTEN
HYPERCHO
 /fixed = MOFROMINDEX AGE BMI DIABETES HYPERTEN HYPERCHO
 /print = solution
 /random = intercept  | subject(ADC)
/random = intercept  | subject(ADC*ID) .
```

SPSS OUTPUT

                                    Warnings

```
Insufficient memory to estimate the model parameters.
Execution of this command stops.
```

Comments: The three-level model did not converge in SPSS. This is not uncommon. The structure of the data and the size of certain subgroup at times make it difficult to converge.

4.5.4 Stata Syntax and Output for Three-Level Mixed Models

The Stata syntax follows:

```
. xtmixed cdrsum mofromindex age bmi diabetes hyperten hypercho
|| adc: || id:
Performing EM optimization:
Performing gradient-based optimization:
Iteration 0:    log likelihood = -106069.09
Iteration 1:    log likelihood = -106069.09
Computing standard errors:
Mixed-effects ML regression              Number of obs  =      45,508
```

Comments: The estimates are obtained using EM optimization.

	No. of Observations per Group			
Group Variable	Groups	Minimum	Average	Maximum
naccadc	35	10	1,300.2	2,955
id	12,258	2	3.7	10

```
                     Wald chi2(4)    =    3961.35
Log      likelihood  =   -106069.09  Prob > chi2 =   0.0000
```

Comments: There are 35 ADCs and 12,238 clusters (patients). The cluster sizes are between 2 and 10. The p-value (Prob > chi2 = 0.0000) suggests that the set of covariates is significant.

CDRSUM	Coef.	Std. Err.	z	P>z	[95% Conf. Interval]	
MOFROMINDEX	0.017	0.001	34.06	0.000	0.016	0.018
AGE	0.057	0.004	14.88	0.000	0.050	0.065
BMI	-0.019	0.005	-3.74	0.000	-0.029	-0.009
DIABETES	0.299	0.062	4.81	0.000	0.177	0.421
HYPERTEN	0.141	0.035	4.05	0.000	0.073	0.209
HYPERCHO	0.118	0.031	3.78	0.000	0.057	0.179
_CONS	-1.016	0.387	-2.63	0.009	-1.774	-0.258

Comments: We find that all six covariates are not significant predictors of CDR-SUM after adjusting for patient and center effect.

Random-Effects Parameters	Estimate	Std. Err.	[95% Conf. Interval]	
adc: Identity				
var(_cons)	1.558	0.398	0.944	2.570
id: Identity				
var(_cons)	15.581	0.213	15.170	16.004
var(Residual)	2.768	0.022	2.726	2.811

Comments: The confidence interval for the patient random effects parameter for the subject level (ID) does not include zero. As such, we support the use of the random effects in patients in the model. In addition, the covariance for the center random intercept has a confidence interval that does not include zero.

4.6 Summary and Discussions

In this chapter, we discuss two key models for the analysis of hierarchical data with continuous outcomes. While both methods analyze the mean of the outcomes of a continuous distribution, they do not address the same question (Hu et al. 1998). The GEE model fits the marginal mean or population-averaged mean, and the random effects model fits the conditional mean. The GEE method accounts for the clustering (correlation) through a working correlation matrix implemented in the random component. Thus GEE has no full like-lihood and relies on quasi-likelihood to obtain the regression coeffi-cient estimates. The random effects model addresses the model in the systematic component. The regression coefficients are obtained from a full likelihood.

We model a three-level structure but with the random effects mod-els, in which we analyzed repeated measures on patients who are nested within centers. Adding additional levels of clustering into the model increases the complexity and can also make the results more difficult to interpret. But Irimata and Wilson (2017) showed that one can use their method or the V^2 method to determine when it is nec-essary to go to the complexity of higher-level hierarchical structure in modeling.

The GEE model and the hierarchical model do not answer the same research question, except if the random effects are not needed. The GEE models tells about the overall mean. The random effect model tells about the conditional mean.

4.7 Exercises

Consider the longitudinal data described in this chapter (http://www.public.asu.edu/~jeffreyw/). We are interested in identifying factors that are associated with change in BMI for patients diag-nosed with AD versus those who are not over time. Accounting for the ADC effect, analyze the association between BMI and a subset of covariates, including AD diagnosis using GEE and a two-level mixed model.

1. Using GEE, write out the model and fit to the data.
   a. Does AD diagnosis (1 = diagnosed with AD, 0 = no AD diag-nosis) have a significant impact on predicting BMI?
   b. Are any of the covariates significant predictors of BMI?
   c. How do results vary using different correlation structures? Do the results suggest that independence is an appropriate assumption?

2. Using a mixed model, write out the model and fit to the data.
   a. Does AD diagnosis (1 = diagnosed with AD, 0 = no AD diagnosis) have a significant impact on predicting BMI?
   b. Are any of the covariates significant predictors of BMI?
   c. Is there a significant patient effect?
   d. Is there a significant center effect?

Chapter 5

Hierarchical Logistic Regression Models

5.1 Motivating Example

This chapter provides a discussion of models used in the analysis of binary outcome data obtained from a hierarchical structure. In chapter 3, we presented generalized linear models (GLMs). In those models, the responses were independent, as there was only one outcome per person. In chapter 4, we introduced the evaluation of continuous responses from hierarchical structures. This type of analysis is used in the cases where a unit (e.g., a subject) is evaluated at different points in time (longitudinal) or units are nested within groups such as centers or sites in a study (clustered) and the outcome is continuous. Since there is more than one outcome per person, the observations are not independent. We now concentrate on the use of hierarchical models for binary responses, such as the presence or absence of a symptom, which are frequently evaluated in neurodegenerative disease research. As such, we investigate the impact of covariates (symptoms) on the binary outcome (the neurodegenerative disease diagnosis) while accounting for the correlation due to the hierarchical structure.

For example, we consider a physician who believes that certain characteristics of her patient play a role in predicting whether her patient will eventually be diagnosed with Alzheimer's disease (AD). The physician's interest leads to some key questions:

1. What is the impact of patient characteristics while controlling for center and patient?
2. How much variation in AD diagnoses is attributable to the effect of the ADC and the patient?
3. Does the influence of patient characteristics on AD diagnosis vary among patients and centers?

She obtains data from the National Alzheimer's Coordinating Center (NACC) on the following covariates: age, BMI, diabetes status, hypertension status (HYPERTEN), hypercholesterolemia status (HYPERCHO), time from the baseline visit (MOFROMINDEX), and whether the patient was diagnosed with AD (DX_AD). She selects patients who have had at least four visits to an ADC, and obtains a dataset with 28,456 records for 5,122 patients from 32 ADCs. A subset of the data is shown in table 5.1.

These data are in a three-level hierarchical structure. Repeated measurements over time are nested within each patient, and the patients are nested within centers. Consider figure 5.1, which provides a pictorial display of the data in its hierarchical form. The data are correlated as time is nested within patient, and thus there are repeated measurements on the patients. Because the same measurements are taken on the patient, we can expect that the outcomes between dif-

Table 5.1 Subset of Data

ADC	ID	MOFROMINDEX	DX_AD	AGE	BMI	DIABETES	HYPERTEN	HYPERCHO
5452	271	0	1	81	21.5	0	0	1
5452	271	12	1	82	21.6	0	0	0
5452	271	23	1	83	20.2	0	0	1
5452	271	37	1	84	20.6	0	0	1
5452	271	64	1	86	20.2	0	0	0
289	385	16	1	82	29	0	1	1
289	385	28	1	83	29	0	0	1
289	385	41	1	84	26.4	0	0	0
289	385	50	1	84	29	0	0	0

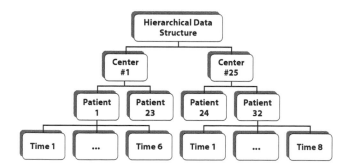

Figure 5.1 Diagram of a three-level hierarchical structure.

ferent visits are related. In addition, the patients are nested within centers, and so we may also expect that patients visiting the same center are related, as they are exposed to the same treatment (such as a husband and wife enrolled in the same ADC). Since each center has its own particular policies or procedures, this may result in correlated outcomes between patients within the center.

In the evaluation of these data, one may attempt to use marginal or subject-specific models. These methods address different but related questions, however. We look at two kinds of models to address such data, generalized estimating equations (GEE) models (marginal) and random effects models (subject-specific).

5.2 Marginal Models for Hierarchical Data

In this section, we use marginal models to address the patient effect. Marginal models are population-averaged models that predict the mean through adjustments to the random component. We present GEEs (Liang and Zeger 1986; Zeger and Liang 1986), a marginal modeling approach, to evaluate these repeated measures data. This technique allows us to analyze the impact of patient characteristics on the probability of an AD diagnosis, while accounting for the inherent correlation due to repeated measurements on patients.

The GEE specifies a working correlation structure, which accounts for the repeated measures in the data. The working correlation structures include independent (IN), compound symmetry (CS), autoregressive (AR), and unstructured (UN), which are also discussed in chapter 4. In our data, patients have between 4 and 10 visits; therefore, we use an overall symmetric matrix of dimension 10 to represent the averaging of the working correlation across patients. If the correlation matrix is an identity matrix, this suggests that all measurements across the visits are independent (no relationship). If we would like to be conservative, we could assume that measurements from any two visits will have the same relationship, which is referred to as compound symmetry or exchangeability. In a form of autoregressive correlation structures, we assume that the correlation between time-points decreases as the time-points become further apart. Alternatively, we could assume the measurements between any two visits have different correlations (unstructured), which will result in $10 \times (10 - 1)/2 = 45$ parameters. While an unstructured correlation structure is flexible, it burdens our model and can result in convergence issues, as was the case in chapter 4 with continuous data. We can evaluate model fit statistics to identify the best working correlation structure for a particular analysis.

The construction of statistical tests and confidence interval depends a great deal on the variance and covariance. Because the observations are correlated, we need to replace the covariance for independent observations with a variance-covariance relation that reflects the correlation. We can do this through the GEE working correlation matrix. The analysis uses the specified covariance matrix structure in place of the independent covariance matrix. The resulting regression coefficients are referred to as the GEE estimates. These are computed in most statistical software packages, including SAS, R, SPSS, and Stata. The GEE method produces consistent estimates even if the working correlation structure is misspecified. Similar to chapter 4, we use GEE to fit models with various working correlation matrices.

Problem: Do age, BMI, diabetes, hypertension, and hypercholesterolemia have an impact on the probability of an AD diagnosis while accounting for the repeated measures?

Solution: We use SAS, R, SPSS, and Stata to address this and related questions. We fit GEE models with various working correlation structures (CS, AR, and UN). The model with a compound symmetry working correlation matrix resulted in the best model fit (lowest Quasilikelihood under the Independence model Criterion (QIC) statistic). QIC can be used to find an acceptable working correlation structure for a given model. But Hardin and Hilbe (2003) recommend the use of QIC only to choose among otherwise equally suitable structures. They provide several guidelines based on the nature of the

Table 5.2 Analysis of GEE Parameter Estimates

Parameter	Estimate	Std Err	p-Value
Intercept	−4.232	0.259	<0.0001
MOFROMINDEX	−0.004	0.000	<0.0001
AGE	0.050	0.004	<0.0001
BMI	−0.006	0.001	<0.0001
DIABETES	0.010	0.014	0.445
HYPERTEN	−0.018	0.005	0.001
HYPERCHO	0.019	0.004	<0.0001

data for selecting suitable structures that should be applied first. The GEE parameter estimates, standard errors, and p-values are reported in table 5.2.

We find that time since the baseline visit (MOFROMINDEX), age, BMI, hypertension, and hypercholesterolemia are significant predictors of an AD diagnosis ($p < 0.05$). Diabetes is not found to be a contributing factor to Alzheimer's disease in this cohort. From these results, we see that older patients (as the estimate is a positive value) and patients with lower BMIs (as the estimate is a negative value) are more likely to have an AD diagnosis. In addition, patients that have hypertension or hypercholesterolemia are more likely to be diagnosed with AD. We obtain these findings from SAS, R, SPSS, and Stata.

5.2.1 SAS Syntax and Output for GEE

Compound Symmetry Working Correlation Matrix

We begin by fitting a GEE model with compound symmetry (or exchangeability) as the working correlation matrix. The response is binary. The SAS syntax follows:

```
¹PROC GENMOD DATA=CHAP5 DESCEND;

²CLASS ID;

³MODEL DX_AD= MOFROMINDEX AGE BMI DIABETES HYPERTEN HYPERCHO/
DIST=BIN;

⁴REPEATED SUBJECT=ID / CORR=CS CORRW;

RUN;
```

[1]To fit GEE models. The DATA= option is used to specify the dataset being evaluated (in this case, the dataset is called CHAP5). The option DESCEND is used for the analysis of binary variables and indicates that the outcome "1" should be modeled (as opposed to the default of "0").

[2]To specify categorical variables, which in this example includes the subject ID (ID).

[3]Defines the outcome = predictors. Outcome follows binomial distribution by the option DIST=BIN.

[4]The repeated statement is used to specify repeated measurements (within the variable SUBJECT=). The working correlation structure is specified using the option CORR=. In this example, we use CORR=CS, where CS is compound symmetry/exchangeability. The CORRW option prints the estimated working correlation structure in the output.

SAS OUTPUT

Model Information

Dataset	WORK.CHAP5
Distribution	Binomial
Link Function	Logit
Dependent Variable	DX_AD

Comments: The model specifies a binomial distribution as the random component and a logit link. The outcome variable is DX_AD, a binary variable indicating whether or not the patient has been diagnosed with Alzheimer's disease.

Response Profile

Ordered Value	DX_AD	Total Frequency
1	1	7980
2	0	20476

PROC GENMOD is modeling the probability that DX_AD='1'.

Comments: Because the DESCEND option was specified in the SAS syntax, we are modeling the outcome DX_AD = 1 (probability of a patient being diagnosed with AD, as opposed to not being diagnosed with AD). The response profile summarizes the number of cases in which DX_AD = 1 and DX_AD = 0. For this dataset, there are 7,980 cases with AD diagnoses (DX_AD = 1).

GEE Model Information	
Correlation Structure	Exchangeable
Subject Effect	ID (5122 levels)
Number of Clusters	5122
Correlation Matrix Dimension	10
Maximum Cluster Size	10
Minimum Cluster Size	4

Comments: The GEE Model Information table summarizes information about the repeated measurements. In this dataset, there are 5,122 patients. Each patient has between 4 (Min Cluster Size) and 10 (Max Cluster Size) visits. The estimated working correlation matrix will be 10×10 (Correlation Matrix Dimension) with a compound symmetry, or exchangeable, correlation structure (Correlation Structure).

Exchangeable Working Correlation	
Correlation	0.922

Comments: Compound symmetry requires only one correlation parameter to be estimated. After fitting the GEE model, we find that the estimated correlation parameter has a value of 0.922.

GEE Fit Criteria	
QIC	32819.547
QICu	32811.154

Comments: The GEE fit criteria are used to compare various model fits. The QIC for this particular model is 32,819.5 and is compared to the

QIC statistic of other models. A lower QIC statistic indicates a better model fit. The simplified QIC (QICu) is similar to the QIC statistic but has a penalization for a larger number of parameters in the model.

Analysis of GEE Parameter Estimates

Empirical Standard Error Estimates

Parameter	Estimate	Standard Error	95% Confidence Limits		Z	Pr > |Z|
Intercept	-4.232	0.259	-4.740	-3.724	-16.320	<.0001
MOFROMINDEX	-0.004	0.000	-0.005	-0.004	-15.100	<.0001
AGE	0.050	0.004	0.043	0.057	14.290	<.0001
BMI	-0.006	0.001	-0.008	-0.003	-4.570	<.0001
DIABETES	0.010	0.014	-0.016	0.037	0.760	0.445
HYPERTEN	-0.018	0.005	-0.028	-0.007	-3.290	0.001
HYPERCHO	0.019	0.004	0.011	0.027	4.700	<.0001

Comments: The results indicated the variables MOFROMINDEX, age, BMI, hypertension, and hypercholesterolemia are highly statistically significant. Older patients, patients with lower BMI, patients without hypertension, and those with hypercholesterolemia are more likely to be diagnosed with AD.

Autoregressive Working Correlation Matrix

The SAS program is altered slightly to conduct the analysis with an autoregressive working correlation matrix. The SAS syntax follows:

```
PROC GENMOD DATA=CHAP5 DESCEND;
CLASS ID;
MODEL DX_AD= MOFROMINDEX AGE BMI DIABETES HYPERTEN HYPERCHO/
DIST=BIN;
1REPEATED SUBJECT=ID / CORR=AR CORRW;
RUN;
```

[1]The correlation structure is changed to use an autoregressive correlation structure by specifying CORR=AR.

SAS OUTPUT

	Col1	Col2	Col3	Col4	Col5	Col6	Col7	Col8	Col9	Col10
					Working Correlation Matrix					
Row1	1.000	0.987	0.974	0.961	0.949	0.936	0.924	0.912	0.900	0.888
Row2	0.987	1.000	0.987	0.974	0.961	0.949	0.936	0.924	0.912	0.900
Row3	0.974	0.987	1.000	0.987	0.974	0.961	0.949	0.936	0.924	0.912
Row4	0.961	0.974	0.987	1.000	0.987	0.974	0.961	0.949	0.936	0.924
Row5	0.949	0.961	0.974	0.987	1.000	0.987	0.974	0.961	0.949	0.936
Row6	0.936	0.949	0.961	0.974	0.987	1.000	0.987	0.974	0.961	0.949
Row7	0.924	0.936	0.949	0.961	0.974	0.987	1.000	0.987	0.974	0.961
Row8	0.912	0.924	0.936	0.949	0.961	0.974	0.987	1.000	0.987	0.974
Row9	0.900	0.912	0.924	0.936	0.949	0.961	0.974	0.987	1.000	0.987
Row10	0.888	0.900	0.912	0.924	0.936	0.949	0.961	0.974	0.987	1.000

GEE Fit Criteria	
QIC	32847.080
QICu	32842.089

Comments: The estimated working correlation matrix and the GEE fit criteria are displayed. In the working correlation matrix, we see that time-points that are further apart have a lower correlation (by definition of the autoregressive structure). For example, the correlation between AD diagnoses at visit 1 and visit 2 (Row1 and Col2 or Col1 and Row2) is 0.987, while the correlation between AD diagnoses at visit 1 and visit 10 is 0.888. In addition, we see that the QIC (32,847.1) is slightly higher than the QIC of the GEE model with compound symmetry (32,819.5). This indicates that the GEE model using a compound symmetry working correlation matrix has a better fit.

			Analysis of GEE Parameter Estimates			
			Empirical Standard Error Estimates			
Parameter	Estimate	Standard Error	95% Confidence Limits		Z	Pr > |Z|
Intercept	-3.895	0.220	-4.327	-3.464	-17.700	<.0001
MOFROMINDEX	-0.004	0.000	-0.004	-0.003	-15.570	<.0001

Parameter	Estimate	Standard Error	95% Confidence Limits		Z	Pr > |Z|
AGE	0.044	0.003	0.038	0.050	14.680	<.0001
BMI	-0.002	0.000	-0.003	-0.001	-4.910	<.0001
DIABETES	0.004	0.005	-0.005	0.013	0.830	0.406
HYPERTEN	-0.005	0.002	-0.008	-0.001	-2.850	0.004
HYPERCHO	0.005	0.001	0.003	0.007	4.550	<.0001

Comments: Similar to the findings using GEE with a compound symmetry working correlation structure, diabetes ($p = 0.406$) is the only factor identified as not significantly affecting the probability of an AD diagnosis.

Unstructured Working Correlation Matrix

We now use SAS to fit GEE with an unstructured (UN) working correlation matrix. The SAS syntax follows:

```
PROC GENMOD DATA=CHAP5 DESCEND;
CLASS ID;
¹MODEL DX_AD= MOFROMINDEX AGE BMI DIABETES HYPERTEN HYPERCHO/
DIST=BIN;
REPEATED SUBJECT=ID / CORR=UN CORRW;
RUN;
```

[1]The working correlation structure is specified as unstructured by the option CORR=UN.

SAS OUTPUT

Working Correlation Matrix

	Col1	Col2	Col3	Col4	Col5	Col6	Col7	Col8	Col9	Col10
Row1	1.000	1.000	1.000	1.000	0.957	0.820	0.706	0.604	0.572	0.553
Row2	1.000	1.000	1.000	1.000	0.957	0.820	0.706	0.604	0.572	0.553
Row3	1.000	1.000	1.000	1.000	0.957	0.820	0.706	0.604	0.572	0.553
Row4	1.000	1.000	1.000	1.000	0.957	0.820	0.706	0.604	0.572	0.553

	Col1	Col2	Col3	Col4	Col5	Col6	Col7	Col8	Col9	Col10
Row5	0.957	0.957	0.957	0.957	1.000	0.820	0.706	0.604	0.572	0.553
Row6	0.820	0.820	0.820	0.820	0.820	1.000	0.706	0.604	0.572	0.553
Row7	0.706	0.706	0.706	0.706	0.706	0.706	1.000	0.604	0.572	0.553
Row8	0.604	0.604	0.604	0.604	0.604	0.604	0.604	1.000	0.572	0.553
Row9	0.572	0.572	0.572	0.572	0.572	0.572	0.572	0.572	1.000	0.553
Row10	0.553	0.553	0.553	0.553	0.553	0.553	0.553	0.553	0.553	1.000

GEE Fit Criteria	
QIC	33714.638
QICu	33717.741

Comments: The working correlation matrix has many parameters to estimate, as opposed to the compound symmetry, where we needed one parameter. We have $10^*(10-1)/2 = 45$ parameters to estimate. One needs many observations to have convergence. Although each correlation parameter should be estimated independently, we see that many of the correlation parameters are reported to be the same to three decimal places. This is an indicator of a convergence issue. The GEE fit criteria for the unstructured correlation structure is the highest of all three models examined and thus is not the best model of the three correlation structures investigated.

Analysis of GEE Parameter Estimates

Empirical Standard Error Estimates

Parameter	Estimate	Standard Error	95% Confidence Limits		Z	Pr > |Z|
Intercept	−1.041	0.033	−1.106	−0.976	−31.37	<.0001
MOFROMINDEX	−0.000	0.000	−0.000	−0.000	−14.56	<.0001
AGE	0.003	0.000	0.002	0.003	14.43	<.0001
BMI	−0.000	0.000	−0.000	−0.000	−3.69	0.000
DIABETES	0.000	0.000	−0.000	0.000	1.24	0.213
HYPERTEN	−0.000	0.000	−0.000	0.000	−0.60	0.552
HYPERCHO	0.000	0.000	−0.000	0.000	1.50	0.134

Comments: For the GEE model with an unstructured (UN) working correlation structure, the variables MOFROMINDEX, AGE, and BMI are identified as significant predictors of an AD diagnosis. DIABETES ($p = 0.213$), HYPERTEN ($p = 0.552$), and HYPERCHO ($p = 0.134$) are not found to have a significant impact on the outcome. This result differs from the other models.

5.2.2 R Syntax and Output for GEE

To use R to fit GEE models in this chapter, we utilize the library geepack (an alternative to the library GEE discussed in chapter 4).

Compound Symmetry Working Correlation Matrix
The R syntax follows:

```
¹library(geepack)

²gee_cs_out <- geeglm(DX_AD ~ MOFROMINDEX + AGE + BMI + DIABETES
+ HYPERTEN + HYPERCHO, id=ID, data=dta, corstr="exchangeable",
family = binomial(link="logit"))
³summary(gee_cs_out)
```

[1]The library geepack contains the function geeglm(), which is used to fit GEE models.
[2]Used to fit GEE models. Outcome (DX_AD) ~ Predictors (MOFROMINDEX + AGE + BMI + DIABETES + HYPERTEN + HYPERCHO). ID indicates repeated measures. The working correlation structure for compound symmetry structure is corstr="exchangeable." Using family determines the distribution and for the binomial link="logit."
[3]Prints the GEE model fit and model parameter estimates.

R OUTPUT

```
summary(gee_cs_out)
##
## Call:
```

```
## geeglm(formula = DX_AD ~ MOFROMINDEX + AGE + BMI + DIABETES +
##     HYPERTEN + HYPERCHO, family = binomial(link = "logit"), data = dta,
##     id = ID, corstr = "exchangeable")
##
##   Coefficients:
##              Estimate Std.err Wald Pr(>|W|)
## (Intercept) -4.231833 0.259286 266.379 < 2e-16 ***
## MOFROMINDEX -0.004392 0.000291 227.842 < 2e-16 ***
## AGE          0.049798 0.003486 204.106 < 2e-16 ***
## BMI         -0.005464 0.001196 20.874 4.90e-06 ***
## DIABETES     0.010378 0.013598 0.582 0.44535
## HYPERTEN    -0.017482 0.005317 10.811 0.00101 **
## HYPERCHO     0.019200 0.004085 22.085 2.61e-06 ***
## ---
## Signif. codes:  0 '***' 0.001 '**' 0.01 '*' 0.05 '.' 0.1 ' ' 1
##
## Estimated Scale Parameters:
##              Estimate Std.err
## (Intercept)    0.9415 0.01726
##
## Correlation: Structure = exchangeable Link  = identity
##
## Estimated Correlation Parameters:
##        Estimate Std.err
## alpha    0.9219 0.01982
## Number of clusters:   5122   Maximum cluster size: 10
```

Comments: The GEE model output indicates that time since baseline (MOFROMINDEX), age, BMI, hypertension, and hypercholesterolemia are identified as statistically significant predictors of AD diagnosis. The estimated correlation parameter for the compound symmetry matrix is 0.922, which is the same as the correlation estimate from SAS.

Autoregressive Working Correlation Matrix

The R syntax follows:

```
1gee_ar_out <- geeglm(DX_AD ~ MOFROMINDEX + AGE + BMI + DIABETES
+ HYPERTEN + HYPERCHO, id=ID, data=dta, corstr="ar1",family =
binomial(link="logit"))
summary(gee_ar_out)
```

[1]Use an autoregressive working correlation matrix, the option corstr="ar1" is used.

R OUTPUT

```
summary(gee_ar_out)
##
## Call:
## geeglm(formula = DX_AD ~ MOFROMINDEX + AGE + BMI + DIABETES +
##     HYPERTEN + HYPERCHO, family = binomial(link = "logit"), data = dta,
##     id = ID, corstr = "ar1")
##
## Coefficients:
##              Estimate   Std.err   Wald Pr(>|W|)
## (Intercept) -4.167586  0.253129 271.07  < 2e-16 ***
## MOFROMINDEX -0.004764  0.000287 276.23  < 2e-16 ***
## AGE          0.048683  0.003411 203.74  < 2e-16 ***
## BMI         -0.004870  0.001039  21.99  2.7e-06 ***
## DIABETES     0.012611  0.013070   0.93  0.33464
## HYPERTEN    -0.015779  0.004778  10.91  0.00096 ***
## HYPERCHO     0.016156  0.003422  22.29  2.3e-06 ***
## ---
## Signif. codes: 0 '***' 0.001 '**' 0.01 '*' 0.05 '.' 0.1 ' ' 1
##
## Estimated Scale Parameters:
##              Estimate Std.err
## (Intercept)     0.942  0.0168
##
```

```
## Correlation: Structure = ar1 Link  = identity
##
## Estimated Correlation Parameters:
##        Estimate Std.err
## alpha      0.96 0.0069
## Number of clusters:   5122   Maximum cluster size: 10
```

Comments: Using an AR(1) correlation structure, all predictors except diabetes ($p = 0.33464$) are found to be statistically significant drivers of an AD diagnosis. The estimated correlation coefficient for the AR(1) structure is 0.96.

Unstructured Working Correlation Matrix
The R syntax follows:

```
1gee_un_out <- geeglm(DX_AD ~ MOFROMINDEX + AGE + BMI + DIABETES
+ HYPERTEN + HYPERCHO, id=ID, data=dta, corstr="unstructured",-
family = binomial(link="logit"))
summary(gee_un_out)
```

[1]Use unstructured working correlation matrix, the option corstr= "unstructured."

R OUTPUT

```
summary(gee_un_out)
##
## Call:
## geeglm(formula = DX_AD ~ MOFROMINDEX + AGE + BMI + DIABETES +
##     HYPERTEN + HYPERCHO, family = binomial(link = "logit"), data = dta,
##     id = ID, corstr = "unstructured")
##
##  Coefficients:
##              Estimate   Std.err   Wald Pr(>|W|)
## (Intercept) -5.082597  0.343096 219.45  < 2e-16 ***
## MOFROMINDEX -0.002236  0.000349  41.12  1.4e-10 ***
```

```
## AGE            0.052376  0.003874 182.78  < 2e-16 ***
## BMI            0.012716  0.005898   4.65   0.0311 *
## DIABETES      -0.034000  0.054434   0.39   0.5322
## HYPERTEN       0.048387  0.018447   6.88   0.0087 **
## HYPERCHO      -0.049646  0.011603  18.31  1.9e-05 ***
## ---
## Signif. codes:  0 '***' 0.001 '**' 0.01 '*' 0.05 '.' 0.1 ' ' 1
##
## Estimated Scale Parameters:
##               Estimate Std.err
## (Intercept)          1  0.0303
##
## Correlation: Structure = unstructured  Link = identity
##
## Estimated Correlation Parameters:
##            Estimate Std.err
## alpha.1:2     1.085  0.0282
## alpha.1:3     1.078  0.0281
## alpha.1:4     1.070  0.0280
## alpha.1:5     0.956  0.0298
## alpha.1:6     0.831  0.0323
## alpha.1:7     0.702  0.0337
## alpha.1:8     0.587  0.0330
## alpha.1:9     0.536  0.0383
## alpha.1:10    0.429  0.0371
## alpha.2:3     1.070  0.0281
## alpha.2:4     1.062  0.0281
## alpha.2:5     0.951  0.0299
## alpha.2:6     0.830  0.0322
## alpha.2:7     0.703  0.0336
## alpha.2:8     0.590  0.0329
## alpha.2:9     0.540  0.0381
## alpha.2:10    0.434  0.0372
## alpha.3:4     1.056  0.0280
## alpha.3:5     0.947  0.0299
```

```
## alpha.3:6      0.828   0.0322
## alpha.3:7      0.704   0.0336
## alpha.3:8      0.593   0.0329
## alpha.3:9      0.543   0.0379
## alpha.3:10     0.437   0.0369
## alpha.4:5      0.942   0.0299
## alpha.4:6      0.827   0.0321
## alpha.4:7      0.705   0.0335
## alpha.4:8      0.596   0.0328
## alpha.4:9      0.548   0.0379
## alpha.4:10     0.442   0.0370
## alpha.5:6      0.826   0.0321
## alpha.5:7      0.707   0.0334
## alpha.5:8      0.600   0.0328
## alpha.5:9      0.551   0.0375
## alpha.5:10     0.448   0.0371
## alpha.6:7      0.708   0.0334
## alpha.6:8      0.603   0.0327
## alpha.6:9      0.554   0.0373
## alpha.6:10     0.452   0.0370
## alpha.7:8      0.606   0.0328
## alpha.7:9      0.559   0.0372
## alpha.7:10     0.458   0.0374
## alpha.8:9      0.563   0.0372
## alpha.8:10     0.463   0.0377
## alpha.9:10     0.468   0.0379
## Number of clusters:   5122   Maximum cluster size: 10
```

Comments: Similar to the GEE model results using the compound symmetry and AR(1) correlation structures in R, we find that MO-FROMINDEX, age, BMI, hypertension, and hypercholesterolemia are significant predictors of the probability of an AD diagnosis. Each of the correlation estimates (alpha) for the unstructured correlation structure are reported in the output. Because the correlation structure is a 10×10 matrix, there are $\dfrac{t(t-1)}{2} = \dfrac{10(9)}{2} = 45$ correlation parameters estimated. The correlation estimate between visits 9 and 10 is alpha.9:10 = 0.458.

5.2.3 SPSS Syntax and Output for GEE

Compound Symmetry Working Correlation Matrix

We begin by fitting a GEE model with compound symmetry (or exchangeability) as the working correlation matrix. The SPSS syntax follows:

```
* Generalized Estimating Equations.
GENLIN DX_AD (REFERENCE=FIRST) WITH BMI AGE MOFROMINDEX
DIABETES HYPERTEN HYPERCHO
  /MODEL BMI AGE MOFROMINDEX DIABETES HYPERTEN HYPERCHO
INTERCEPT=YES
DISTRIBUTION=BINOMIAL LINK=LOGIT
  /CRITERIA METHOD=FISHER(1) SCALE=1 MAXITERATIONS=100
MAXSTEPHALVING=5 PCONVERGE=1E-006(ABSOLUTE)
    SINGULAR=1E-012 ANALYSISTYPE=3(WALD) CILEVEL=95
LIKELIHOOD=FULL
  /REPEATED SUBJECT=ID SORT=YES CORRTYPE=EXCHANGEABLE
ADJUSTCORR=YES COVB=ROBUST
    MAXITERATIONS=100 PCONVERGE=1e-006(ABSOLUTE) UPDATECORR=1
  /MISSING CLASSMISSING=EXCLUDE
  /PRINT MODELINFO FIT SUMMARY SOLUTION.
```

SPSS OUTPUT

Dependent Variable	DX_AD
Probability Distribution	Binomial
Link Function	Logit
Subject Effect 1	ID
Working Correlation Matrix Structure	Exchangeable

a. The procedure models 1 as the response, treating 0 as the reference category.

Comments: The random component of the model is binomial with a logit link function. The binary outcome variable is DX_AD, which is an indicator for Alzheimer's disease. The working correlation matrix is specified as exchangeable (or compound symmetry).

Parameter	B	Std. Error	95% Wald Confidence Interval		Hypothesis Test	
			Lower	Upper	Wald Chi-Square	Sig.
(Intercept)	-4.229	.260	-4.738	-3.720	265.517	.000
BMI	-.005	.001	-.008	-.003	20.809	.000
AGE	.050	.004	.043	.056	202.484	.000
MOFROMINDEX	-.004	.000	-.005	-.004	232.790	.000
DIABETES	.015	.011	-.007	.036	1.835	.176
HYPERTEN	-.001	.005	-.011	.008	.087	.767
HYPERCHO	.021	.0048	.014	.028	30.702	.000
(Scale)	1					

Comments: The variables BMI, age, MOFROMINDEX, and hypercholesterolemia are identified as statistically significant predictors of the probability of an AD diagnosis (p-values < 0.05). In other words, older patients, patients with lower BMIs, and patients with hypercholesterolemia are more likely to have AD in our cohort. Diabetes and hypertension are not identified as significant contributing factors to the probability of having AD.

Autoregressive Working Correlation Matrix

We alter the following syntax in SPSS to use an autoregressive working correlation matrix (AR(1)):

```
/REPEATED SUBJECT=ID SORT=YES CORRTYPE=AR(1) ADJUSTCORR=YES
COVB=ROBUST MAXITERATIONS=100
```

SPSS OUTPUT

Parameter Estimates

| Parameter | B | Std. Error | 95% Wald Confidence Interval | | Hypothesis Test | | |
			Lower	Upper	Wald Chi-Square	df	Sig.
(Intercept)	-3.896	.2202	-4.328	-3.465	313.252	1	.000
BMI	-.002	.0004	-.002	-.001	23.436	1	.000
AGE	.044	.0030	.038	.050	214.871	1	.000
MOFROMINDEX	-.004	.0002	-.004	-.003	244.527	1	.000
DIABETES	.006	.0041	-.002	.014	2.111	1	.146
HYPERTEN	-.001	.0016	-.004	.002	.229	1	.633
HYPERCHO	.007	.0012	.004	.009	31.569	1	.000
(Scale)	1						

Comments: Using an autoregressive structure, we find that BMI, age, MOFROMINDEX, and hypercholesterolemia are highly statistically significant (p-values are nearly 0). We find that diabetes and hypertension do not contribute to the probability of an AD diagnosis, however.

Unstructured Working Correlation Matrix

To use an unstructured working correlation matrix, we change the following syntax in SPSS:

```
/REPEATED SUBJECT=ID SORT=YES CORRTYPE=UNSTRUCTURED
ADJUSTCORR=YES COVB=ROBUST
```

SPSS OUTPUT

| Parameter | B | Std. Error | 95% Wald Confidence Interval | | Hypothesis Test | |
			Lower	Upper	Wald Chi-Square	Sig.
(Intercept)	-1.041	0.033	-1.106	-0.976	983.737	0.000
BMI	0.000	0.000	0.000	0.000	13.225	0.000

| Parameter | B | Std. Error | 95% Wald Confidence Interval | | Hypothesis Test | |
			Lower	Upper	Wald Chi-Square	Sig.
AGE	0.003	0.000	0.002	0.003	208.100	0.000
MOFROMINDEX	0.000	0.000	0.000	0.000	212.404	0.000
DIABETES	0.000	0.000	0.000	0.000	1.900	0.168
HYPERTEN	0.000	0.000	0.000	0.000	0.002	0.964
HYPERCHO	0.000	0.000	0.000	0.000	2.939	0.086
(Scale)	1					

Comments: In the unstructured (UN) correlation structure, we now identify that hypercholesterolemia is not a contributing factor to the probability of an AD diagnosis (in addition to diabetes and hypertension). BMI, age, and time since baseline are identified as statistically significant.

5.2.4 Stata Syntax and Output for GEE

Compound Symmetry Working Correlation Matrix
The Stata syntax follows:

```
XTGEE DX_AD BMI AGE MOFROMINDEX DIABETES HYPERTEN HYPERCHO,
FAMILY(BINOMIAL 1) LINK(LOGIT) CORR(EXCHANGEABLE)
```

STATA OUTPUT

```
Iteration 1: tolerance = .22625777
Iteration 2: tolerance = .02344641
Iteration 3: tolerance = .00060854
Iteration 4: tolerance = .00003
Iteration 5: tolerance = 2.089e-06
Iteration 6: tolerance = 1.896e-07
GEE population-averaged  model      Number of obs   =   28,456
Group variable:              id     Number of groups =    5,122
```

```
Link:                        logit    Obs per group:
Family:              binomial                    min =    4
Correlation:  exchangeable                       avg =    5.6
                                                 max =    10
                                        Wald chi2(6) =    230.88
Scale parameter:         1              Prob > chi2 =    0.0000
```

Comments: The distribution (family) of the outcome is specified as binomial, with a logit link function. We use an exchangeable, or compound symmetry, correlation structure for the GEE model (CORR(EXCHANGEABLE)). The Stata output summarizes the number of observations (28,456), the number of individuals with repeated measures (5,122), as well as the minimum (4), average (5.6), and maximum (10) number of measurements. The iterations report the tolerance calculations (model fit) for each model. We obtain convergence after six iterations.

DX_AD	Coef.	Std. Err.	z	P>z	[95% Conf. Interval]	
BMI	−0.005	0.003	−2.000	0.045	−0.011	0.000
AGE	0.050	0.003	14.810	0.000	0.043	0.056
MOFROMINDEX	−0.004	0.000	−13.820	0.000	−0.005	−0.004
DIABETES	0.010	0.036	0.280	0.776	−0.061	0.082
HYPERTEN	−0.017	0.019	−0.930	0.352	−0.054	0.019
HYPERCHO	0.019	0.016	1.160	0.244	−0.013	0.052
_CONS	−4.232	0.262	−16.130	0.000	−4.746	−3.718

Comments: The output table indicates that age and MOFROMINDEX are significant covariates. The variables BMI, diabetes, hypertension, and hypercholesterolemia are not contributing factors to the probability of having AD in our cohort.

Autoregressive Working Correlation Structure

The Stata syntax to use an autoregressive working correlation structure (AR 1) follows:

```
XTGEE DX_AD BMI AGE MOFROMINDEX DIABETES HYPERTEN HYPERCHO,
FAMILY(GAUSSIAN) LINK(IDENTITY) CORR(AR 1)
```

STATA OUTPUT

```
GEE population-averaged  model    Number of obs        =  28,456
Group and time vars: id  visitnum  Number of groups =    5,122
Link:                     logit    Obs per group:
Family:                   binomial              min  =      4
Correlation:              AR(1)                 avg  =     5.6
                                                max  =     10
                                     Wald chi2(6)   =  197.02
Scale parameter:             1        Prob > chi2   =   0.0000
```

Comments: The output is altered slightly to report that an AR(1) correlation structure is used in this analysis.

DX_AD	Coef.	Std. Err.	z	P>z	[95% Conf. Interval]	
BMI	−0.002	0.002	−1.180	0.239	−0.005	0.001
AGE	0.044	0.003	13.870	0.000	0.038	0.050
MOFROMINDEX	−0.004	0.000	−12.600	0.000	−0.004	−0.003
DIABETES	0.004	0.021	0.180	0.860	−0.038	0.045
HYPERTEN	−0.005	0.010	−0.440	0.657	−0.025	0.015
HYPERCHO	0.005	0.009	0.590	0.553	−0.012	0.022
_CONS	−3.897	0.238	−16.400	0.000	−4.363	−3.432

Comments: The GEE model with an autoregressive (AR) working correlation structure suggests that the covariates AGE and MOFRO-MINDEX are statistically significant predictors of AD diagnosis.

Unstructured Working Correlation Structure

The Stata syntax using an unstructured working correlation structure follows:

. XTGEE DX_AD BMI AGE MOFROMINDEX DIABETES HYPERTEN HYPERCHO,
FAMILY(GAUSSIAN) LINK(IDENTITY) CORR(UNSTRUCTURED)

STATA OUTPUT

DX_AD	Coef.	Std. Err.	z	P>z	[95% Conf. Interval]	
BMI	-0.010	0.004	-2.800	0.005	-0.017	-0.003
AGE	0.050	0.003	14.560	0.000	0.043	0.057
MOFROMINDEX	-0.005	0.000	-14.690	0.000	-0.006	-0.004
DIABETES	0.031	0.047	0.660	0.507	-0.061	0.123
HYPERTEN	-0.032	0.025	-1.250	0.211	-0.081	0.018
HYPERCHO	0.041	0.023	1.790	0.073	-0.004	0.086
_CONS	-4.176	0.277	-15.060	0.000	-4.720	-3.633

convergence not achieved r(430);

Comments: The model did not converge. Thus we cannot comment on the results.

CONCLUSIONS AND COMPARISONS

We conduct a fit of GEE models using different statistical programs. With each of these statistical programs, we utilize compound symmetry, autoregressive, and unstructured working correlation structures. The model fits for the different correlation structures across the four statistical programs give conflicting results. A summary of the nonsignificant covariates from each of the models is reported in table 5.3.

This highlights the differences in the use of statistical programs and the working correlation matrix. The working correlation matrix within the same program presents different results. These programs use a different means of estimation that is sensitive to the working correlation matrix.

Table 5.3 Identifying Nonsignificant Covariates by Working Correlation Structure

	Working Correlation Structure		
Program	Exchangeability	AR(1)	Unstructured
SAS	Diabetes	Diabetes	Diabetes Hypertension Hypercholesterolemia
R	Diabetes	Diabetes	Diabetes
SPSS	Diabetes Hypertension	Diabetes Hypertension	Diabetes Hypertension Hypercholesterolemia
Stata	BMI Diabetes Hypertension Hypercholesterolemia	BMI Diabetes Hypertension Hypercholesterolemia	Did not converge

5.3 Two-Level Random Effects Models

Because there is correlation in the data from the repeated measures and the clustering, we are unable to use a standard regression model. The challenge with correlation is that it contributes to an increase in the standard error. Recall from chapter 2 that test statistics are constructed using a form of the standard error in the denominator. Small standard errors will result in larger test statistics and thus smaller p-values. Small p-values suggest that the covariate is statistically significant. Thus neglecting to account for correlation in the model results in identifying covariates as significant, when in fact they are not.

This correlation between measurements in the hierarchy is referred to as intraclass correlation. In the case when the intraclass correlation is strong, we need to use an appropriate correlated model such as generalized estimating equations, discussed in section 5.2, or a hierarchical regression model. The hierarchical model is often referred to as a mixed model or a regression model with random effects. The random effects in the model measure the effects of the grouping or clusters, which may represent centers, families, or repeated measurements. These random effects capture differences between the clusters, which may otherwise be unmeasurable.

Random effects are used to account for variation between groups in a nested structure. We assume that random effects are normally distributed with a mean of 0 and a variance σ^2. This indicates on average that a particular individual or group does not have an impact on the outcome. But to measure the amount of variation we see in the impacts of particular individuals or groups, we estimate σ^2. Large estimates of the variance indicate that there is large variation in the impact of the group, whereas small estimates of the variance suggest little to no variation in the impact of the groups on the outcome. The group effect is estimated, which reveals the impact that a particular group has on the outcome. For example, in the analysis of AD diagnoses, if an ADC has a positive estimate for the random effect, this indicates that the center is more likely to have AD diagnoses. Alternatively, ADCs with negative estimates tend to be less likely to have AD diagnoses.

Statistical Model: We start by focusing on a two-level model, such as the evaluation of the repeated measures on each patient. The two-level mixed model with a random intercept for a binary outcome with a logit link is:

$$\log\left(\frac{P_{event}}{P_{nonevent}}\right) = \beta_0 + \beta_1 X_1 + \cdots + \beta_p X_p + \gamma,$$

where P_{event} and $P_{nonevent}$ are the probabilities of the event of interest occurring and the event of interest not occurring, respectively. The terms β_i are the regression coefficients for the fixed effects given by the covariates X_i and γ is the random effect at the first level. This model determines the impact of the covariates on the outcome while controlling for the level 1 patient random effects. In this model, the random effect measures the variation between the level 1 units through the intercept. This identifies any baseline differences between the units that may have been unaccounted for while controlling for the covariates.

In order to calculate the intraclass correlation for the data, we start by fitting the model without the covariates:

$$\log\left(\frac{P_{\text{event}}}{P_{\text{nonevent}}}\right) = \beta_0 + \gamma,$$

where β_0 is the constant (fixed intercept term) and γ is the random effects due to the first level of clustering. The intraclass correlation is calculated as $\dfrac{\gamma}{\epsilon + \gamma}$, where $\epsilon = 3.29$, which is the estimated error variance of the random effects model for binary data with a logit link. This measures the variation within the first level of clustering. In the case of longitudinal data, large values of the intraclass correlation indicate strong correlation between the time measurements (units) within each patient (cluster), while small values of the intraclass correlation indicate a weak correlation between the time measurements within each patient.

Problem: In the evaluation of repeated measures data, do MOFRO-MINDEX, age, BMI, diabetes, hypertension, and hypercholesterolemia affect the probability of an AD diagnosis?

Solution: To demonstrate the use of a binary two-level model with random intercept, we evaluate a subset of data from NACC. We wish to determine whether the time since the baseline visit (MOFROMIN-DEX), BMI, age, diabetes, hypertension, and hypercholesterolemia affect the probability of an AD diagnosis while adjusting for the patient's effects through random effects (identified by the subject ID). The two-level model of interest, which includes the covariates above, is:

$$\log\left(\frac{P_{\text{AD}}}{P_{\text{no AD}}}\right) = \beta_0 + \beta_1 X_{\text{MOFROMINDEX}} + \beta_2 X_{\text{BMI}} + \beta_3 X_{\text{AGE}} + \beta_4 X_{\text{DIABETES}}$$
$$+ \beta_5 X_{\text{HYPERTEN}} + \beta_6 X_{\text{HYPERCHO}} + \gamma_{\text{ID}},$$

where P_{AD} is the probability of having AD and $P_{no\,AD}$ is the probability of a non–AD diagnosis. The regression coefficients β_i for $i = 1, 2, 3, 4, 5, 6$ represent the effects of each covariate. The random effect γ_{ID} measures the variation within the measurements at the patient level. We report on the analysis of these data using statistical software. While we report results using SAS and R, the size of the data and the complexity of the cluster sizes did not allow convergence when we used SPSS and Stata. We provide the syntax for those who may have a similar problem but a different data configuration.

The random effects for patients (capturing variation between the measurements at different visits) are assumed to follow a normal distribution with mean zero and variance σ_{ID}^2, where this variable represents the variation between patients (differentiated using the variable ID). A test of the variance gives $10.9174/0.2967 = 36.80 > 1.96$. Thus, because the variance is statistically significant (more than 1.96 standard deviations away from the mean), it makes sense to include a random intercept representing the patient effect. Table 5.4 reports the two-level mixed model parameter estimates for the fixed effects.

Using a mixed model with a random intercept, we find that time since baseline, age, BMI, hypertension, and hypercholesterolemia are statistically significant predictors of an AD diagnosis. The results also indicate that older patients, patients with lower BMIs, patients without hypertension (remote/inactive/absent hypertension), and patients with recent/active hypercholesterolemia are more likely to have an AD diagnosis. Diabetes is not identified as a contributing factor to the probability of having AD.

Table 5.4 Two-Level Mixed Model Results

Parameter	Estimate	Std Err	p-Value
Intercept	−6.790	0.584	<0.0001
MOFROMINDEX	−0.016	0.001	<0.0001
AGE	0.091	0.006	<0.0001
BMI	−0.042	0.011	0.0002
DIABETES	0.187	0.170	0.2712
HYPERTEN	−0.265	0.106	0.0120
HYPERCHO	0.346	0.098	0.0004

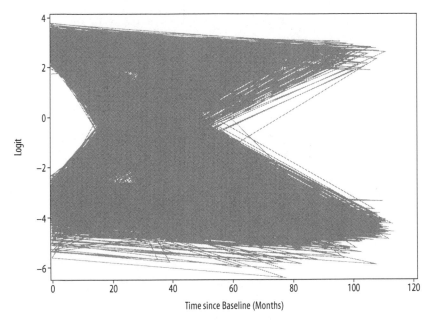

Figure 5.2 Logit of Alzheimer's diagnosis versus time since baseline (months).

A plot of the logit $\left(\log\left(\dfrac{P_{AD}}{P_{no\,AD}}\right)\right)$ by MOFROMINDEX shows variation and different patterns in the responses for each patient over time through the different lines (fig. 5.2).

5.3.1 SAS Syntax and Output for Two-Level Hierarchical Data

We fit a two-level hierarchical model with PROC GLIMMIX in SAS using the following syntax:

```
¹PROC GLIMMIX DATA=CHAP5 PCONV = 1E-4;
²CLASS ID;
³MODEL DX_AD(EVENT='1') = MOFROMINDEX AGE BMI DIABETES HYPERTEN
HYPERCHO/DIST=BIN LINK=LOGIT DDFM=RESIDUAL S;
⁴RANDOM INTERCEPT /SUBJECT=ID;
RUN;
```

[1]PROC GLIMMIX is used for fitting generalized linear mixed models for correlated data. The data are stored in the SAS dataset CHAP5, and the option PCONV = is used to set the parameter estimate convergence criterion.

[2]The class statement is used to specify categorical variables, which includes the patient ID.

[3]The model statement defines the outcome (DX_AD) = predictors. For binary outcomes, the value for the outcome of interest is set using EVENT=. Since we would like to model the probability of an AD diagnosis, we model EVENT=1. We specify a binomial distribution (DIST=BIN) and logit link function (LINK=LOGIT). We select the residual degrees of freedom method, and S is used to print the parameter estimates for the fixed effects.

[4]The random statement identifies the random effects (in this case, we specify a random intercept). SUBJECT= is used to specify the level of the random effects. For this example, we look at associations between measurements on a patient (identified by ID).

SAS OUTPUT

```
                    The GLIMMIX Procedure
                      Model Information
```

Data Set	WORK.CH5DATA
Response Variable	DX_AD
Response Distribution	Binomial
Link Function	Logit
Variance Function	Default
Variance Matrix Blocked By	ID
Estimation Technique	Residual PL
Degrees of Freedom Method	Residual

Comments: The model has a binomial random component and a logit link. The binary variable is DX_AD, which is an indicator for an AD diagnosis.

Dimensions	
G-side Cov. Parameters	1
Columns in X	7
Columns in Z per Subject	1
Subjects (Blocks in V)	5122
Max Obs per Subject	10

Comments: The hierarchical model has seven fixed effects (Columns in X) and one random effect (Columns in Z per Subject). There are 5,122 patients evaluated in this dataset, which have up to 10 visits (repeated measurements).

Convergence criterion (PCONV=0.0001) satisfied.

Comments: The model converged, and so we can continue with interpreting the results.

Fit Statistics	
-2 Res Log Pseudo-Likelihood	160583.1
Generalized Chi-Square	4630.30
Gener. Chi-Square / DF	0.16

Comments: The fit statistics reveal that the model is a good fit, as Gener. Chi-Square/DF is 0.16, less than 1 (which is the guideline for a good model fit).

Covariance Parameter Estimates			
Cov Parm	Subject	Estimate	Standard Error
Intercept	ID	10.917	0.297

Comments: The random effect is assumed to follow a normal distribution with mean zero and variance σ_{ID}^2. A test of the variance gives estimate/standard error $= 10.9174/0.2967 = 36.80 > 1.96$. Thus, we have evidence that patients should be included as a random effect in our cohort.

		Standard			
Effect	Estimate	Error	DF	t Value	Pr > |t|
Intercept	−6.790	0.584	28449	−11.62	<.0001
MOFROMINDEX	−0.016	0.001	28449	−11.22	<.0001
AGE	0.091	0.006	28449	13.99	<.0001
BMI	−0.042	0.011	28449	−3.77	0.0002
DIABETES	0.187	0.170	28449	1.10	0.2712
HYPERTEN	−0.265	0.106	28449	−2.51	0.0120
HYPERCHO	0.346	0.098	28449	3.52	0.0004

Solutions for Fixed Effects

Comments: The variables MOFROMINDEX, age, BMI, hypertension, and hypercholesterolemia are highly statistically significant. Diabetes is not found to be a significant driver of an AD diagnosis.

5.3.2 R Syntax and Output for Two-Level Hierarchical Data

The R syntax follows:

```
¹library(lme4)
²mm_1_out <- glmer(DX_AD ~ MOFROMINDEX + AGE + BMI + DIABETES +
HYPERTEN + HYPERCHO + (1 | ID), family =
binomial(link="logit"), data = dta)
³ds <- dta
⁴ds[c("MOFROMINDEX","AGE","BMI")] <- scale(ds[c("MOFROMINDEX","A
GE","BMI")])
⁵ss <- getME(mm_1_out,c("theta","fixef"))
⁶m1s <- update(mm_1_out,data=ds,start=ss,control=glmerControl(op
tCtrl=list(maxfun=2e4)))
summary(m1s)
```

[1]Used to fit mixed models using the glmer() function.
[2]Used to fit mixed models as outcome ~ predictors + random effects. The random component is specified as a binomial distribution with

the family = option. For the data in this example, there is a convergence issue warning printed when this syntax is run. We resolve this issue by rescaling the continuous variables (3 and 4) and updating the starting values and convergence options (5 and 6).

[3]Create data frame called ds, same as dta (the original data). Scale the variable.

[4]Scale continuous variables MOFROMINDEX, AGE, and BMI in the data frame ds.

[5]The getME() function saves specified values from the mixed model output. In this case, we reference the first model fit (mm_1_out) to save the values of theta (the random effects) and the values of fixef (the fixed effects) into the vector ss.

[6]We rerun the mixed model by using the function update(). Update() is used to update previous model results (mm_1_out), using new options. We update the previous model fit to use the data frame ds (which contains the scaled continuous variables), to use the starting values for the random and fixed effects from the previous fit (saved in the vector ss) and to specify the maximum number of iterations.

R OUTPUT

```
summary(m1s)
## Generalized linear mixed model fit by maximum likelihood (Laplace
##     Approximation) [glmerMod]
##   Family: binomial  ( logit )
## Formula:
## DX_AD ~ MOFROMINDEX + AGE + BMI + DIABETES + HYPERTEN + HYPERCHO +
##     (1 | ID)
##     Data: ds
## Control: glmerControl(optCtrl = list(maxfun = 20000))
##
##      AIC      BIC   logLik deviance df.resid
##     5244     5310    -2614     5228    28448
##
```

```
## Scaled residuals:
##      Min       1Q    Median       3Q      Max
## -0.00244 -0.00109 -0.00083  0.02519  0.04559
##
## Random effects:
##  Groups Name        Variance Std.Dev.
##  ID     (Intercept) 4177     64.6
## Number of obs: 28456, groups:  ID, 5122
##
## Fixed effects:
##               Estimate Std. Error z value Pr(>|z|)
## (Intercept)   -13.819      0.319  -43.36   <2e-16 ***
## MOFROMINDEX    -0.392      0.135   -2.91   0.0037 **
## AGE             0.543      0.185    2.94   0.0033 **
## BMI            -0.136      0.173   -0.79   0.4310
## DIABETES        0.162      0.503    0.32   0.7479
## HYPERTEN       -0.215      0.325   -0.66   0.5086
## HYPERCHO        0.278      0.306    0.91   0.3633
## ---
## Signif. codes:  0 '***' 0.001 '**' 0.01 '*' 0.05 '.' 0.1 ' ' 1
##
## Correlation of Fixed Effects:
##             (Intr) MOFROM AGE    BMI    DIABET HYPERT
## MOFROMINDEX  0.139
## AGE         -0.050 -0.304
## BMI          0.184  0.008  0.164
## DIABETES    -0.064 -0.015 -0.017 -0.157
## HYPERTEN    -0.372  0.003 -0.222 -0.179 -0.112
## HYPERCHO    -0.401 -0.047  0.044 -0.069 -0.122 -0.204
```

Comments: The glmer() output includes fit statistics (Akaike Information Criterion (AIC), Bayesian Information Criterion (BIC), log likelihood (logLik), deviance, and residual degrees (df.resid)), the estimate for the random effect, and the estimates for the fixed effects.

Although we achieved model convergence after scaling the variables and adjusting the model options, we see that the results may not be reliable. The estimate for the variance of the random effect is 4,177, which is highly unusual (as this value is extremely large). In addition, the model indicates that MOFROMINDEX and age are the only significant predictors. These findings differ from the results we obtained using GEE as well as the mixed model results from SAS.

5.3.3 Stata Syntax and Output for Two-Level Hierarchical Data

In Stata, we can use the xtmelogit command to estimate a mixed effects logistic regression model with time since baseline, age, BMI, diabetes, hypertension, and hypercholesterolemia as predictors. The random intercept for the patient is inserted using the patient's ID (ID). The Stata syntax follows:

```
.MELOGIT DX_AD AGE BMI DIABETES HYPERTEN HYPERCHO MOFROMINDEX
|| ID:
```

Comments: The model does not run.

5.4 Three-Level Models with Multiple Random Intercepts

In the cases of higher-level hierarchical data, with more than two levels, we are interested in evaluating the impact of the random effects at the various level of nesting. For example, measurements across time (level 1) are collected on each patient (level 2), and patients are nested within ADCs (level 3). In the two-level model, we evaluated the grouping effect of patients through a random intercept, which measures the impact of each patient on the individual measurements at each time-point. For the three-level model, we wish to capture the grouping impact of patients as well as centers. We can have models with more than three levels.

We have hierarchical binary outcome data with three levels, based on repeated measures on the presence/absence of AD with risk factors. Times are nested within patients, and patients are nested within centers. One important aspect of modeling in such data analysis is the correlation that occurs at each level of the data. The intraclass correlation has an important role in identifying significant clustering in higher-level models. In parametric modeling, accounting for higher-level clustering increases the complexity of the model but addresses the correlation. Irimata and Wilson (2017) developed a measure of intraclass correlation at each stage of a three-level nested structure and presented guidelines for determining when the clustering in hierarchical models needs to be taken into account. They provide a simple rule of thumb to assist researchers faced with the challenge of choosing an appropriately complex model when analyzing hierarchical binary data. In general, we find that the intraclass correlation within clusters tends to decrease as we move up the hierarchy. Thus higher-level clusters tend to have less correlation compared to lower-level clusters.

Statistical Model: We present a statistical model for three-level hierarchical models with random effects. For random intercept models, we incorporate two random effects representing levels 2 and 3 of the data. A statistical model for three-level hierarchical data with covariates is:

$$\log\left(\frac{P_{\text{event}}}{P_{\text{nonevent}}}\right) = \beta_0 + \beta_1 X_1 + \cdots + \beta_p X_p + \gamma_1 + \gamma_2,$$

where β_i represents the regression coefficient associated with the ith covariates X_i, γ_1 is the random effect representing the first level of clustering assumed to be normally distributed a mean of zero and variance of σ_1^2, and γ_2 is the random effect representing the second level of clustering, which is assumed to be normally distributed with a mean of zero and variance of σ_2^2.

The strength of the intraclass correlation is evaluated by fitting the model with no covariates:

$$\log\left(\frac{P_{\text{event}}}{P_{\text{nonevent}}}\right) = \beta_0 + \gamma_1 + \gamma_2.$$

This model calculates the covariance of the random effects (σ_1^2 and σ_2^2) without the impact of the fixed effects. The total variance is composed of the level 1 variance σ_1^2, level 2 variance σ_2^2, and the residual error of a logistic regression model, which is assumed to be 3.29. Thus the intraclass correlation for the level 1 grouping (e.g., center) is found as $\dfrac{\sigma_1^2}{\sigma_1^2 + \sigma_2^2 + 3.29}$, and the intraclass correlation for the level 2 grouping (e.g., patients within centers) is $\dfrac{\sigma_2^2}{\sigma_1^2 + \sigma_2^2 + 3.29}$. If the estimates of the intraclass correlation are close to zero, this indicates there is not strong correlation within the specified level of clustering.

Problem: Do MOFROMINDEX, age, BMI, diabetes, hypertension, and hypercholesterolemia affect an Alzheimer's disease diagnosis after adjusting for the person's unmeasurable characteristics and center effects?

Solution: We are interested in examining the impact of BMI, age, diabetes, hypertension, and hypercholesterolemia on an AD diagnosis. In the two-level model, we adjusted for the patient impact through a random effect. In the three-level model, we wish to additionally account for the effect of the ADC.

The generalized linear mixed model to address our research question is:

$$\log\left(\frac{P_{AD}}{P_{no\,AD}}\right) = \beta_0 + \beta_1 X_{MOFROMINDEX} + \beta_2 X_{AGE} + \beta_3 X_{BMI} + \beta_4 X_{DIABETES}$$

$$+ \beta_5 X_{HYPERTEN} + \beta_6 X_{HYPERCHO} + \gamma_{ID} + \gamma_{ADC},$$

where P_{AD} is the probability of an AD diagnosis, $P_{no\,AD}$ is the probability of no AD, and the regression coefficients $\beta_0 - \beta_6$ represent the effects of each covariate. The random intercept γ_{ID} measures patient-level variation, while the additional term γ_{ADC} is a random intercept

Table 5.5 Three-Level Mixed Model Results

Parameter	Estimate	Std Err	p-Value
Intercept	−7.139	0.655	<0.0001
MOFROMINDEX	−0.017	0.002	<0.0001
AGE	0.098	0.007	<0.0001
BMI	−0.048	0.011	<0.0001
DIABETES	0.180	0.174	0.301
HYPERTEN	−0.191	0.109	0.080
HYPERCHO	0.302	0.101	0.003

for the grouping owing to the center and measures any variation between the centers. In the model, we fit $\log\left(\dfrac{P(DX\_AD=1)}{P(DX\_AD=0)}\right)$.

The estimate of the random effect variance for the patient level is 10.238, with a standard error of 0.2854. Thus, because the ratio $10.238/0.285 = 35.923$ is larger than 1.96, the random intercept at the patient level is statistically significant. Hence, modeling the patient as a random effect was a wise choice. Similarly, the estimated variance of the random effects for center is 1.817, with standard error 0.494. The ratio $1.817/0.494 = 3.708$ is larger than 1.96, which signifies that it is also statistically significant, and it is important to include center as a random effect in the model. The estimates for the random effects in the three-level mixed model are reported in table 5.5.

Comments: From the model results, which account for the patient and center clustering effects through random intercepts, we find that time since baseline (MOFROMINDEX), age, BMI, and hypercholesterolemia are statistically significant predictors of the probability of an AD diagnosis. Diabetes and hypertension are not identified as statistically significant drivers of AD.

5.4.1 SAS Syntax and Output for Three-Level Hierarchical Data

A three-level hierarchical mode with patient effect and center effect was fitted using SAS PROC GLIMMIX. One can also run these models with PROC NLMIXED.

```
¹PROC GLIMMIX DATA=LONGITUDINAL NOCLPRINT PCONV = 1E-4;
²CLASS ADC ID;
³MODEL DX_AD(EVENT='1') = MOFROMINDEX AGE BMI DIABETES HYPERTEN
HYPERCHO /DIST=BIN LINK=LOGIT DDFM=RESIDUAL S;
⁴RANDOM INTERCEPT /SUBJECT=ID(ADC);
⁵RANDOM INTERCEPT/SUBJECT=ADC;
RUN;
```

[1]SAS PROC GLIMMIX fits mixed models for the specified dataset DATA=. The option NOCLPRINT suppresses the class-level output for categorical variables. The option PCONV is used to specify the convergence criterion for parameter estimates.

[2]The CLASS statement is used to specify the categorical variables in the model.

[3]The MODEL statement specifies the outcome in terms of the predictors. A logit link function (LINK=LOGIT) is specified, and the responses are a binomial (DIST=BIN).

[4]This random statement fits a random intercept term for the patient level (ID).

[5]This random statement fits a random intercept for the center (ADC).

SAS OUTPUT

```
                    The GLIMMIX Procedure
                     Model Information
```

Data Set	WORK.SURVIVAL
Response Variable	DX_AD
Response Distribution	Binomial
Link Function	Logit
Variance Function	Default
Variance Matrix Blocked By	ADC
Estimation Technique	Residual PL
Degrees of Freedom Method	Residual

Comments: The Model Information output summarizes the dataset and model assumptions. We see that the response variable, DX_AD, is distributed as binomial, and the model is fit using a logit link. The variances (Variance Matrix Blocked by) are given at the center level. The estimation technique utilized is the residual profile likelihood (Residual PL).

	Dimensions
G-side Cov. Parameters	2
Columns in X	7
Columns in Z per Subject	353
Subjects (Blocks in V)	32
Max Obs per Subject	2321

Comments: There are two random effects parameters, as noted in the G-side Cov. Parameters row. One represents the patients as the random effects, and the other represents the center. These covariate parameters are tested to be zero. If each random effect is not different from zero, we conclude it is not necessary to include the random effects in the model. There are seven parameters representing the fixed effects in the model, which are often referred to as the predictors in the model.

Cov Parm	Subject	Estimate	Standard Error
Intercept	ID(ADC)	10.2375	0.285
Intercept	ADC	1.817	0.494

Comments: An estimate of the variance of the responses from one patient to the next is 10.238, with a standard error of 0.285. Since the ratio $10.238/0.285 = 35.923$ is larger than 1.96, this indicates the random intercept at the patient level is statistically significant. Hence modeling the patient as a random effect was a wise choice. Similarly, the variance of the responses from one center to the next is 1.817, with a standard error of 0.494. The ratio $1.817/0.494 = 3.708$ is larger than 1.96, which signifies it is also statistically significant, and it is important to include center as a random effect in the model.

		Standard			
Effect	Estimate	Error	DF	t Value	Pr > |t|
Intercept	−7.139	0.655	28449	−10.90	<.0001
MOFROMINDEX	−0.017	0.002	28449	−11.02	<.0001
AGE	0.098	0.007	28449	14.40	<.0001
BMI	−0.048	0.011	28449	−4.20	<.0001
DIABETES	0.180	0.174	28449	1.04	0.3006
HYPERTEN	−0.191	0.109	28449	−1.75	0.0797
HYPERCHO	0.302	0.101	28449	2.98	0.0029

Solutions for Fixed Effects

Comments: The Solution for Fixed Effects table reports the parameter estimates, standard errors, and *p*-values. The significant variables include MOFROMINDEX, age, BMI, and hypercholesterolemia.

5.4.2 R Syntax and Output for Three-Level Hierarchical Data

The R syntax follows:

```
¹mm_2_out <- glmer(DX_AD ~ MOFROMINDEX + AGE + BMI + DIABETES +
HYPERTEN + HYPERCHO + (1 | ID) + (1 | ADC), family =
binomial(link="logit"), data = dta)
²ss <- getME(mm_2_out,c("theta","fixef"))
³m2s <- update(mm_2_out,data=ds,start=ss,control=glmerControl(op
timizer="bobyqa", optCtrl=list(maxfun=2e5)))
summary(m2s)
```

[1]The glmer() function in the R library lme4 fits mixed models. We have a convergence issue (which is shown in the output) and resolve this issue by refitting the model using a scaled dataset and adjusting the optimization options.[2,3]
[2]The estimates of the random effects (theta) and fixed effects (fixef) are saved in the vector ss using the getME() function.
[3]The mixed model is refit by updating the previous output using the scaled dataset created in section 5.3.2 (ds) and the bobyqa optimizer.

R OUTPUT

```
summary(m2s)
## Generalized linear mixed model fit by maximum likelihood (Laplace
##    Approximation) [glmerMod]
##  Family: binomial  ( logit )
## Formula:
## DX_AD ~ MOFROMINDEX + AGE + BMI + DIABETES + HYPERTEN + HYPERCHO +
##     (1 | ID) + (1 | ADC)
##    Data: ds
## Control:
## glmerControl(optimizer = "bobyqa", optCtrl = list(maxfun = 2e+05))
##
##      AIC      BIC   logLik deviance df.resid
##     5238     5312    -2610     5220    28447
##
## Scaled residuals:
##      Min       1Q   Median       3Q      Max
## -0.00373 -0.00105 -0.00076  0.02458  0.04542
##
## Random effects:
##  Groups Name        Variance Std.Dev.
##  ID     (Intercept) 4289.8   65.50
##  ADC    (Intercept)    2.8    1.67
## Number of obs: 28456, groups:  ID, 5122; ADC, 32
##
## Fixed effects:
##              Estimate Std. Error z value Pr(>|z|)
## (Intercept)   -14.648      0.453  -32.33   <2e-16 ***
## MOFROMINDEX    -0.396      0.135   -2.94   0.0032 **
## AGE             0.539      0.188    2.86   0.0042 **
## BMI            -0.164      0.174   -0.94   0.3465
## DIABETES        0.147      0.507    0.29   0.7717
## HYPERTEN       -0.205      0.327   -0.63   0.5297
## HYPERCHO        0.260      0.308    0.84   0.3986
```

```
## ---
## Signif. codes:  0 '***' 0.001 '**' 0.01 '*' 0.05 '.' 0.1 ' ' 1
##
## Correlation of Fixed Effects:
##             (Intr) MOFROM AGE    BMI    DIABET HYPERT
## MOFROMINDEX  0.108
## AGE         -0.049 -0.312
## BMI          0.177  0.005  0.161
## DIABETES    -0.045 -0.013 -0.022 -0.156
## HYPERTEN    -0.276  0.007 -0.217 -0.173 -0.118
## HYPERCHO    -0.273 -0.046  0.037 -0.073 -0.120 -0.199
```

Comments: Although we achieve convergence after refitting the model, we suspect there is an issue with convergence, as the variance for the patient random effect is large (4,289.8). In addition, we find that only MOFROMINDEX and age are significant covariates, which differs from our previous findings.

5.4.3 SPSS Syntax and Output for Three-Level Hierarchical Data

To fit a three-level model, two random subcommands are needed. The subcommands are listed in the order of nesting, from the highest to lowest levels. In our example, the first random subcommand inserts a random intercept for center (the second level), and the second random subcommand inserts a random intercept for the patient (the first level). The SPSS syntax follows:

```
GET FILE ="C:\USER\DOCUMENTS\DATA\CHAP5.SAV "
GENLINMIXED
   /DATA_STRUCTURE SUBJECTS=ID
   /FIELDS TARGET=DX_AD TRIALS=NONE OFFSET=NONE
   /TARGET_OPTIONS DISTRIBUTION=BINOMIAL LINK=LOGIT
   /FIXED  EFFECTS=MOFROMINDEX  AGE BMI DIABETES HYPERTEN
HYPERCHO USE_INTERCEPT=TRUE
   /RANDOM USE_INTERCEPT=TRUE COVARIANCE_TYPE=VARIANCE_COMPONENTS
```

```
 /BUILD_OPTIONS TARGET_CATEGORY_ORDER=ASCENDING INPUTS_
CATEGORY_ORDER=ASCENDING MAX_ITERATIONS=100 CONFIDENCE_LEVEL=95
DF_METHOD=RESIDUAL COVB=MODEL PCONVERGE=0.000001(ABSOLUTE)
SCORING=0 SINGULAR=0.000000000001
 /EMMEANS_OPTIONS SCALE=ORIGINAL PADJUST=LSD.
```

Comments: There is no output. These models do not converge in SPSS.

5.4.4 Stata Syntax and Output for Three-Level Hierarchical Data

To estimate a three-level logistic model with two random intercepts (for patients and centers), we use the following command:

```
MELOGIT DX_AD BMI AGE MOFROMINDEX DIABETES HYPERTEN HYPERCHO,
 || ID:  ||ADC:  , COVARIANCE(EXCHANGEABLE)
```

Comments: These models do not converge in Stata.

5.5 Marginal versus Subject Specific Models

In this chapter, we discuss generalized estimating equations and random effects models. GEE is a marginal modeling approach, which allows us to draw conclusions about the population. For example, when we evaluated the NACC data, we identified factors that contribute to an AD diagnosis. In the interpretation of this model result, we can conclude that, on average, factors such as age, BMI, hypertension, and hypercholesterolemia affect the probability of an AD diagnosis in our dataset. We cannot predict whether a specific individual will have an AD diagnosis, however.

Alternatively, random effect models are subject-specific models. These models allow one to draw conclusions about a certain subject, given information about random variation due to the subject or cluster. In addition, random effects models allow one to draw conclusions about the impact of the nested structures at a population level, rather than being limited only to the specific groups evaluated in the sample (Hox and Kreft 1994). Although we only evaluated a subset of 32

ADCs in this study, the random effects model allows us to discuss the impact of centers in general, including ADCs that were not considered in our analysis. Thus the interpretation between GEE and mixed models differs.

We focused on modeling with random intercepts, as these are common in generalized linear mixed models. But it is also possible to evaluate random slopes. By random slope, we mean measure of the differential impact that a certain covariate has across the groups. The random slope model is:

$$\log\left(\frac{P_{event}}{P_{nonevent}}\right) = \beta_0 + (\beta_1 + \gamma_1)X_1 + \cdots + \beta_p X_p,$$

where P_{event} is the probability of the event of interest, $P_{nonevent}$ is the probability of nonevent, β_i is the regression coefficient for the fixed effects due to covariates X_i, and γ_1 is the random slope due to the covariate X_1. We can fit the model and evaluate if the variance of the random slope suggests significant variation between the impact of X_1 on the outcome across groups.

5.6 Summary and Discussions

In this chapter, we discuss two- and three-level mixed models with random intercepts for binary outcomes using a logit link. This chapter provides an important discussion on evaluating the correlation within groups using the intraclass correlation, and accounting for various levels of nesting through higher-order models. We evaluate data on AD diagnosis to demonstrate these methods. We pursue the building of two types of models, marginal and subject-specific models for binary data, which address different research questions.

5.7 Exercises

We are interested in evaluating the binary outcome diabetes status (where 0 denotes absent and 1 denotes present). Patient-level variables used in this study include age, gender (SEX), diagnosis, and hypertension status. The primary interest is to investigate the impact of certain characteristics of patient and center-level variables on a patient's likelihood of having diabetes. Therefore, using visit level as the observational level, and patient and center levels as secondary and primary levels, respectively, we investigate the relationship between diabetes and the list of predictors. Using one of the four statistical programs discussed (SAS, R, SPSS, or Stata), answer the following questions. The NACC dataset is available at http://www.public.asu.edu/~jeffreyw/.

1. What is the probability of patient having diabetes at a typical visit?
2. Does diabetes status vary across patients and centers?
3. What is the relationship between gender and the likelihood of diabetes while controlling for age and diagnosis?
4. What is the relationship between gender and the likelihood of diabetes while controlling for visit and patient characteristics?
5. What is the probability of being diabetic, given a particular center?

Chapter 6

Bayesian Regression Models

6.1 Motivating Example

In chapter 5, we fit frequentist logistic regression models with generalized estimating equations (GEEs) and random effects models using maximum and restricted maximum likelihood methods. In some cases, however, one may have prior information concerning the outcome of interest to incorporate in the model. Bayesian models allow us to incorporate information that may be available from prior studies or other sources. For example, in a study of Alzheimer's disease (AD), it would make sense to incorporate the information that there is a negligible probability of someone younger than 39 years of age having sporadic Alzheimer's disease (i.e., not having a mutation that causes the disease or a risk factor).

We revisit data analyzed in chapter 5, in which we analyzed longitudinal data for 5,122 patients with four or more visits, representing 32 Alzheimer's Disease Centers (ADCs). A total of 28,456 records are contained in this dataset. We analyze these data using a Bayesian logistic regression model and a Bayesian hierarchical logistic regression methods. In both models, we consider several predictors that simultaneously affect the probability of an AD diagnosis (DX_AD). A subset of the data is given (table 6.1). The table includes center ID (ADC), patient's ID (ID), BMI, age, and the binary predictors, hypertension, diabetes, and hypercholesterolemia. We fit these Bayesian models using the statistical software SAS, R, and Stata.

6.2 What Is Bayesian Analysis?

Bayesian analysis is a statistical approach that estimates parameters through the use of probability distributions. This approach addresses

Table 6.1 Subset of Chapter 6 Data

ADC	ID	MOFROMINDEX	DX_AD	AGE	BMI	DIABETES	HYPERTEN	HYPERCHO
5452	271	0	1	81	21.5	0	0	1
5452	271	12	1	82	21.6	0	0	0
5452	271	23	1	83	20.2	0	0	1
5452	271	37	1	84	20.6	0	0	1
5452	271	64	1	86	20.2	0	0	0
289	385	16	1	82	29	0	1	1
289	385	28	1	83	29	0	0	1
289	385	41	1	84	26.4	0	0	0
289	385	50	1	84	29	0	0	0

the following questions: What is the probability that treatment A is more cost-effective than treatment B for AD? What is the probability that a patient's Clinical Dementia Rating Scale Sum of Boxes (CDR-SUM) score decreases if she or he is given drug A? What is the probability that a person will develop AD if she or he has an APOE 4 allele? These types of questions and others are common, as Bayesian analysis assumes that all parameters are random quantities. Bayesian approaches are often useful in studies quantifying risk. In the classical frequentist method, all parameters are assumed to have fixed values. Alternatively, in Bayesian analysis, the parameters are assumed to follow a statistical distribution rather than a fixed value. In this chapter, we concentrate on estimating the distribution of the parameter of interest, referred to as the posterior distribution. The posterior distribution is the key to Bayesian analysis.

6.3 Bayes Probability, Priors, and Posteriors

Bayesian analyses are derived from Bayes' theorem. Consider that for some events A and B, Bayes' theorem states

$$P(A|B) = \frac{P(B|A)P(A)}{P(B)},$$

where $P(A)$ is the probability of event A, $P(B)$ is the probability of event B, $P(B|A)$ is the conditional probability of event B given that event A is true, and $P(A|B)$ is the conditional probability of event A given that the event B is true. For example, let event B represent that the patient has diabetes. Let event A represent that a patient is diagnosed with AD. Then, given information about the probability of patients with AD and the probability of patients with diabetes (prior), as well as information about the probability that a patient with AD has diabetes (likelihood), we can then determine the probability that a patient has AD given that the patient has diabetes (posterior).

Bayesian inference is focused on the posterior distribution. The posterior distribution provides information about the parameter based on the observed data (the data we have collected and are evaluating). We use the posterior distribution to form various summaries for the model parameters, including point estimates such as posterior means, medians, percentiles, and interval estimates known as credible intervals. The posterior distribution depends on the chosen prior distribution and the likelihood. It is obtained through analytical or approximate methods. One key method of approximation is the Markov Chain Monte Carlo (MCMC) method (Berger 1985).

The parameters in a Bayes model are random quantities that have distributions, as opposed to the frequentist model parameters of classical statistics. The statistical inferences in the Bayesian approach are obtained from summary measures of the posterior distribution. We obtain point and interval estimates for the mean or median of a posterior distribution, and quantiles provide credible intervals. These credible intervals are known as credible sets and are analogous to the confidence intervals in frequentist analysis.

The great aspects of Bayesian analysis include incorporating prior information in the analysis. This leads to interpretation of credible intervals as fixed ranges to which a parameter is known to belong with a prespecified probability. Moreover, there is the assignment of actual probability to any hypothesis of interest. Bayesian analysis typically consists of three steps:

1. Write the likelihood function of the data.
2. Select prior distributions for all the unknown parameters.

3. Use Bayes' theorem to find the posterior distribution over all parameters.

We follow these steps through the analysis of binary data in section 6.5.

6.4 Advantages and Disadvantages

The Bayesian analysis is an alternative approach to the frequentist methods of analyses. Although both methods (frequentist and Bayes) are used in the estimation of model parameters, each method has advantages and disadvantages. Some advantages of a Bayesian approach over a frequentist approach are:

1. Bayesian methods utilize known information about a parameter that was previously collected (the prior).
2. Exact inference is used and does not require asymptotic approximation for small sample sizes.
3. It follows Bayes' principle, which indicates that all information from the data for inference on the model parameters are contained in the likelihood function.
4. Computationally, Bayesian methods are more flexible and able to estimate many complex models, including hierarchical models with higher levels of clustering.
5. Model selection methods, such as the Bayesian Information Criterion (BIC), are often superior to frequentist model fit comparisons.

Some of the disadvantages to using a Bayesian analysis include:

1. There is no "correct" choice of a prior, and it may be difficult to express the past information in terms of a prior.
2. The posterior distribution, which is used to draw inferences, is influenced by the choice of priors.
3. Bayesian methods have a high computational cost, particularly when there are a large number of parameters.
4. In statistical software, frequentist analyses are often easier to set up and perform.

While there are advantages and disadvantages to Bayesian and frequentist approaches, many of the differences are philosophical. Both approaches require preliminary review of the data to understand the data collection methods, its structure, correlation, and missing data. We need these to allow us to make inferences about model parameters and associations between covariates. Ultimately, the selection of the estimation approach is the choice of the researcher.

6.5 Bayesian Logistic Regression Models

Although Bayesian approach applies to any type of model, in this chapter, we concentrate on fitting Bayesian logistic regression models. In frequentist regression models, we were interested in estimating the regression parameters. In Bayesian regression models, our interest is similar.

1. We start with the likelihood function. We have the binary outcomes that vary depending on subject's covariates; thus the ith individual in the likelihood gives

$$\text{likelihood}_i = (P_{\text{individual}|\text{covariates}})^y \, (1 - P_{\text{individual}|\text{covariates}})^{1-y},$$

where $P_{\text{individual}|\text{covariates}}$ is the probability that subject i has covariates $x_{i,}$ and y_i is 1 if the event has occurred and 0 otherwise. As the patients provide independent observations, we take the product of the likelihoods over a dataset of n patients. Therefore the joint likelihood (a product) is

$$\text{joint}_{\text{likelihood}} = \prod_{i=1}^{n} [(P_{\text{individual}|\text{covariates}})^{y_i} (1 - P_{\text{individual}|\text{covariates}})^{1-y_i}].$$

Consider an example of a model with five covariates $X_1, X_2, \ldots, X_5$ (for an outcome such as the probability of AD diagnosis against the covariates age, BMI, diabetes, hypertension, and hypercholesterolemia). Then, the probability

$$P_{\text{individual}|\text{covariates}} = \frac{\exp^{\beta_0 + \beta_1 X_1 + \cdots \beta_5 X_5}}{1 + \exp^{\beta_0 + \beta_1 X_1 + \cdots \beta_5 X_5}}.$$

This leads to a joint likelihood,

$$\text{joint}_{\text{likelihood}} = \Pi_{1=1}^{n} \left[\left(\frac{\exp^{\beta_0 + \beta_1 X_{1i} + \cdots \beta_5 X_{5i}}}{1 + \exp^{\beta_0 + \beta_1 X_{1i} + \cdots \beta_5 X_{5i}}} \right)^{y_i} \right. $$
$$\left. \times \left(1 - \frac{\exp^{\beta_0 + \beta_1 X_{1i} + \cdots \beta_5 X_{5i}}}{1 + \exp^{\beta_0 + \beta_1 X_{1i} + \cdots \beta_5 X_{5i}}} \right)^{1-y_i} \right].$$

2. Select the prior distributions for our unknown parameters $\beta_0, \beta_1, \ldots, \beta_5$. We need a prior distribution on each of these parameters. If we have no information or little is known about the coefficients, we can settle for the choice of a "diffuse" or "noninformative" priors. When informative prior distributions are desired, it is often difficult to give such information on the logistic scale, that is, on the parameters directly. In addition, we prefer to provide prior information on the odds ratio scale and then compute what it would be on the logit scale. It is customary to choose normal priors for the betas such that $\beta_j \sim \aleph(0, \sigma_j^2)$, however. The variance σ_j^2 is usually chosen to be large enough (between 100 and 10,000) to be considered noninformative.

3. We determine the posterior distribution using Bayes' theorem. The posterior distribution is derived by multiplying the prior distribution over all parameters by the full likelihood function, so that the posterior is

$$= \Pi_{1=1}^{n} \left[\left(\frac{\exp^{\beta_0 + \beta_1 X_{1i} + \cdots \beta_5 X_{5i}}}{1 + \exp^{\beta_0 + \beta_1 X_{1i} + \cdots \beta_5 X_{5i}}} \right)^{y_i} \left(1 - \frac{\exp^{\beta_0 + \beta_1 X_{1i} + \cdots \beta_5 X_{5i}}}{1 + \exp^{\beta_0 + \beta_1 X_{1i} + \cdots \beta_5 X_{5i}}} \right)^{1-y_i} \right]$$
$$\times \Pi_{j=0}^{p} - \frac{1}{2\pi^{0.5}} \exp \left(\frac{\beta_j}{\sigma_j} \right)^2.$$

The posterior has no closed form expression and is even; if it did, we would need multiple integration to obtain the marginal distribution for each coefficient. The Bayesian approach is to use the Gibbs sampler as implemented by the statistical software WinBUGS, the Windows version of BUGS (Bayesian Inference Using Gibbs Sampling) (Lunn et al. 2000), to provide an approximation of the properties of the marginal posterior distributions for each parameter.

When the response variable is binary, the traditional approach is to perform a logit transformation on the variable to address in a linear form. The question in this setting is: Can this random variable (such as the probability of an AD diagnosis) be sufficiently captured in the binomial likelihood, or is there correlation in the data caused by one factor or another that needs to be addressed?

LOGISTIC REGRESSION MODEL

We model the binary outcome Y with probability p_{ij} such that

$$Y \sim \text{binomial } (n_{ij}, p_{ij}).$$

We use the logistic link function to link the covariates of each patient to the probability of success (the outcome of interest),

$$p_i = \frac{e^{\beta_0 + \beta_1 X_1 + \cdots + \beta_p X_p}}{1 + e^{\beta_0 + \beta_1 X_1 + \cdots + \beta_p X_p}}$$

$$\text{logit } (p_i) = \beta_0 + \beta_1 X_1 + \cdots + \beta_p X_p,$$

where the beta parameters $\beta_0, \beta_1, \ldots, \beta_p$ are model parameters. There are many options for prior distributions, although if we do not have any prior information about the parameter, we may select a noninformative prior, such as $\beta_i \sim \aleph(0, 100{,}000)$ for $i = 0, 1, \ldots, p$. A normal distribution with a large variance is a flat, noninformative prior.

Problem: Do age, BMI, diabetes, hypertension, and hypercholesterolemia affect the diagnosis (AD or no AD)? We previously considered this research problem in chapter 3, and now address the question using a Bayesian approach. The posterior mean, standard deviation, and lower and upper bounds for the 95% highest posterior density (HPD) intervals are reported in table 6.2.

Table 6.2 Bayesian Model Results

Parameter	Alpha	Equal-Tail Interval		HPD Interval	
		Posterior Intervals			
Intercept	0.050	−4.1235	−2.7627	−4.1063	−2.7491
BMI	0.050	0.0435	0.0582	0.0437	0.0583
AGE	0.050	−0.0550	−0.0268	−0.0550	−0.0268
HYPERTEN	0.050	−0.1048	0.3357	−0.1084	0.3318
DIABETES	0.050	−0.2775	−0.00673	−0.2763	−0.00588
HYPERCHO	0.050	0.1534	0.4134	0.1526	0.4120

Solution: We analyze the data using SAS, R, and Stata. The posterior summary information obtained is given in table 6.2. BMI, age, diabetes, and hypercholesterolemia are identified as significant in explaining an Alzheimer's disease diagnosis. To obtain the odds ratios for each covariate, we can calculate the exponential of the HPD interval.

6.5.1 SAS Syntax and Output for Bayesian Logistic Regression

We use the Bayes' option in PROC GENMOD in SAS to fit Bayesian logistic regression models. The process generates a Markov chain. Its stationary distribution is the desired posterior distribution. We check its convergence before we accept the resulting posterior statistics. There is no definitive way of determining that you have convergence, but there are a number of diagnostic tools. The built-in Bayesian procedures provide a number of convergence diagnostic tests and tools, such as Gelman-Rubin, Geweke, Heidelberger-Welch, and Raftery-Lewis tests. The following SAS syntax fits the data from the baseline visits:

```
¹PROC GENMOD DATA=CHAP6 DESCENDING;
²MODEL DX_AD = AGE BMI DIABETES HYPERTEN HYPERCHO / DIST=BIN
LINK=LOGIT;
³BAYES SEED=1 CPRIOR=NORMAL(VAR=1E6) OUTPOST=NEUOUT PLOTS=TRACE
NMC=20000;
⁴WHERE MOFROMINDEX=0;
RUN;
```

[1]Options to implement Bayesian generalized linear models.

[2]Outcome = predictors specifies a binomial distribution with a logit link function.

[3]The Bayes statement consists of a random seed (used to replicate results) and the specification of the assumed prior distribution (CPRIOR=). We can specify the number of iterations after burn-in using NMC=. The option PLOTS=TRACE gives the trace plots, and OUTPOST= is used to save an SAS dataset containing the posterior samples.

[4]WHERE statement to select the baseline visits (that have MOFROMINDEX=0).

SAS OUTPUT

The GENMOD Procedure

Bayesian Analysis

Model Information

Data Set	WORK.CHAP6
Burn-In Size	2000
MC Sample Size	20000
Thinning	1
Sampling Algorithm	Gamerman
Distribution	Binomial
Link Function	Logit
Dependent Variable	DX_AD

Number of Observations Read	4882
Number of Observations Used	4882
Number of Events	1541
Number of Trials	4882

Comments: The Model Information table reports key information about the model fit. We use a burn-in size of 2,000, which is the number of iterations we do not consider. We assume an underling binomial distribution for the outcome. We have a dataset with 4,882 observations, containing baseline measurements for patients.

	Response Profile	
Ordered Value	DX_AD	Total Frequency
1	0	1541
2	1	3341

PROC GENMOD is modeling the probability that DX_AD = 1.

Comments: PROC GENMOD is modeling the probability that DX_AD = 1 (AD diagnosis) as we specify the DESCENDING option in the PROC statement.

		Analysis of Maximum Likelihood Parameter Estimates			
Parameter	DF	Estimate	Standard Error	Wald 95% Confidence Limits	
Intercept	1	-3.4372	0.3469	-4.1171	-2.7573
BMI	1	0.0507	0.0038	0.0434	0.0581
AGE	1	-0.0407	0.0071	-0.0546	-0.0268
HYPERTEN	1	0.1185	0.1121	-0.1011	0.3382
DIABETES	1	-0.1419	0.0698	-0.2786	-0.0052
HYPERCHO	1	0.2836	0.0664	0.1533	0.4138
Scale	0	1.0000	0.0000	1.0000	1.0000

Comments: BMI, age, diabetes, and hypercholesterolemia are significant. These are the results we obtain if we were to use the frequentist approach.

Independent Normal Prior for Regression Coefficients		
Parameter	Mean	Precision
Intercept	0	1E-6
BMI	0	1E-6
AGE	0	1E-6
HYPERTEN	0	1E-6
DIABETES	0	1E-6
HYPERCHO	0	1E-6

Algorithm converged.

Initial Values of the Chain

Chain	Seed	Intercept	BMI	AGE	HYPERTEN	DIABETES	HYPERCHO
1	1	-3.437	0.051	-0.041	0.119	-0.142	0.284

Comments: In the analysis, we assume independent normal distributions as the prior distributions for each regression coefficient. The maximum likelihood parameter estimates (from the frequentist approach) are used as the initial values of the chain for MCMC.

Posterior Summaries

Parameter	N	Mean	Standard Deviation	Percentiles 25%	50%	75%
Intercept	20000	-3.4396	0.3463	-3.6730	-3.4370	-3.2062
BMI	20000	0.0508	0.00374	0.0482	0.0508	0.0533
AGE	20000	-0.0408	0.00714	-0.0455	-0.0408	-0.0360
HYPERTEN	20000	0.1172	0.1124	0.0405	0.1184	0.1942
DIABETES	20000	-0.1417	0.0694	-0.1888	-0.1416	-0.0955
HYPERCHO	20000	0.2835	0.0662	0.2392	0.2837	0.3282

Comments: The Posterior Summaries table reports the means of the posterior distributions (parameter estimates) as well as the standard deviations and percentiles. We note that the mean and median (50th percentile) appear to be similar for all parameters.

Posterior Intervals

Parameter	Alpha	Equal-Tail Interval		HPD Interval	
Intercept	0.050	-4.1235	-2.7627	-4.1063	-2.7491
BMI	0.050	0.0435	0.0582	0.0437	0.0583
AGE	0.050	-0.0550	-0.0268	-0.0550	-0.0268
HYPERTEN	0.050	-0.1048	0.3357	-0.1084	0.3318
DIABETES	0.050	-0.2775	-0.00673	-0.2763	-0.00588
HYPERCHO	0.050	0.1534	0.4134	0.1526	0.4120

Comments: The posterior intervals report the predicted intervals. The HPD interval suggests that BMI, age, diabetes, and hypercholesterolemia are highly influential (as 0 is not included in the interval) predictors of an AD diagnosis.

Posterior Correlation Matrix

Parameter	Intercept	BMI	AGE	HYPERTEN	DIABETES	HYPERCHO
Intercept	1.000	-0.844	-0.624	0.058	0.212	-0.038
BMI	-0.844	1.000	0.132	-0.001	-0.208	0.012
AGE	-0.624	0.132	1.000	-0.121	-0.209	-0.076
HYPERTEN	0.058	-0.001	-0.121	1.000	-0.136	-0.093
DIABETES	0.212	-0.208	-0.209	-0.136	1.000	-0.229
HYPERCHO	-0.038	0.012	-0.076	-0.093	-0.229	1.000

Comments: The Posterior Correlation Matrix shows the correlations between each of the covariates. It contains relatively low correlations between the covariates (e.g., the correlation between BMI and age is 0.132).

Posterior Autocorrelations

Parameter	Lag 1	Lag 5	Lag 10	Lag 50
Intercept	0.1298	0.0087	0.0017	-0.0254
BMI	0.1318	0.0104	-0.0034	-0.0243
AGE	0.1326	-0.0052	0.0105	-0.0086
HYPERTEN	0.1348	-0.0032	-0.0058	-0.0007
DIABETES	0.1132	0.0086	-0.0111	0.0105
HYPERCHO	0.1140	0.0053	-0.0048	-0.0003

Comments: Autocorrelation measures the dependency among the Markov chain samples, and high correlations can indicate poor mixing. We see that in our data these values tend to decline over time.

Geweke Diagnostics		
Parameter	z	Pr > |z|
Intercept	0.5591	0.5761
BMI	-0.2127	0.8316
AGE	-0.7224	0.4700
HYPERTEN	0.6872	0.4920
DIABETES	-0.2503	0.8023
HYPERCHO	0.0412	0.9671

Comments: The Geweke statistic compares means from early and late parts of the Markov chain to see whether they have converged.

Effective Sample Sizes			
Parameter	ESS	Autocorrelation Time	Efficiency
Intercept	15391.8	1.2994	0.7696
BMI	15180.3	1.3175	0.7590
AGE	15807.8	1.2652	0.7904
HYPERTEN	15416.3	1.2973	0.7708
DIABETES	15762.3	1.2689	0.7881
HYPERCHO	16287.9	1.2279	0.8144

Comments: The effective sample size (ESS) is particularly useful, as it provides a numerical indication of mixing status. The closer ESS is to $n = 20,000$ (the number of iterations after burn-in), the better the mixing in the Markov chain. In general, an ESS of approximately 1,000 is adequate for estimating the posterior density.

Comments: Figures 6.1 and 6.2 are the trace plots for the intercept, age, BMI, diabetes, hypertension, and hypercholesterolemia. The trace plots are plots of the estimated values of a parameter versus the number of iterations. Visual examination of these plots is one method of assessing convergence. Plots containing many estimates around the mode of the distribution that lack a trend indicate convergence. The plots above support model convergence in our current example.

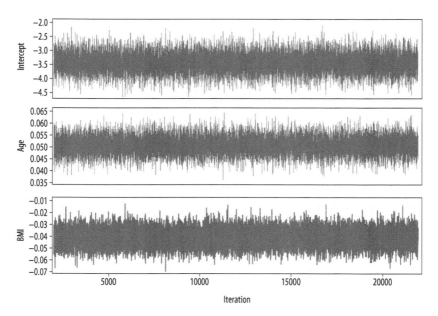

Figure 6.1 Trace plots for the intercept, age, and BMI.

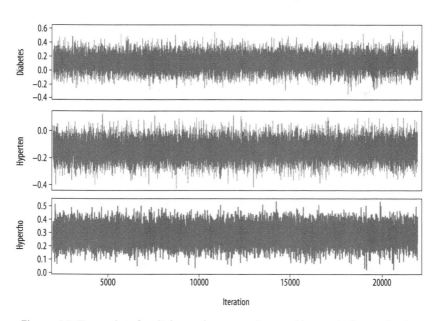

Figure 6.2 Trace plots for diabetes, hypertension, and hypercholesterolemia.

6.5.2 R Syntax and Output for Bayesian Logistic Regression

There are many R packages for Bayesian modeling and data analysis, some of which are called WinBUGS. We introduce the package MC-MCpack (Martin et al. 2011), which is a standalone R package for Bayesian data analysis. The R syntax follows:

```
1library(MCMCpack)
2chap6baseline <- chap6[chap6$MOFROMINDEX==0,]
3mcmcfit <- MCMClogit(DX_AD~AGE + BMI + DIABETES + HYPERTEN +
HYPERCHO, data=chap6baseline, burnin=1000, mcmc=21000)

4summary(mcmcfit)
5plot(mcmcfit)
```

[1]The MCMCpack library is one package used to fit Bayesian models.
[2]The chap6 dataset is a subset to create a dataset containing the baseline visits (chap6baseline), where MOFROMINDEX=0.
[3]The function MCMClogit() is used to fit the Bayesian logistic regression model for the baseline visits. The model is specified as outcome ~ predictors, where the number of discarded burn-in iterations is specified using burnin=, and the number of estimation iterations is specified using mcmc=. The model output is saved in the object mcmcfit.
[4]The summary() function is used to print a summary of the model fit and parameter estimates.
[5]The plot() function is used to output the diagnostic plots for Bayesian modeling, including the trace and density plots for each parameter.

R OUTPUT

```
summary(mcmcfit)
##
## Iterations = 1001:22000
## Thinning interval = 1
## Number of chains = 1
```

```
## Sample size per chain = 21000
##
## 1. Empirical mean and standard deviation for each variable,
##    plus standard error of the mean:
##
##                  Mean       SD  Naive SE Time-series SE
## (Intercept) -3.45594 0.342329 2.362e-03      0.0105863
## AGE          0.05090 0.003741 2.582e-05      0.0001162
## BMI         -0.04063 0.007065 4.875e-05      0.0002183
## DIABETES     0.12571 0.111776 7.713e-04      0.0034582
## HYPERTEN    -0.13860 0.071383 4.926e-04      0.0022674
## HYPERCHO     0.28381 0.065549 4.523e-04      0.0019962
##
## 2. Quantiles for each variable:
##
##                  2.5%      25%      50%      75%      97.5%
## (Intercept) -4.14841 -3.68057 -3.46270 -3.21995 -2.785833
## AGE          0.04339  0.04832  0.05090  0.05339  0.058222
## BMI         -0.05423 -0.04529 -0.04068 -0.03602 -0.026295
## DIABETES    -0.09013  0.04795  0.12655  0.20062  0.342492
## HYPERTEN    -0.27791 -0.18637 -0.13954 -0.09078  0.006172
## HYPERCHO     0.15034  0.23920  0.28339  0.33005  0.411474
```

Comments: The means and the standard deviations, along with the quantiles, for the posterior distributions of each parameter are reported. Using the 2.5% and 97.5% quantiles, we can evaluate the 95% HPD interval. We find that age, BMI, and hypercholesterolemia are statistically significant predictors of the probability of AD.

```
plot(mcmcfit)
```

Comments: The trace plots and density plots in figures 6.3 and 6.4 for each covariate are reported above. The trace plots do not show a trend, and the estimates center around the mode of the posterior distribution. Thus we conclude we have convergence in our model.

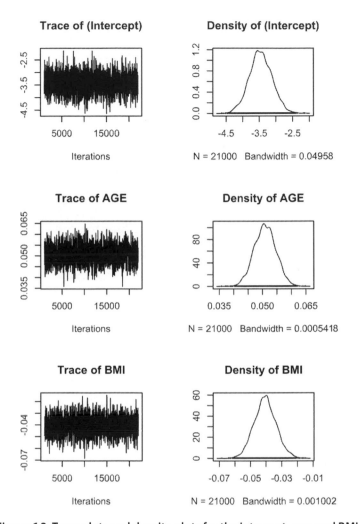

Figure 6.3 Trace plots and density plots for the intercept, age, and BMI.

6.5.3 Stata Syntax for Bayesian Logistic Regression

The Stata syntax follows:

```
if mofromindex>0 then delete
. bayes, coef search(repeat(1000)) : logistic  dx_ad   age      bmi
diabetes  hyperten     hypercho
```

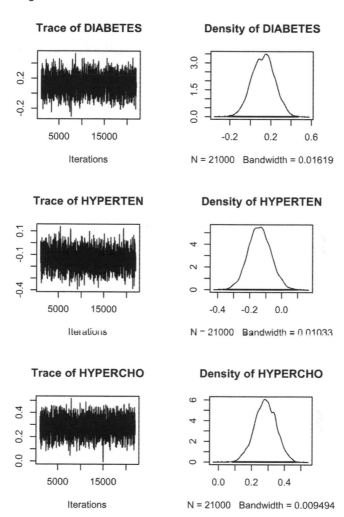

Figure 6.4 Trace plots and density plots for diabetes, hypertension, and hypercholesterolemia.

STATA OUTPUT

```
Likelihood: dx_ad ~ logistic(xb_dx_ad)
Prior: {dx_ad:age bmi diabetes hyperten hypercho _cons} ~
normal(0,10000)          (1)
(1) Parameters are elements of the linear form xb_dx_ad.
Bayesian logistic regression              MCMC iterations = 12,500
```

```
Random-walk Metropolis-Hastings sampling Burn-in         = 2,500
                                         MCMC sample size = 10,000
                                         Number of obs    = 4,882
                                         Acceptance rate  = .141
                                         Efficiency: min  = .002262
                                                     avg  = .009618
Log marginal likelihood = -2953.82                   max  = .03337
```

DX_AD	Mean	Std. Dev.	MCSE	Median	[95% Cred. Interval]	
AGE	.0496	.003	.00041	.0495331	.0438,	.0550825
BMI	-.0425	.006	.000331	-.0423465	-.055011	-.0305562
DIABETES	.152	.104	.015279	.1508927	-.0692269	.3557106
HYPERTEN	-.148	.066	.006994	-.1461369	-.2864882	-.0210332
HYPERCHO	.293	.068	.011503	.2948529	.1602693	.4300821
_CONS	-3.308	.194	.040826	-3.312829	-3.656066	-2.902616

Comments: The output reports the mean, standard deviation, Markov Chain standard error (MCSE), median, and the 95% credible interval. The interval suggests that BMI, age, hypercholesterolemia, and hypertension are highly influential (as 0 is not included in the interval).

The Stata syntax for diagnostic plots follows:

```
. bayesgraph diagnostics {dx_ad:age} {dx_ad:bmi} {dx_ad:age}
{dx_ad:hyperten} {dx_ad:hypercho}
```

STATA OUTPUT

Figures 6.5–6.9 report the diagnostic plots for each covariate. Each output displays the trace plot, histogram, autocorrelation, and density.

6.6 Bayesian Hierarchical Logistic Regression Models

We model the binary outcome, $Y_i \sim$ binomial (n_{ij}, p_{ij}). We use the logistic link function to link the covariates of each patient to the probability of interest,

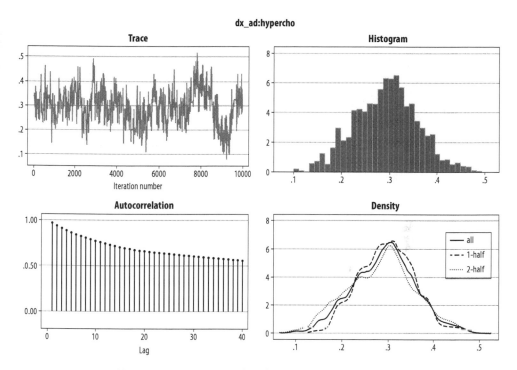

Figure 6.5 Diagnostics plots for hypercholesterolemia.

$$p_{ij} = \exp[\beta_0 + \beta_1 X_1 + \cdots + \beta_p X_p + \gamma]/[1 + \exp[\beta_0 + \beta_1 X_1 + \cdots + \beta_p X_p + \gamma]]$$

$$\text{Prob}(Y) = \text{logistic } (p_i + \gamma)$$

where γ is the random effect, which is assumed to be a normally distributed, $\gamma \sim N(0, \sigma^2)$. The beta parameters β_0, β_1, . . . , β_p and the variance of the random effect are model parameters. We can use available information about the impact of the covariates on the outcome to select the prior distributions, or we may implement noninformative priors.

Problem: Do age, BMI, diabetes, hypertension, and hypercholesterolemia have an impact on the probability of an AD diagnosis while accounting for the repeated measures for each patient?

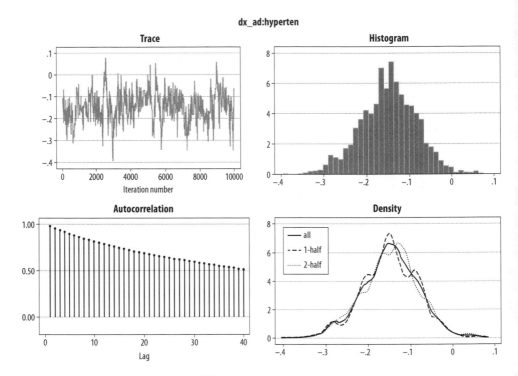

Figure 6.6 Diagnostic plots for hypertension.

Solution: We examined this research question in chapter 5, and now we apply a Bayesian estimation approach to obtain parameter estimates. The model estimates are reported in table 6.3.

6.6.1 SAS Syntax and Output for Bayesian Hierarchical Logistic Regression

The SAS syntax follows:

```
¹PROC MCMC DATA=CHAP6 OUTPOST=POSTOUT SEED=332786 NMC=20000
PROPCOV=QUANEW;
²PARMS BETA0-BETA6 S2 1;
³PRIOR BETA: ~ NORMAL(0,VAR=1E6);
³PRIOR S2 ~ GENERAL(0, LOWER=0);
```

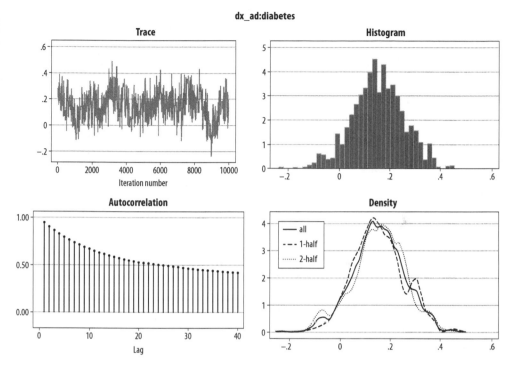

Figure 6.7 Diagnostic plots for diabetes.

```
4MU = BETA0 + BETA1*MOFROMINDEX + BETA2*AGE + BETA3*BMI +
BETA4*DIABETES+BETA5*HYPERTEN + BETA6*HYPERCHO;
5RANDOM DELTA ~ NORMAL(0, VAR=S2) SUBJECT=ID;
6P = LOGISTIC(MU + DELTA);
7MODEL DX_AD ~ BINARY(P);
RUN;
```

[1]The PROC MCMC statement specifies the input (DATA=) and output (OUTPOST=) datasets, sets a seed for the random number generator (SEED=), and specifies the simulation size (NMC=). The option PROPCOV=QUANEW uses a numerical approximation to estimate the covariance matrix for the posterior distribution.

[2]The PARMS statement declares the model parameters and the starting values. In this case, there are eight model parameters (intercept,

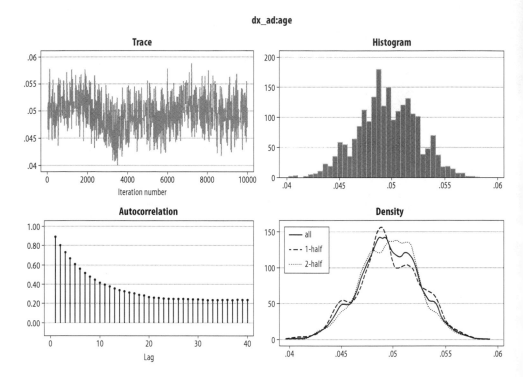

Figure 6.8 Diagnostic plots for age.

six covariates, and the variance of the random effect S2). The start-ing value for the parameter can be provided after the parameter name (if unspecified, the default value is 0).

[3]The PRIOR statements specify the prior distributions for the given parameters. In this case, the first statement specifies the distribution for each of the betas (BETA:), and the second statement specifies the distribution for the random effect variance (S2).

[4]This statement calculates the regression mean, which is stored as the value MU. This is a function of the regression parameters and covariates.

[5]The RANDOM statement specifies the distribution of the random effect. In our example, DELTA is assumed to follow a normal prior distribution, with mean 0 and variance S2. The SUBJECT= option in-dicates the group index for the random effects parameters.

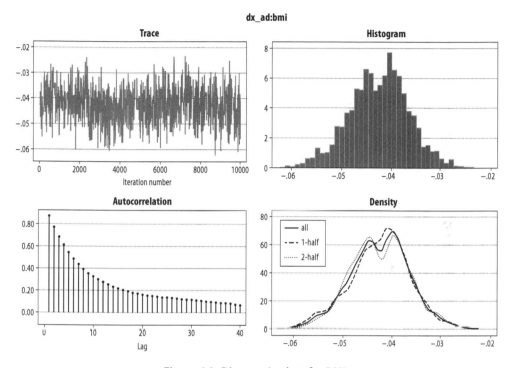

Figure 6.9 Diagnostic plots for BMI.

Table 6.3 Bayesian Model Results

Parameter	Alpha	Posterior Intervals Equal-Tail Interval		HPD Interval	
Intercept	0.050	−166.8	−123.2	−168.3	−125.8
MOFROMINDEX	0.050	−0.177	−0.133	−0.175	−0.132
AGE	0.050	1.460	1.901	1.455	1.895
BMI	0.050	−0.536	−0.058	−0.539	−0.061
DIABETES	0.050	−6.860	−0.534	−6.190	−0.213
HYPERTEN	0.050	−3.661	−1.126	−3.623	−1.121
HYPERCHO	0.050	−0.408	2.641	−0.486	2.494
Variance	0.050	2,968.0	3,991.6	2,963.8	3,985.5

[6]This statement calculates P, which is the logit transformation of MU and DELTA.

[7]The MODEL statement specifies the response variable (DX_AD) as binary with probability P.

Parameters

Block	Parameter	Sampling Method	Initial Value	Prior Distribution
1	BETA0	N-Metropolis	0	normal(0, SD=1000)
	BETA1	N-Metropolis	0	normal(0, SD=1000)
	BETA2		0	normal(0, SD=1000)
	BETA3		0	normal(0, SD=1000)
	BETA4		0	normal(0, SD=1000)
	BETA5		0	normal(0, SD=1000)
	BETA6		0	normal(0, SD=1000)
	S2		1.0000	general(0, lower=0)

Comments: The prior distribution for the regression parameters β_i is $N(0, 1{,}000^2)$. A normal distribution with a large variance is a flat, noninformative prior. For the variance of the random effect S2, we also specify a noninformative prior.

Random Effect Parameters

Parameter	Sampling Method	Subject	Number of Subjects	Subject Values	Prior Distribution
DELTA	N-Metropolis	ID	5122	NACC000271 NACC000385 NACC000875 NACC000920 NACC000959 NACC001006 NACC001075 NACC001412 NACC001504 NACC001628 NACC002043 NACC002128 NACC002171 NACC002720 NACC002855 NACC002865 NACC003052 NACC003112 NACC003807 NACC003952...	normal(0, VAR=S2)

Comments: The parameter delta represents the random effect for the subjects (denoted by the variable ID). The random effect is distributed normal $(0, S^2)$, where S^2 follows a noninformative prior.

Posterior Summaries

Parameter	N	Mean	Standard Deviation	Percentiles		
				25	50	75
BETA0	20000	−144.1	11.7750	−154.4	−143.3	−134.7
BETA1	20000	−0.1520	0.0117	−0.1602	−0.1501	−0.1433
BETA2	20000	1.6635	0.1283	1.5551	1.6450	1.7728
BETA3	20000	−0.2770	0.1209	−0.3517	−0.2684	−0.1947
BETA4	20000	−3.3683	1.6129	−4.4046	−3.2283	−2.2309
BETA5	20000	−2.3808	0.6794	−2.8754	−2.3830	−1.8935
BETA6	20000	1.0305	0.7753	0.4923	1.0117	1.5180
S2	20000	3495.0	269.2	3333.7	3494.7	3692.2

Comments: The posterior summary has evidence of nonconvergence, as there are large parameter estimates for the variance and intercept. Checking the diagnostic plots, we see that there is significant auto-correlation, and thus the parameter estimates may not be reliable. We also had convergence issues when evaluating the two-level mixed model using frequentist approaches in chapter 5.

Posterior Intervals

Parameter	Alpha	Equal-Tail Interval		HPD Interval	
BETA0	0.050	−166.8	−123.2	−168.3	−125.8
BETA1	0.050	−0.177	−0.133	−0.175	−0.132
BETA2	0.050	1.460	1.901	1.455	1.895
BETA3	0.050	−0.536	−0.058	−0.539	−0.061
BETA4	0.050	−6.860	−0.534	−6.190	−0.213
BETA5	0.050	−3.661	−1.126	−3.623	−1.121
BETA6	0.050	−0.408	2.641	−0.486	2.494
S2	0.050	2968.0	3991.6	2963.8	3985.5

Comments: The diagnostic plots for model parameters BETA0, BETA1, BETA2, BETA3, BETA4, BETA5, BETA6, and S2 (figs. 6.10, 6.11, 6.12, 6.13, 6.14, 6.15, 6.16, and 6.17, respectively) indicate that there are convergence issues with the model. For some of the predictors, the

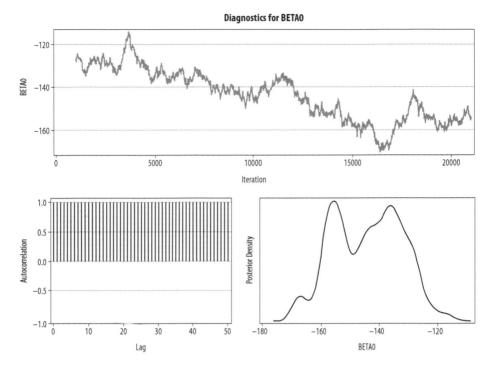

Figure 6.10 Diagnostic plots for the intercept.

trace plot displays a trend. In addition, the autocorrelation plots show there is high autocorrelation after 50 lags.

6.6.2 R Syntax and Output for Bayesian Hierarchical Logistic Regression

The R syntax follows:

```
1library(MCMCpack)
2mcmcfit2 <- MCMChlogit(fixed=DX_AD ~ MOFROMINDEX + AGE + BMI +
DIABETES + HYPERTEN + HYPERCHO, random=~1,
group="ID",data=chap6, burnin=1000, mcmc=21000,r=1,
R=diag(c(1)))
3summary(mcmcfit2$mcmc)
4plot(mcmcfit2$mcmc)
```

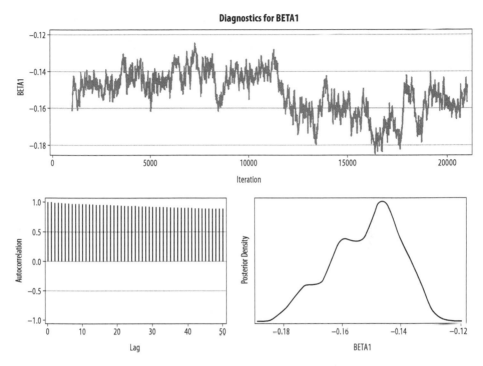

Figure 6.11 Diagnostic plots for time since baseline.

[1]The MCMChlogit() function in the MCMCpack library is used to fit hierarchical logistic Bayesian models.

[2]The MCMChlogit() function specifies the fixed effects model outcome ~ predictors and the random effects model as ~ predictors. The option burnin= specifies the number of burn-in iterations, and mcmc= specifies the number of estimation iterations. The options r and R, which are the shape and scale parameters, respectively, of the Inverse-Wishart prior distribution for the random effect variance, must be specified. The output is saved in the object mcmcfit2.

[3]The summary() function is used to print a summary of the model fit and parameter estimates using $mcmc from the model output. In this case, we look at the summary of mcmcfit2$mcmc.

[4]The plot() function is used to output the diagnostic plots for Bayesian modeling, including the trace and density plots for each parameter.

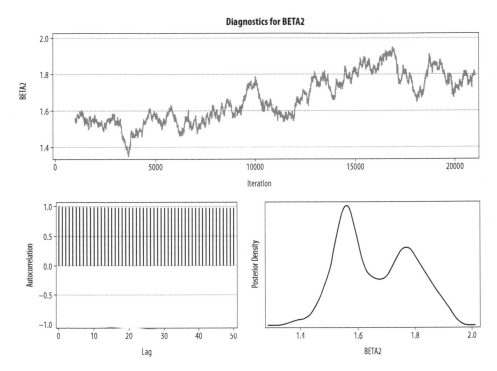

Figure 6.12 Diagnostic plots for age.

R OUTPUT

```
summary(mcmcfit2$mcmc)
##
## Iterations = 1001:21991
## Thinning interval = 10
## Number of chains = 1
## Sample size per chain = 2100
##
## 1. Empirical mean and standard deviation for each variable,
##    plus standard error of the mean:
##
##                          Mean        SD  Naive SE Time-series SE
## beta.(Intercept)    -6.724e+00 5.379e-01 1.174e-02      1.507e-01
## beta.MOFROMINDEX    -1.384e-02 1.178e-03 2.570e-05      3.536e-04
```

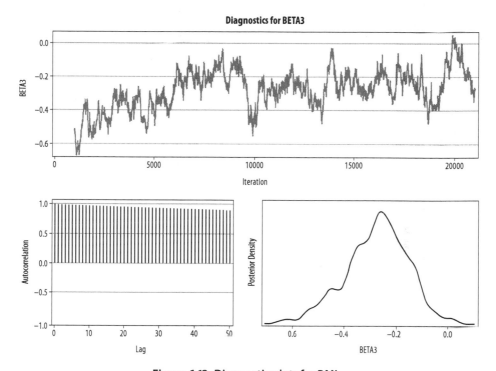

Figure 6.13 Diagnostic plots for BMI.

```
## beta.AGE                      8.779e-02 6.291e-03 1.373e-04      9.900e-04

## beta.BMI                     -3.719e-02 4.368e-03 9.532e-05      1.230e-03

## beta.DIABETES                 2.055e-01 1.605e-01 3.502e-03      1.239e-01

## beta.HYPERTEN                -2.476e-01 4.202e-02 9.170e-04      1.525e-02

## beta.HYPERCHO                 2.650e-01 4.287e-02 9.354e-04      1.531e-02

## b.(Intercept).100063          3.635e+00 1.123e+00 2.451e-02      6.132e-01

## b.(Intercept).100115          4.153e+00 6.804e-01 1.485e-02      1.980e-01

[bu8]

## b.(Intercept).999675          1.010e+00

## b.(Intercept).999854         -1.265e+00

## VCV.(Intercept).(Intercept)  1.255e+01

## sigma2                        2.104e-02

## Deviance                      6.187e+03
```

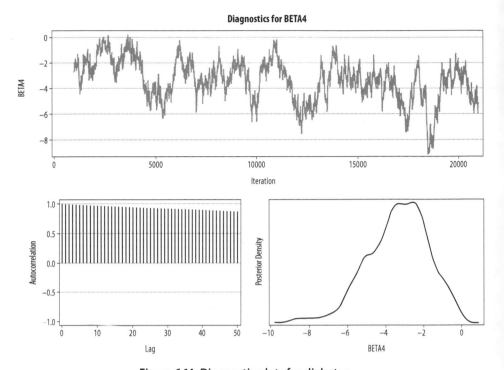

Figure 6.14 Diagnostic plots for diabetes.

Comments: The diagnostic plots (not shown) indicate that there may be issues with convergence, so we cannot interpret the model parameter estimates and covariate relationships. But we do see that the MCMChlogit output contains the posterior mean, standard deviation, and HPD interval estimates for each parameter.

6.6.3 Stata Syntax and Output for Bayesian Hierarchical Logistic Regression

The Stata syntax follows:

```
. melogit dx_ad age bmi diabetes hyperten hypercho mofromindex
||      id:
```

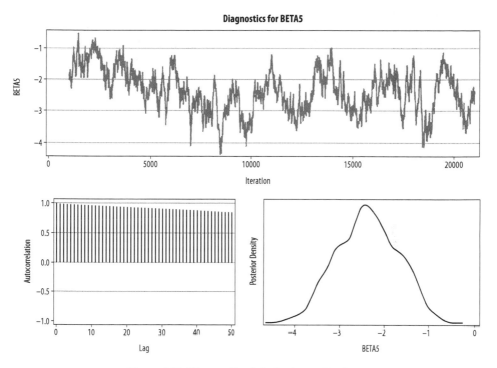

Figure 6.15 Diagnostic plots for hypertension.

STATA OUTPUT

```
Fitting fixed-effects model:
Iteration 0:    log likelihood=-15948.764
Iteration 1:    log likelihood=-15927.683
Iteration 2:    log likelihood=-15927.681
Iteration 3:    log likelihood=-15927.681
Refining starting values:
Grid node 0:    log likelihood=-10671.358
Fitting full model:
Iteration 0:    log likelihood=-10671.358
Iteration 1:    log likelihood=-6144.3514
Iteration 2:    log likelihood=-5008.891
Iteration 3:    log likelihood=-3974.9181
```

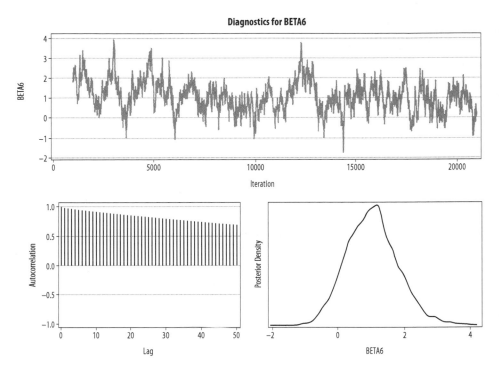

Figure 6.16 Diagnostic plots for hypercholesterolemia.

```
Iteration 4:    log likelihood = -3303.5735
Iteration 5:    log likelihood = -3179.4252      (not concave)
Iteration 6:    log likelihood = -3153.6083      (not concave)
Iteration 7:    log likelihood = -3165.8123      (not concave)
Iteration 8:    log likelihood = -3149.9408      (not concave)
Iteration 9:    log likelihood = -3166.9346      (not concave)
Iteration 10:   log likelihood = -3175.2604      (not concave)
Iteration 11:   log likelihood = -3185.6066      (not concave)
Iteration 12:   log likelihood = -3198.9876      (not concave)
Iteration 13:   log likelihood = -3222.9269
Iteration 14:   log likelihood = -3207.5677
Iteration 15:   log likelihood = -3227.7955
Iteration 16:   log likelihood = -3195.8401
Iteration 17:   log likelihood = -3162.3956
```

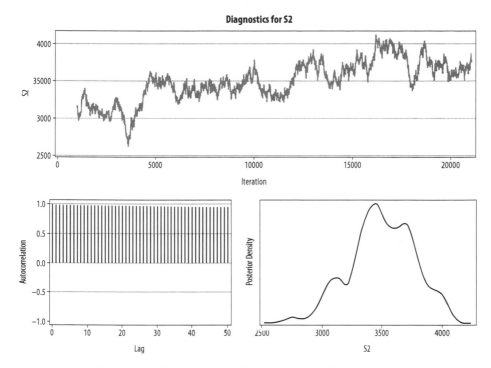

Figure 6.17 Diagnostic plots for the random effect variance.

```
Iteration 18:   log likelihood = -3123.4655
Iteration 19:   log likelihood = -3083.7586
Iteration 20:   log likelihood = -3045.2863
Iteration 21:   log likelihood = -2994.2223
Iteration 22:   log likelihood = -2921.3082
Iteration 23:   log likelihood = -2884.841
Iteration 24:   log likelihood = -2866.8976
Iteration 25:   log likelihood = -2854.3559
Iteration 26:   log likelihood = -2839.2044
Iteration 27:   log likelihood = -2828.8342
Iteration 28:   log likelihood = -2817.1106
Iteration 29:   log likelihood = -2809.7955
Iteration 30:   log likelihood = -2798.8567
Iteration 31:   log likelihood = -2789.7393
```

```
Iteration 32:   log likelihood = -2784.7835

Iteration 33:   log likelihood = -2777.1123

Iteration 34:   log likelihood = -2773.7482

Iteration 35:   log likelihood = -2768.5904

Iteration 36:   log likelihood = -2767.4166

Iteration 37:   log likelihood = -2764.6996

Iteration 38:   log likelihood = -2762.7725

Iteration 39:   log likelihood = -2760.828

Iteration 40:   log likelihood = -2758.7622

Iteration 41:   log likelihood = -2758.7392

Iteration 42:   log likelihood = -2758.3527

Iteration 43:   log likelihood = -2758.3408

Iteration 44:   log likelihood = -2758.3047

Iteration 45:   log likelihood = -2758.269

Iteration 46:   log likelihood = -2758.2493

Iteration 47:   log likelihood = -2758.2484

Iteration 48:   log likelihood = -2758.2447

Iteration 49:   log likelihood = -2758.2428

Iteration 50:   log likelihood = -2758.2433

Iteration 51:   log likelihood = -2758.2416

Iteration 52:   log likelihood = -2758.2414  (not concave)

Iteration 53:   log likelihood = -2758.2414
```

Comments: There are many iterations, and we see that the model does not converge.

```
Mixed-effects logistic regression    Number of obs   = 28,456

Group variable:          id          Number of groups =  5,122

                                     Obs per group:

                                                  min =      4

                                                  avg =    5.6

                                                  max =     10

Integration method:    ghermite     Integration pts. =      7

                                     Wald chi2(6)     =   0.00

Log likelihood = -2758.2414              Prob > chi2  = 1.0000
```

Comments: The model does not converge. The Wald Chi is 0, and the *p*-value is 1.

DX_AD	Coef.	Std. Err.	z	P>z	[95% Conf.	Interval]
AGE	-.0146	42.813	-0.00	1.000	-83.927	83.897
BMI	.007	70.067	0.00	1.000	-137.323	137.336
DIABETES	.139	1827.202	0.00	1.000	-3581.112	3581.389
HYPERTEN	.038	669.676	0.00	1.000	-1312.502	1312.578
HYPERCHO	.403	2251.322	0.00	1.000	-4412.107	4412.912
MOFROMINDEX	.001	14.828	0.00	1.000	-29.06191	29.062
_CONS	-869.376	10151.25	-0.09	0.932	-20765.47	19026.71
ID						
VAR(_CONS)		2.59e+07		7.40e-13	1.98e+24	
1209897						

Comments: All the *p*-values are 1. These are all signs of nonconvergence.

```
LR test vs. logistic model: chibar2(01) = 26,338.88
Prob >= chibar2 = 0.0000
```

Note: The above coefficient values are the result of nonadaptive quadrature because the adaptive parameters could not be computed.

Comments: This last remark is given by the program.

6.7 Summary and Discussion

In this chapter, we cover basic concepts of the Bayesian approach to analyze correlated binary response data, including obtaining parameter estimates and making inferences. We illustrate Bayesian logistic regression modeling and Bayesian hierarchical logistic regression modeling using data from chapter 5 to address the differences in the probability of an AD diagnosis. We use SAS, R, and Stata to obtain results.

The increasing number of dementia studies provides a range of historic information. This information can easily be incorporated in the choice of informative Bayesian priors. In cases where the historical data are not as rich, however, the Bayesian approach can still be applied with less informative or more diffuse priors.

6.8 Exercises

Consider the binary outcome diabetes status (data located at http://www.public.asu.edu/~jeffreyw/). Fit a Bayesian logistic regression model to address the probability of diabetes based on the patient-level variables. The data are obtained with age, gender, race, and hypertension status. We consider longitudinal data with repeated measures across visits for each patient.

1. What is the probability of diabetes accounting for age, gender, race, hypertension, and patient effect?
2. Do diabetes rates differ across patients?
3. What is the impact of the patient's characteristics after adjusting for patient as a random effect?
4. What is the relationship between gender and the likelihood of diabetes while controlling for age, gender, race, and hypertension?

Chapter 7

Multiple-Membership Models

7.1 Motivating Example

In chapters 4, 5, and 6, we considered hierarchical structured data in which members of a lower level of hierarchy (patients) are completely nested within higher levels of the hierarchy (centers). In those chapters, patients were completely nested within Alzheimer's Disease Centers (ADCs). In fact, in our dataset, each patient belongs to one and only one center, having single membership. But there are cases when a unit (i.e., a patient) may be nested within more than one higher level of the hierarchical structure. In medical and health studies, we often experience such membership. For example, the patient may see more than one doctor, or the doctor may serve more than one hospital. The patient may visit multiple centers. The patient may have more than one neurodegenerative disease diagnosis. These scenarios are all cases of multiple membership (fig. 7.1).

In this chapter, we describe and analyze multiple-membership data. In neurodegenerative diseases, disease heterogeneity is common (Armstrong et al. 2005; Schneider et al. 2007; Dugger et al. 2014; Kawas et al. 2015). We analyze a subset of data obtained from the National Alzheimer's Coordinating Center (NACC) website for patients having one or more of four clinical diagnoses: Alzheimer's disease (AD), dementia with Lewy bodies (DLB), frontotemporal dementia (FTD), and vascular dementia (VaD). This subset of the data consists of 5,185 patients, representing 39 ADCs, who have up to three clinical diagnoses. Most (87.16%) had one clinical diagnosis, while 12.30% had two diagnoses, and 0.54% had three diagnoses. We address the question of how age, BMI, diabetes, hypertension, and hypercholesterolemia (the covariates) affect the Clinical Dementia Rating Scale Sum of Boxes

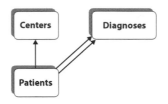

Figure 7.1 Multiple-membership, multiple-classification of patients, centers, and diagnoses.

Table 7.1 Subset of Data Used in Multiple-Membership Models

ID	CDRSUM	AGE	BMI	DIABETES	Mix_AD	Mix_DLB	Mix_FTD	Mix_VaD
000095	5.5	87	25.5	0	1	0	0	0
000245	6.5	78	24.1	0	1	0	0	1
000290	12	78	21.6	0	1	0	0	0
000449	0.5	83	33.4	0	1	0	0	0
000480	9	52	22.8	0	1	1	0	0
000731	4	82	33.8	0	1	0	0	0
000998	4	76	27	0	1	0	0	0
001095	6	49	18.7	0	1	1	0	0
001118	1.5	71	23.9	0	0	0	0	1
001300	3.5	75	29.7	0	1	0	0	0

(CDR-SUM) (the outcome). But center, patient, and disease/diagnosis are random effects that must be accounted for in our deliberation. Patients and centers are single membership, while disease is multiple membership. Accounting for disease, as these diseases can have certain profiles of CDR-SUM, would help physicians better understand the differences in the conditional mean CDR-SUM score based on the patient, the center, and the disease. A subset of the data, including predictors, is given in table 7.1.

The variables Mix_AD, Mix_DLB, Mix_FTD, and Mix_VaD are binary indicator variables indicating which dementia subtypes contribute to the patient's dementia diagnosis (for AD, DLB, FTD, and VaD, respectively).

7.2 Background

Hierarchical, nested, or clustered data contain extra sources of correlation that must be addressed. The hierarchical models used to analyze such data usually consist of a single membership, as measurements are nested within patients, and patients nested within centers. In these examples (chaps. 4, 5, and 6), patients had one diagnosis (AD or no AD), and patients did not attend more than one ADC. The data were single membership, and thus the data were completely nested. It is not uncommon to have multiple membership, however. For example, it is common for a patient to see more than one doctor, or for a patient to have more than one disease. Furthermore, a patient may visit multiple centers or hospitals. If a patient has more than one disease, it should be factored into the model, as this can potentially affect treatment outcomes and interventions. In this chapter, we address including this aspect of the data into the model.

In multiple-membership data, lower-level units belong to more than one higher-level unit. Therefore lower-level units are nested within multiple higher-level units from the same classification. For example, patients (lower-level units) may visit multiple doctors (higher-level units), and so patients are nested within more than one doctor. There are cases when the design may be even more complicated and contain two or more membership structures. An important feature of multiple-membership data structures is the degree to which each lower-level unit belongs to each higher-level unit. The model must address this factor of the data. These types of models bring a certain degree of complexity but can greatly improve the model fit and predictive performance. We fit multiple-membership, multiple-classification regression models to appropriately address correlation in nonhierarchical nested structures. This is necessary because fitting a single-membership model when a multiple-membership model is appropriate results in biased estimates of the regression coefficients and standard errors for the random effects (Chung and Beretvas 2012).

7.2.1 Types of Multiple Membership

Multiple-membership, multiple-class models are a general class of models used for various complex data structures. While our focus in this chapter is on multiple membership, we discuss different types of multiple-membership, multiple-class data.

Multiple-membership data describe data in which each unit is associated with multiple factors from the nesting within multiple clusters. For example, if a patient visits multiple doctors, we may wish to understand how each doctor affects the patient. In addition, patients may have multiple diagnoses, and we would like to test how the diagnoses affect the patient.

Cross-classified multilevel data describe clustered data where there are multiple factors, but the factors are crossed rather than in a hierarchical structure. For example, we may be interested in studying the impact of doctors and centers on a patient. The data are not hierarchical, however, as some doctors work at multiple centers.

7.2.2 Weights in Multiple Membership

A multiple-membership regression model accounts for the multiplicity through weights. Weights are determined on the basis of the information available in the data. In our analysis of dementia data, patients may have one or more diagnoses. We may choose to define the multiple-membership weights according to the proportion of time the patient has had each diagnosis (e.g., a patient may have had VaD for five years, and in the past year was diagnosed with AD). These weights reflect the fact that we might expect one of the diagnoses to be more influential in determining the patient's CDR-SUM score if the patient has had the diagnosis longer. The weights may also be based on previous knowledge of how the disease may alter the CDR-SUM score. In VaD, there may not be large changes in CDR-SUM over time; however, with AD, there may be a more drastic change in CDR-SUM over time. Other weighting schemes may equally be applied, and it is interesting to explore a range of weighting schemes as part of a sensitivity analysis for the model. If no additional information is available, we may choose to weight the diagnoses proportional to the number of diagnoses each patient has. Ignoring the fact that patients are multiple members of diagnoses will typically lead us to underestimate the standard errors on the diagnosis level. We assume there are known weights that represent the degree of membership for a patient for each of the diagnoses.

7.3 Single Hierarchical Membership Model

In the analysis of continuous data, we distinguish between the modeling independent and correlated observations. When the outcomes are obtained independently, one usually fits the standard regression model with k covariates such that

$$E(Y|X) = \beta_0 + \beta_1 x_1 + \beta_2 x_2 + \cdots + \beta_k x_k,$$

where β_i are regression coefficients for the covariates x_i and $i = 1, 2, \ldots, k$. It is customary to obtain estimates of the regression coefficients $\hat{\beta}_i$ based on a method of maximum likelihood. In the analysis of nested data, however, the independence assumption is no longer applicable. Because this analysis ignores the intraclass correlation inherent to the nested structure, the standard regression model is not appropriate. The data structure demands a model that incorporates the correlation that arises from the hierarchical structure of the data and the multiple membership present. A hierarchical model accounts for correlation inherent at the different levels of the hierarchy. A standard model ignores clustering, and as such is likely to make unreliable conclusions regarding the parameter estimates. Thus the inferences made are not valid, which is further reviewed in Stroup (2012) and Irimata and Wilson (2017). While chapters 4 and 5 considered fitting single-membership regression models, the models in this chapter allow one to account for multiple sources of variation owing to the multiple levels of the hierarchy that may affect the response but are not directly measured (Zhu 2014).

A single-membership regression model with patient as random effects,

$$E(Y \mid X) = \beta_0 + \beta_1 X_{1i} + \beta_2 X_{2i} + \cdots + \beta_k X_{ki} + \gamma_j,$$

where patient i is nested within center j, β_0 is the fixed intercept term, β_1, β_2, . . . , β_k are the coefficients of the patient time-level covariates X_{1i}, X_{2i}, . . . , X_{ki}, γ_j is the center-level random effect distributed as $N(0, \sigma_\gamma^2)$, and σ_γ^2 represents the variance among the patient of the random intercept γ_j. A measure of the intraclass correlation at the patient level (Zhu 2014) is

$$\text{corr}(y_{i|j}), (y_{i'|j}) = \frac{\sigma_\gamma^2}{\sigma_\gamma^2 + \sigma_\varepsilon^2},$$

where σ_γ^2 is the variance for center-level units, and σ_ε^2 is the variance at the patient level. The intraclass correlation $\text{corr}(y_{i|j}, y_{i'|j})$ where $i \neq i'$ provides a measure of the strength of the correlation between measurements for a particular patient.

7.4 Multiple-Membership Models

Although the multiple-membership structure is common, it is often ignored owing to the added complexity of requiring theoretical derivation. We address multiple-membership, multiple-classification (MMMC) models. We fit a model with complete nesting within centers but multiple membership within diagnoses. Figure 7.1 reveals that patients are completely nested within centers (one patient per center) but not completely nested into diagnoses (patients may have more than one diagnosis).

The structure gives rise to the MMMC regression model,

$$E(Y|X) = \beta_0 + \beta_1 X_{1i} + \cdots + \beta_K X_{ki} + \theta_m^{(2)} + \sum_{j \in \text{diagnoses}(i)} w_{ij}^{(3)} \gamma_j^{(3)},$$

showing the impact of the random effects on diagnoses $(\gamma_j^{(3)})$ and random effects on centers $(\theta_m^{(2)})$, with k fixed effects $(X_{1i}, \ldots, X_{ki})$ at the patient level $i = 1, \ldots, n$, where there are $m = 1, \ldots, M$ centers and $j = 1, \ldots, J$ diagnoses. The term $E(Y|X)$ is the mean of the CDR-SUM score that patient i has a certain outcome, given the random effects in diagnoses and centers for each patient. Diagnoses(i) is the set of diagnoses that patient i received, $w_{ij}^{(3)}$ is the weight corresponding to diagnosis j on patient i, the superscript denotes that the diagnosis is at level 3 in the combined design analysis that patient i received, and $\gamma_j^{(3)}$ is the random effect associated with diagnosis j, such that $\gamma_j^{(3)} \sim N(0, \sigma_\gamma^2)$ with $\theta_m^{(2)}$ considered for centers as random effect and distributed as $\theta_m^{(2)} \sim N(0, \sigma_\theta^2)$. In this model, it is assumed that the random effects for diagnoses and centers are independent; also, the residuals are assumed to follow a normal distribution with mean 0 and variance σ_ε^2. Thus the mean CDR-SUM score for patient i with diagnoses $1, \ldots, J$ in center m is

$$E(\text{CRDSUM})_{i \,|\, \text{diagnosis}(i), m} = \beta_0 + \beta_1 X_{1i} + \cdots + \beta_K X_{Ki} + \theta_m^{(2)}$$
$$+ \sum_{j \in \text{diagnosis}(i)} w_{ij}^{(3)} \gamma_j^{(3)}.$$

Then the total response variance for patient i is

$$\text{var}((Y_{i \,|\, \text{diagnosis}(i), m})) = \sigma_\rho^2 \sum_{j \in \text{diagnosis}(i)} (w_{ij}^{(3)})^2 + \sigma_\theta^2 + \sigma_\varepsilon^2.$$

This total variance is used to compute the intraclass correlation coefficient between two different measures on the same patient.

7.5 Fit of Multiple-Membership Models

Problem: Is a patient's CDR-SUM score affected by factors including age, BMI, diabetes, hypertension, and hypercholesterolemia, while adjusting for random effects for center and disease?

Solution: We evaluate patients with up to three concurrent dementia diagnoses. Table 7.2 shows a summary of the dementia diagnoses by frequency, including random effects in disease.

We evaluate this research question using a multiple-membership model, accounting for each of the contributing dementia diagnoses for patients with mixed dementia. We assign weights to each diagnosis proportional to the number of diagnoses the patient had. Table 7.3 reports the model fit results.

Table 7.2 Frequency of Clinical Dementia Diagnoses

Disease	Frequency	Relative Frequency (%)
AD	3,657	70.53
FTD	583	11.24
AD, VaD	312	6.02
VaD	165	3.18
AD, DLB	156	3.01
DLB	151	2.91
AD, FTD	114	2.20
AD, DLB, VaD	16	0.31
DLB, VaD	13	0.25
FTD, VaD	6	0.12
DLB, FTD	5	0.10
AD, DLB, FTD	5	0.10
AD, FTD, VaD	2	0.04

Table 7.3 Multiple-Membership Parameter Estimates

Parameter	Estimate	Std Err	p-Value
AGE	5.919	1.025	<0.0001
BMI	0.033	0.007	<0.0001
DIABETES	−0.058	0.013	<0.0001
HYPERTEN	0.071	0.191	0.708
HYPERCHO	−0.386	0.138	0.005

We find that age, BMI, diabetes, and hypercholesterolemia are statistically significantly in the CDR-SUM score for patients with mixed dementia.

Hedeker (2014) discussed these models in a talk at the University of Illinois at Chicago and provided code to fit these models in SAS, SPSS, and Stata. Vazquez and Wilson (2019) fitted logistic regression multiple-membership models in SAS models using Bayes' estimates. To fit multiple-membership models in R, users must purchase a license for the multilevel-modeling software package MLwiN (Rasbash et al. 2009). The package R2MLwiN allows R to call MLwiN to fit multiple-membership models. While analyses using R are not discussed in this chapter, Zhang et al. (2016) provide a guide to using R2MLwiN and describes how to fit multiple-membership and cross-classified models in R.

Hedeker (2014) provides a simple but straightforward way to model multiple memberships. His approach, which we adopted in our analyses, accounts for only one of the memberships. In the SAS approach, we account for a maximum of three memberships but account for only one membership when we fit SPSS and Stata.

7.5.1 SAS Syntax and Output for Multiple Membership

The SAS syntax follows:

```
¹DATA CHAP7;
²SET CHAP7;
³SUM_DX = MIX_AD+MIX_DLB+MIX_FTD+MIX_VAD;
⁴P1=MIX_AD/(SUM_DX);
 P2=MIX_DLB/(SUM_DX);
 P3=MIX_FTD/(SUM_DX);
 P4=MIX_VAD/(SUM_DX);
⁵CONS=1;
RUN;
/*FIT NULL MULTIPLE MEMBERSHIP MODEL*/
⁶PROC MIXED DATA= CHAP7 COVTEST METHOD=REML;
⁷CLASS CONS ADC;
⁸MODEL CDRSUM = / S;
⁹RANDOM P1-P4 / SUBJECT=CONS TYPE=TOEPLITZ(1);
RUN;
/*FIT MULTIPLE MEMBERSHIP MODEL WITH COVARIATES*/
PROC MIXED DATA= CHAP7 COVTEST METHOD=ML;
CLASS CONS ADC;
¹⁰MODEL CDRSUM = AGE BMI DIABETES HYPERTEN HYPERCHO / S;
RANDOM P1-P4 / SUBJECT=CONS TYPE=TOEPLITZ(1);
RUN;
```

[1]We use a DATA step to create additional variables in the multiple-membership evaluation.

[2]Additions to the dataset to be created are specified in lines (3)–(5).

[3]We create the variable Sum_DX by adding the indicator variables for each diagnosis.

[4]We create the weights for multiple membership, equally based on number of diagnoses.

[5]We need to create a constant variable named CONS, which is equal to 1 for all values.

[6]We begin with a fit of the null model to estimate the intraclass correlation.

PROC MIXED fits linear mixed models. We use maximum likelihood estimation (METHOD=ML). The option COVTEST tests for the significance of the random effects.

[7]The CLASS statement identifies categorical variables. CONS (the variable defined in (5)) and ADC are categorical variables.

[8]We fit the null model, and S prints the estimates for the fixed effects (intercept only in this case).

[9]We identify the random effects in the data through SUBJECT=. A Toeplitz matrix is the correlation structure, which assumes constant correlation on the diagonals of the matrix.

[10]We fit a second multiple-membership model in which we specify the covariates (AGE BMI DIABETES HYPERTEN HYPERCHO) as fixed effects.

SAS OUTPUT

Null Multiple-Membership Model

The Mixed Procedure

Model Information

Data Set	WORK.CHAP7
Dependent Variable	CDRSUM
Covariance Structures	Variance Components, Banded Toeplitz
Subject Effects	ADC(cons), cons
Estimation Method	REML
Residual Variance Method	Profile
Fixed Effects SE Method	Model-Based
Degrees of Freedom Method	Containment

Comments: The dependent variable is CDR-SUM, a continuous variable. The covariance matrix is a Toeplitz structure with a banded structure (the diagonals that are parallel to the main diagonal are constant). A model-based method is used to estimate the fixed effects standard error (SE).

	Dimensions
Covariance Parameters	3
Columns in X	1
Columns in Z per Subject	43
Subjects	1
Max Obs per Subject	5185

Comments: This model has no predictors, only an intercept term, as the value in the Columns in X row is equal to 1. The three covariance parameters are for the variance of errors, variance of the center, and variance of the diseases.

		Covariance Parameter Estimates			
Cov Parm	Subject	Estimate	Standard Error	Z Value	Pr > Z
Intercept	ADC(cons)	2.915	0.801	3.640	0.000
Variance	cons	2.357	1.983	1.190	0.117
Residual		20.608	0.407	50.690	<.0001

Comments: The variance for the constant (cons) measures the variance for the mixed diagnoses, while the variance for ADC(cons) is for the center. We find that the effects of mixed diagnoses are not statistically significant ($p = 0.117$), while the center effect is statistically significant. The residual measures the random error in the data, which is found to be statistically significant ($p < 0.0001$). Thus the center accounts for $[2.915/(2.915 + 2.357 + 20.608)] = 11.3\%$ of the variation in the CDR-SUM score. Diseases account for 9.1%.

		Solution for Fixed Effects			
Effect	Estimate	Standard Error	DF	t Value	Pr > |t|
Intercept	6.266	0.827	38	7.58	<.0001

Comments: The likelihood ratio test for the null model (model with no covariates) statistically tests whether the outcome (CDR-SUM) is different than 0. We see that the CDR-SUM mean for our data is statistically significantly different than 0 (p-value < 0.0001). This is not very informative, but this model fit allows us to estimate the intraclass correlation using the covariance estimates.

```
              Multiple-Membership Model with Covariates
                        The Mixed Procedure
                             Dimensions
```

Covariance Parameters	3
Columns in X	6
Columns in Z per Subject	43
Subjects	1
Max Obs per Subject	5185

Comments: Because we are now evaluating covariates (age, BMI, diabetes, hypertension, and hypercholesterolemia) in this model, the Columns in X row has six values (intercept plus five covariates). We still have three covariance parameters, a random for center, a random effect for the mixed dementia, and the error term. We evaluate the same dataset, containing 5,185 observations.

```
                    Convergence criteria met.
```

Comments: We see that convergence was achieved, so we can continue with interpreting our results.

```
                 Covariance Parameter Estimates
```

Cov Parm	Subject	Estimate	Standard Error	Z Value	Pr > Z
Intercept	ADC(cons)	2.778	0.765	3.630	0.000
Variance	cons	2.244	1.888	1.190	0.117
Residual		20.244	0.400	50.660	< .0001

Comments: The estimates for the variance components are similar to the null model (the covariance for ADC was previously estimated as 2.915, and the covariance for cons was estimated as 2.357). The center effect is significant (p-value = 0.0000), and thus we should address the center effect through this model.

		Solution for Fixed Effects			
Effect	Estimate	Standard Error	DF	t Value	Pr > |t|
Intercept	5.919	1.025	38	5.77	<.0001
AGE	0.033	0.007	5138	4.80	<.0001
BMI	-0.058	0.013	5138	-4.65	<.0001
DIABETES	0.071	0.191	5138	0.37	0.708
HYPERTEN	-0.386	0.138	5138	-2.80	0.005
HYPERCHO	-0.636	0.135	5138	-4.73	<.0001

Comments: The fixed effect covariates are reported in the Solution for Fixed Effects table. Age, BMI, hypertension, and hypercholesterolemia are significant factors in explaining the variation in CDR-SUM. Older patients with low BMI and who are not hypertensive nor have hypercholesterolemia tend to have higher CDR-SUM scores, even after accounting for centers and multiple diagnostic groups.

7.5.2 SPSS Syntax and Output for Multiple Membership
MULTIPLE-MEMBERSHIP NULL MODEL

The SPSS syntax follows:

```
¹COMPUTE CONS=1.
²MIXED
³CDRSUM BY ADC Disease
⁴/FIXED =
⁵/METHOD = ML
⁶/PRINT = SOLUTION TESTCOV
⁷/RANDOM ADC DISEASE.
```

SPSS OUTPUT

```
            Null Multiple-Membership Model
                Mixed Model Analysis
                  Model Dimension
```

		Number of Levels	Covariance Structure	#Parameters
Fixed Effects	Intercept	1		1
Random Effects	ADC + Disease	52	Variance Components	2
Residual				1
Total		53		4

Comments: The dependent variable is CDR-SUM, a continuous variable. There are two random effects, the single membership in an ADC and the multiple membership in disease.

```
                Information Criteria
```

-2 Log Likelihood	30443.566
Akaike's Information Criterion (AIC)	30451.566
Hurvich and Tsai's Criterion (AICC)	30451.573
Bozdogan's Criterion (CAIC)	30481.780
Schwarz's Bayesian Criterion (BIC)	30477.780

Comments: These are measures of the fit of the model. We can use these criteria to compare the fit between models. For these criteria, smaller values indicate better model fit.

```
            Estimates of Fixed Effects
```

						95% Confidence Interval	
Parameter	Estimate	Std. Error	df	t	Sig.	Lower Bound	Upper Bound
Intercept	7.055	.650	16.676	10.855	.000	5.682	8.428

Comments: In this example, we are fitting the null model (intercept only). We are testing whether the mean of the outcome (CDR-SUM) is different than 0, and we find that it is significantly different (Sig. = 0.000).

Estimates of Covariance Parameters

Parameter		Estimate	Std. Error	Wald Z	Sig.	95% Confidence Interval Lower Bound	Upper Bound
Residual		20.249	.340	50.649	.000	19.481	21.048
ADC	Variance	2.826	.773	3.654	.000	1.653	4.832
Disease	Variance	3.393	1.689	2.008	.045	1.278	9.003

Comments: The variance for Disease measures the variance for the mixed diagnoses. They are not statistically significant ($p = 0.045$). Residual measures the random error in the data, which is found to be statistically significant ($p < 0.0001$). Thus ADC accounts for [2.826/ (20.249 + 2.826 + 3.393)] = 10.7% of the variation in CDR-SUM, while diseases accounts for 12.8%.

MULTIPLE-MEMBERSHIP MODEL WITH COVARIATES

The SPSS syntax follows:

```
MIXED
CDRSUM WITH AGE BMI DIABETES HYPERTEN HYPERCHO by ADC Disease
/FIXED = AGE BMI DIABETES HYPERTEN HYPERCHO
/METHOD = ML
/PRINT = SOLUTION TESTCOV
/RANDOM ADC DISEASE.
```

SPSS OUTPUT

Estimates of Fixed Effects

Parameter	Estimate	Std. Error	df	t	Sig.	95% Confidence Interval	
						Lower Bound	Upper Bound
Intercept	6.825	0.888	67.826	7.690	0.000	5.054	8.596
AGE	0.030	0.007	5173.308	4.340	0.000	0.016	0.043
BMI	-0.055	0.012	5149.422	-4.400	0.000	-0.079	-0.030
DIABETES	0.075	0.189	5149.597	0.399	0.690	-0.295	0.446
HYPERTEN	-0.406	0.137	5146.254	-2.967	0.003	-0.675	-0.138
HYPERCHO	-0.642	0.133	5148.471	-4.817	0.000	-0.904	-0.381

Comments: The fixed effect covariates are reported in the Estimates of Fixed Effects table. Age, BMI, hypertension, and hypercholesterolemia are significant factors in explaining the variation in CDR-SUM. From the output, we see that older patients (positive coefficient for age) with low BMI (negative coefficient) without hypertension or hypercholesterolemia (which have negative coefficients) tend to have higher CDR-SUM scores. Diabetes is not found to significantly contribute to the predicted CDR-SUM score.

Estimates of Covariance Parameters

Parameter	Estimate	Std. Error	Wald Z	Sig.	95% Confidence Interval	
					Lower Bound	Upper Bound
Residual	19.894	0.393	50.650	0.000	19.139	20.679
ADC	2.693	0.738	3.647	0.000	1.573	4.609
Disease -MM	3.098	1.546	2.004	0.045	1.165	8.237

Comments: MM stands for multiple membership. The estimates for the variance components in the table above are similar to the estimates of the variance components in the null model (20.249, 2.826, and 3.393 for the residual, ADC, and disease, respectively). The center effects are significant (Sig. = 0.000), and thus it is important to address the center random effects.

7.5.3 Stata Syntax and Output for Multiple Membership

MULTIPLE-MEMBERSHIP NULL MODEL

The syntax of the multiple-membership model in Stata follows:

```
xtmixed cdrsum || _all: R.Disease || adc:, reml
```

STATA OUTPUT

```
Performing EM optimization:
Performing gradient-based optimization:
Iteration 0:    log restricted-likelihood = -15221.279
Iteration 1:        log restricted-likelihood = -15221.279
```

Comments: The program stopped after one iteration, as it achieved convergence.

```
Computing standard errors:
Mixed-effects REML regression    Number of obs =   5,185
Log restricted-likelihood  =   -15221.279
```

		Solution for Fixed Effects				95% CI	
Effect	Estimate	Standard Error	DF	t Value	Pr > |t|	Lower	Upper
_Cons	7.071	0.671	38.000	10.540	0.000	5.756	8.385

Comments: The program uses mixed-effects restricted maximum likelihood (REML) regression to estimate the model parameters. The null model identifies that the mean of the outcome (CDR-SUM) is significantly different than 0 (*p*-value = 0.000). While this is not informative, the null model provides a means of measuring the intraclass correlation.

Covariance Parameter Estimates

	Estimate	Std. Err.	[Lower 95%	Upper 95%]
Disease	1.925	0.493	1.165	3.182
Center (ADC)	1.687	0.232	1.288	2.208
Residual	4.450	0.044	4.414	4.588

LR test vs. linear model: chi2(2) = 423.33   Prob > chi2 = 0.0000

Comments: The random effects are statistically significant for center and for multiple membership in diseases (confidence intervals are strictly positive). The residual measures the random error in the data, which is found to be statistically significant ($p < 0.000$). Thus we find that center accounts for $[1.687/(1.925 + 1.687 + 4.450)] = 20.9\%$ of the variation in the CDR-SUM score, while disease accounts for 23.9%. The combined random effects are significant (Prob > chi2 = 0.0000).

MULTIPLE-MEMBERSHIP MODEL WITH COVARIATES

The Stata syntax follows:

```
XTMIXED CDRSUM AGE BMI DIABETES HYPERTEN HYPERCHO || _ALL:
R.DISEASE || ADC:, REML
                                    Wald chi2(5)   =   94.28
Log restricted-likelihood= -15185.09   Prob > chi2   =   0.0000
```

CDRSUM	Coef.	Std. Err	z	P>z	[95% Conf. Interval]	
AGE	0.030	0.007	4.340	0.000	.0162	.043
BMI	-0.055	0.012	4.400	0.000	-.079	-.030
DIABETES	0.076	0.189	0.400	0.689	-.295	.447
HYPERTEN	-0.406	0.137	2.960	0.003	-.674	-.138
HYPERCHO	-0.642	0.133	4.810	0.000	-.904	-.381
_CONS	6.839	0.902	7.580	0.000	5.072	8.607

Comments: The fixed effect covariates are reported in the table above. Age, BMI, hypertension, and hypercholesterolemia are significant factors in explaining the variation in CDR-SUM. Older patients with low BMI or who are not hypertensive or have hypercholesterolemia tend to have higher CDR-SUM scores.

Random-effects Parameters	Estimate	Std. Err.	[95% Conf. Interval]	
Disease	1.840	0.472	1.112	3.042
Center	1.647	0.227	1.257	2.157
Residual	4.462	0.044	4.377	4.550

LR test vs. linear model: chi2(2) = 418.27   Prob > chi2 = 0.0000

Note: LR test is conservative and provided only for reference.

Comments: LR denotes likelihood ratio. The estimates for the variance components are similar to the null model. The center effects and the disease effects appear to have an impact. It is important to have addressed the center random effects.

7.6 Summary and Discussions

We address multiple-membership, multiple-classification models. These models expand on single membership, which we examined in chapters 4, 5, and 6. We consider the case where a subject or unit is not fully nested in one cluster but may belong to more than one cluster. These types of data structure are not uncommon, but they introduce a certain amount of correlation that must be accounted for.

In previous analyses, we assumed that each patient had one dementia diagnosis. In this chapter, we model cases when patients have more than one diagnosis (AD, DLB, FTD, and/or VaD). We find that age, BMI, hypertension, and hypercholesterolemia are significant predictors of CDR-SUM, even after accounting for multiple dementia diagnoses. Center remained a significant random effect. Diseases also had an effect but were not statistically significant.

7.7 Exercises

Consider the dataset analyzed in chapter 2 (to obtain file, please go to http://www.public.asu.edu/~jeffreyw/) for patients with an AD diagnosis versus normal subjects. Patients have multiple cardiovascular risk factors in the data and belong to different centers.

1. Model the probability of an AD diagnosis, adjusting for the demographic information while accounting for center.
2. Model the probability of an AD diagnosis, adjusting for the demographic information and center while accounting for the multiple cardiovascular risk factor.
3. Are the demographic factors significant predictors of an AD diagnosis in both the single-membership model (1) and the multiple-membership model (2)?
4. Is the multiple-membership factor significant? Is the center effect statistically significant?

Chapter 8

Survival Data Analysis

8.1 Motivating Example

This chapter provides methods to model the time to the occurrence of an event. The time to event describes the time to the onset of a certain symptom or the time to death. Imagine that one is interested in the time to the onset of dementia, and one has a specific demographic profile (such as APOE 4 allele and diabetes). In linear regression, as an example, we were interested in studying how risk factors drive the mean of continuous measurements, such as the Mini-Mental State Examination (MMSE) score. In logistic regression, for example, we are interested in studying how risk factors affect the presence or absence of a disease. In survival analysis, however, we are interested in how risk factors affect time to an event, time to disease, or time to death. The time to an event (Y) may vary greatly between patients (fig. 8.1).

Survival analysis is a method to analyze the time until the occurrence of an event of interest. We measure the time to event and refer to it as the survival time, a failure time, or an event time (Cox and Oakes 1984). The time is measured in units such as days, weeks, or years, as is appropriate for the study. For example, in dementia research, we are interested in studying the time (years) until a person develops a certain dementia diagnosis. Such studies are typically longitudinal in nature, as we follow the subjects over time to see if the event of interest, such as dementia, occurs.

We consider a dataset with 16,539 patients from 37 Alzheimer's disease centers (ADCs). There are 7,073 patients diagnosed with Alzheimer's disease (AD), 315 patients with dementia with Lewy bodies (DLB), 165 patients with frontotemporal dementia (FTD), 1,128 patients with vascular dementia (VaD), and 7,858 subjects who are

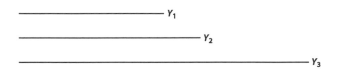

Figure 8.1 Diagram of time until an event occurs for three patients.

Table 8.1 Subset of Data

ID	AGE	SMOKYRS	DIABETES	HYPERTEN	HYPERCHO	SURVIVAL_TIME	DIED
000034	79	0	0	1	0	16	0
000144	79	0	0	1	1	61	0
000184	69	0	0	0	0	13	0
000271	81	36	0	0	1	64	0
000287	79	0	0	1	0	14	0
000385	80	15	0	0	1	105	1
000403	80	28	0	0	0	24	0
000618	63	30	0	1	0	107	1
000792	73	0	0	1	1	52	0
000818	73	27	0	0	0	36	0

nondemented (normal). We are interested in studying the time to death for these patients. In the data, 2,487 patients (15.04%) have expired. A subset of the data, including some of the covariates evaluated in this chapter, is shown in table 8.1. The variable DIED is the status variable denoting censored or uncensored, and SURVIVAL_TIME is the time to the event (months).

8.2 Background

Survival analysis gets its name from the fact that it is often used to look at how long people will live, and which factors influence the time until death (Lee 1992). This model evaluates the time to an event. It is used to answer questions such as:

1. Do women get dementia later than men do?
2. Do Alzheimer's patients without diabetes live longer than Alzheimer's patients with diabetes?
3. Is the length of time that a patient stays in a state of mild cognitive impairment before becoming demented affected by the patient's age?

The survival time response is a continuous measure and is greater than or equal to zero (as one cannot have negative time). In some cases, we will have complete information where we know the exact time that a subject experienced a certain event of interest. In other cases, we may only know that they did not experience the event at a certain time but do not have any further information about the subject. When the information is incomplete, we refer to those observations as censored. This may occur if a subject is lost to follow-up or a clinical trial ends before the event occurs. If there is no censoring (all records are complete), we are free to use other regression procedures. In the case of censoring, however, we use survival analyses to evaluate the data.

Censoring is a key concept in survival analysis. A censored observation indicates that we have not observed the outcome of interest. Censoring can occur for a number of reasons. A study may end before the subject experiences the event, and so we will not have a record of when the subject does experience the event (if they ever do). A subject may choose to withdraw from a study. In the case of longer studies, it is possible to lose a subject to follow-up. In dementia research, we are conducting a study to determine the time to onset of AD. If a patient does not develop AD before the end of the study, we know that the time to dementia onset is at least longer than the course of the study. But we do not have any additional information about the time to AD onset for the subject and consider this record censored.

Survival analysis is an important type of analysis. Although we typically consider linear regression when we are evaluating a continuous outcome (such as time), linear regression is not appropriate for discussing survival times, as survival times are strictly positive. In addition, linear regression is not able to handle censored observations. In many of the regression models we have explored previously (logistic regression, regression, probit regression, among others), records with missing values are excluded from the analysis because we do not have the information we need. In survival analysis, we are able to incorporate information from both the censored and uncensored data to estimate our model parameters and to understand the time to event. Thus two key variables used in survival models are the time to event and the censoring variable.

8.2.1 Definitions and Notation

We begin by presenting some key definitions of terms used in survival models. Time to event and censoring are both used in determining the survival function and the hazard function, which are key components of survival analysis.

Define the time to event as t_E and the time that the subject is censored as t_C. If the event is observed, which means that we have the information t_E, we can set the censoring variable C equal to 1 (event occurred). If the patient is censored before we observed the event ($t_C < t_E$), then we set $C = 0$ (censored). In the data, we record the minimum survival times. If a patient experiences the event, then the survival time is the time between the beginning of the study and the event. If the patient was censored, we can use the time between the beginning of the study and the last patient visit (but we note that the patient is censored).

The survival function measures the probability that a subject will experience the event after some time t. Thus the survival function is defined as $S(t) = P(t_E > t)$, where t_E is the time of the event. This function always stays the same or decreases as time progresses (it is not possible for the probability of survival to increase). Using a survival function in dementia studies allows us to make statements about the probability of the event occurring. For example, given some information about a subject, we predict that the probability of the subject developing dementia after 10 years is 0.64 (64%).

The hazard function, an important function in survival analysis, measures the potential that an event will occur. The hazard function $h(t) = \lim_{\Delta t \to 0} \dfrac{(Pr(t < T \leq t + \Delta t \mid T > t))}{\Delta t}$ measures the rate of the event occurring at a specified time given that the event has not already occurred. Hazard ratios are used to compare the risk between different covariate values or groups. For example, if the hazard ratio (relative risk) of dementia onset for smokers compared to nonsmokers is 1.05, then we believe the rate of dementia onset is 5% more for smokers compared to nonsmokers. The outcome, hazard ratios, is also known as a relative risk.

The survival and hazard functions are closely related. Both are utilized in survival studies to estimate survival times and to understand the impact of certain factors on the time to event.

8.2.2 Types of Survival Models

There are different types of survival models. Models are nonparametric, semiparametric, or parametric.

NONPARAMETRIC SURVIVAL MODELS

Nonparametric survival models do not require distributional assumptions for the hazard function. Nonparametric techniques are typically limited to descriptive methods rather than regression approaches, since we cannot incorporate predictors into the analyses. For example, we determine whether time to dementia is significantly different for women and men. But we cannot account for other contributing factors such as race or cardiovascular risk factors or diagnoses. Common nonparametric techniques include the Kaplan Meier estimator and life tables.

SEMIPARAMETRIC SURVIVAL MODELS

Semiparametric survival models do not require the strict distributional assumptions of parametric techniques, but they still have some underlying assumptions. Semiparametric analyses cannot predict survival times but can account for covariate differences between groups. For example, we can compare the hazard ratios (relative risk) of a dementia diagnosis given gender, race, and cardiovascular risk factor diagnoses. The most popular semiparametric survival analysis approach is the Cox proportional hazards model. The Cox regression model does not require an assumption on the distribution of the hazard function, but it does have an assumption about proportional hazards (which is further discussed in section 8.4).

PARAMETRIC SURVIVAL MODELS

Parametric survival methods assume that the survival times follow a certain probability distribution. In parametric techniques, we must use maximum likelihood to estimate the unknown parameters of the underlying distribution, and we use this information to calculate the likelihood for all patients. This type of analysis allows us to make predictions about a patient's time to event, such as time to dementia onset, given information about the patient. Although we do not address parametric methods in this chapter, common statistical distributions used in the analysis of survival data include the exponential, Weibull, and log-normal distributions (McCullagh and Nelder 1989).

8.3 The Kaplan Meier Method

The Kaplan Meier method of evaluating survival analysis data is a popular nonparametric technique (Kaplan and Meier 1958). This survival method focuses on descriptive statistics, such as the median survival time, to compare the time to event between two or more groups.

In this approach, the Kaplan Meier estimator is used to evaluate survival probabilities over time. We compare the time to event, such as time to dementia diagnosis, across different groupings such as patients with diabetes versus without diabetes, smokers versus nonsmokers, and males versus females. The differences between the survival curves are tested using chi-square tests. Common statistical tests used for the comparison of survival times include the log rank (Mantel 1966), the generalized Wilcoxon (Gehan 1965; Breslow 1970), and the Tarone-Ware tests (Tarone and Ware 1977). Survival curves visualizing the survival probabilities across groups are often paired with this analysis.

Table 8.2 Frequency Table of Diabetes by Censoring

Diabetes	Died	
	0 (Censored)	1 (Death)
0 (remote/inactive/absent)	12,480	2,254
1 (active/recent)	1,572	233

Problem: Compare the time to death for patients with and without diabetes using nonparametric survival analysis techniques. Obtain the Kaplan Meier curves for time to death.

Solution: In our sample of 16,539 patients, 1,805 patients have recent/active diabetes (10.9%). A contingency table (table 8.2) provides a cross-classification of distribution of patients with diabetes and the patients censored.

From the Kaplan Meier analysis, we conclude that the time to death is not significantly different for diabetic and nondiabetic patients (p-value $= 0.612$). The Kaplan Meier curves are plotted. The estimated survival curves (with confidence bands) overlap for diabetic and nondiabetic patients and do not indicate significant differences. We evaluate the time to death between patients with recent/active diabetes and remote/inactive/absent diabetes using SAS, R, SPSS, and Stata.

8.3.1 SAS Syntax and Output for Kaplan Meier Analysis

The SAS syntax follows:

```
¹PROC LIFETEST DATA=CHAP8 ATRISK PLOTS=SURVIVAL(ATRISK CB);
²STRATA DIABETES;
³TIME SURVIVAL_TIME*DIED(0);
RUN;
```

¹PROC LIFETEST performs nonparametric techniques, including the Kaplan Meier estimator. The option ATRISK allows the number of patients at risk (of having the event) to be included and confidence bands (CB).

[2]The STRATA option specifies the different groups. Diabetes is our comparison group of interest, which has the values present or absent (binary).

[3]The TIME option is used to specify the survival time (time to event) along with the censoring variable. We include the syntax to represent a censored observation (in this case, 0).

SAS OUTPUT

The LIFETEST Procedure

Stratum 1: DIABETES = 0

Product-Limit Survival Estimates

SURVIVAL_ TIME	Number at Risk	Observed Events	Survival	Failure	Survival Standard Error	Number Failed	Number Left
0.000	14734	0	1.0000	0	0	0	14734
2.000 *	14734	0	.	.	.	0	14733
3.000 *	14733	0	.	.	.	0	14732
6.000 *	.	0	.	.	.	0	14731
6.000 *	14732	0	.	.	.	0	14730
7.000 *	.	0	.	.	.	0	14729
143.000 *	9	0	.	.	.	2254	4
144.000 *	.	0	.	.	.	2254	3
144.000 *	.	0	.	.	.	2254	2
144.000 *	4	0	.	.	.	2254	1
145.000 *	1	0	0.475	.	.	2254	0

Comments: This output table is split by stratum (diabetes = 0). For each time period (SURVIVAL_TIME), the table reports the Kaplan Meier estimates of the survival function used in plotting the survival curves (Survival). This is a measure of the probability of surviving a certain number of months. Then, the table reports the number of subjects who have experienced the event, as well as the number at risk (Number Left) and the number of subjects who have not experienced the event (Number Failed).

Stratum 1: DIABETES = 0

Summary Statistics for Time Variable SURVIVAL_TIME

Quartile Estimates

Percent	Point Estimate	Transform	95% Confidence Interval [Lower	Upper)
75	.	LOGLOG	.	.
50	133.000	LOGLOG	129.000	.
25	77.000	LOGLOG	75.000	79.000

Mean	Standard Error
107.592	0.504

Comments: The mean survival time and its standard error were underestimated because the largest observation was censored and the estimation was restricted to the largest event time. The point estimates of the mean, standard error, and the first and second quartiles are shown (the third quartile estimate is missing). The mean time to death for nondiabetic patients is 107.592 months, while the median time to death is 133 months.

Stratum 2: DIABETES = 1

Product-Limit Survival Estimates

SURVIVAL_ TIME	Number at Risk	Observed Events	Survival	Failure	Survival Standard Error	Number Failed	Number Left
0.000	1805	0	1.0000	0	0	0	1805
6.000 *	1805	0	.	.	.	0	1804
8.000 *	.	0	.	.	.	0	1803
8.000 *	1804	0	.	.	.	0	1802
9.000 *	.	0	.	.	.	0	1801
9.000 *	.	0	.	.	.	0	1800
9.000 *	1802	0	.	.	.	0	1799
136.000 *	4	0	.	.	.	233	3
137.000 *	3	0	.	.	.	233	2
142.000 *	.	0	.	.	.	233	1
142.000 *	2	0	0.4897	.	.	233	0

Comments: The marked survival times are censored observations. For DIABETES = 1, the output table contains the Kaplan Meier survival estimates, failure rate, standard error, as well as the number of subjects who have experienced the event (Number Failed) and the number of patients who have not experienced the event (Number Left) in the current time period for recent/active diabetes group.

Stratum 2: DIABETES = 1

Summary Statistics for Time Variable SURVIVAL_TIME

Quartile Estimates

| | | | 95% Confidence Interval | |
| | Point | | | |
Percent	Estimate	Transform	[Lower	Upper)
75	.	LOGLOG	.	.
50	126.000	LOGLOG	119.000	.
25	77.000	LOGLOG	73.000	81.000

	Mean	Standard Error
	101.272	1.356

Comments: The mean survival time and its standard error were underestimated because the largest observation was censored and the estimation was restricted to the largest event time. These are summary statistics for the time variable SURVIVAL_TIME for patients with DIABETES = 1. The mean time to event is 101.272 months, and the median time to event is 126 months.

Summary of the Number of Censored and Uncensored Values

| | | | | | Percent |
Stratum	DIABETES	Total	Failed	Censored	Censored
1	0	14734	2254	12480	84.70
2	1	1805	233	1572	87.09
Total		16539	2487	14052	84.96

Comments: There are 1,805 diabetic patients and 14,734 nondiabetic patients in our cohort. The Censored column reports the number of patients (diabetic and nondiabetic) where DIED = 0. The Failed column records the number of patients for which the event (death) occurred (DIED = 1). There are 2,254 subjects without diabetes and 233 subjects with diabetes who have died.

Testing Homogeneity of Survival Curves
for SURVIVAL_TIME over Strata

Rank Statistics

DIABETES	Log-Rank	Wilcoxon
0	-7.237	-50988
1	7.237	50988

Covariance Matrix for the Log-Rank Statistics

DIABETES	0	1
0	203.999	-203.999
1	-203.999	203.999

Covariance Matrix for the Wilcoxon Statistics

DIABETES	0	1
0	1.24E10	-1.24E10
1	-1.24E10	1.24E10

Test of Equality over Strata

Test	Chi-Square	DF	Pr > Chi-Square
Log-Rank	0.257	1	0.612
Wilcoxon	0.210	1	0.647
-2Log(LR)	0.635	1	0.426

Comments: The Test of Equality over Strata output reports the statistical test for differences between strata. The p-value for the Log-Rank test is $0.612 > 0.05$, and so we conclude there is not a significant difference in the survival times of diabetic and nondiabetic patients.

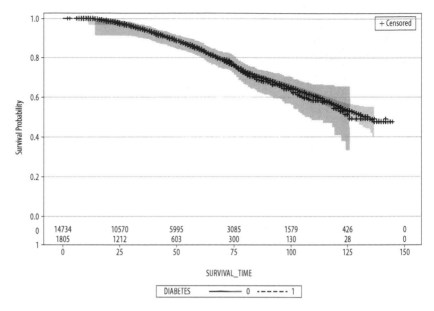

Figure 8.2 Survival plot for time to death by diabetes status.

There is also the Wilcoxon and G^2 test statistics. They support the no-difference conclusion.

Comments: The survival function describes the probability of survival (nonoccurrence of event of interest) (fig. 8.2). This plot is a useful visual to understand how the probability of survival changes over time. The plot above has survival curves plot for both groups (dark gray is nondiabetes, and light gray is diabetes). The x-axis is the length in months of survival time, while the y-axis is the calculated survival probability. Because the confidence bounds overlap for both groups, we cannot conclude that the time to event differs significantly between the diabetic and nondiabetic groups.

8.3.2 R Syntax and Output for Kaplan Meier Analysis

The R syntax follows:

```
¹library(survival)
²y <- Surv(chap8$SURVIVAL_TIME, chap8$DIED)
```

```
³kmfit <- survfit(y~DIABETES,data=chap8)
⁴summary(kmfit)
⁵survdiff(y~DIABETES,data=chap8)
⁶library(survminer)
⁷ggsurvplot(kmfit,data=chap8,risk.table=TRUE)
```

[1]The survival library contains functions to perform survival analyses.
[2]The outcome of the survival analysis (called "y" in this example) is created using the Surv() function and specifying the time to event variable and the censoring variable.
[3]The survfit() function is used to perform a Kaplan Meier analysis. The outcome (created using the Surv() function) is specified in terms of the variable to stratify by. The data frame containing the covariates is specified using the data= option.
[4]The summary() function prints a summary of the survival analysis output.
[5]The survdiff() function is used to perform statistical testing to check whether the time to event variables significantly by strata.
[6]The survminer library contains functions to plot the Kaplan Meier curves.
[7]The ggsurvplot() function produces a plot of the Kaplan Meier curves. The input includes the Kaplan Meier fit (produced by survfit) and the R data frame. The risk.table=TRUE option prints the number of patients at risk for each strata below the plot.

R OUTPUT

```
summary(kmfit)
## Call: survfit(formula = y ~ DIABETES, data = chap8)
##
##                 DIABETES=0
##  time n.risk n.event survival  std.err lower 95% CI upper 95% CI
##    11  14597       2    1.000 9.69e-05        1.000        1.000
##    12  14339       4    1.000 1.70e-04        0.999        1.000
##    13  13459       7    0.999 2.60e-04        0.999        1.000
```

```
##     14   12874        16    0.998 4.04e-04            0.997            0.999
##     15   12494        11    0.997 4.83e-04            0.996            0.998
##     16   12207        18    0.995 5.94e-04            0.994            0.997
  .  .  .
##    131     261         2    0.509 1.14e-02            0.487            0.532
##    132     230         3    0.502 1.19e-02            0.479            0.526
##    133     167         1    0.499 1.22e-02            0.476            0.524
##    135     104         2    0.490 1.37e-02            0.463            0.517
##    136      83         1    0.484 1.48e-02            0.456            0.513
##    137      58         1    0.475 1.67e-02            0.444            0.509
##
##                       DIABETES=1
##   time n.risk n.event survival   std.err lower 95% CI upper 95% CI
##     14    1534        2    0.999 0.000921            0.997            1.000
##     15    1478        6    0.995 0.001890            0.991            0.998
##     16    1438        1    0.994 0.002011            0.990            0.998
##     17    1408        3    0.992 0.002349            0.987            0.996
##     18    1370        5    0.988 0.002844            0.983            0.994
##     19    1340        4    0.985 0.003195            0.979            0.992
  .  .  .
##    114      69        1    0.574 0.028274            0.521            0.632
##    118      55        1    0.564 0.029625            0.509            0.625
##    119      53        2    0.543 0.032100            0.483            0.609
##    122      42        1    0.530 0.033835            0.467            0.600
##    124      30        1    0.512 0.037028            0.444            0.590
##    126      23        1    0.490 0.041573            0.415            0.578
```

Comments: The survfit() output contains tables for each level of strata (DIABETES = 0 and DIABETES = 1). The tables contain the time period, the number of subjects at risk who have not had the event occur (n.risk), the number of subjects who have had the event occur (n.event), the survival function estimate (survival), as well as the standard error and confidence interval estimates.

```
survdiff(y~DIABETES,data=chap8)
## Call:
## survdiff(formula = y ~ DIABETES, data = chap8)
##
##                    N Observed Expected (O-E)^2/E (O-E)^2/V
## DIABETES=0 14734     2254     2261    0.0232    0.257
## DIABETES=1  1805      233      226    0.2320    0.257
##
##   Chisq= 0.3  on 1 degrees of freedom, p= 0.6
```

Comments: The output reports the statistical testing to compare the time to death for the recent/active diabetes and inactive/remote/inactive diabetes groups. We see that the p-value is $0.6 > 0.05$, and thus we conclude that the time to death is not statistically significantly different for the two groups.

```
ggsurvplot(kmfit,data=chap8,risk.table=TRUE)
```

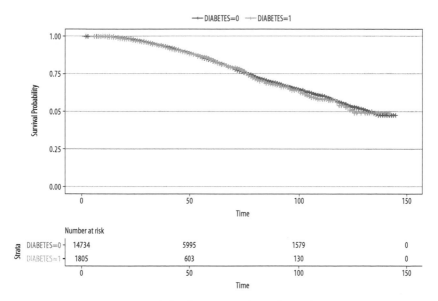

Figure 8.3 Survival plot for time to death by diabetes status.

Comments: The ggsurvplot() function in figure 8.3 plots the survival curves for both groups over time (months). The table under the plot summarizes the number of subjects at risk (who have not experienced the event) for the two groups over time.

8.3.3 SPSS Syntax and Output for Kaplan Meier Analysis

The SPSS syntax follows:

```
KM Survival time BY DIABETES
        /ID=ID
        /STATUS=died(1)
        /PRINT TABLE MEAN
        /PLOT SURVIVAL
        /TEST LOGRANK BRESLOW TARONE
        /COMPARE OVERALL POOLED
        /SAVE SURVIVAL HAZARD.
```

SPSS OUTPUT

DIABETES	Total N	N of Events	Censored	
			N	Percent
0	14734	2254	12480	84.7%
1	1805	233	1572	87.1%
Overall	16539	2487	14052	85.0%

Overall Comparisons

	Chi-Square	df	Sig.
Log Rank (Mantel-Cox)	.257	1	.612
Breslow (Generalized Wilcoxon)	.210	1	.647
Tarone-Ware	.212	1	.645

Test of equality of survival distributions for the different levels of DIABETES

Comments: The output reports a frequency distribution table for diabetes and censoring. The Overall Comparisons table reports the test statistics (Chi-Square) and *p*-values (Sig.) to test whether the survival

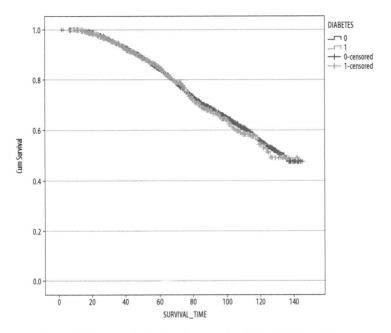

Figure 8.4 Survival plot for time to death by diabetes status.

functions for the two groups are equal. All three statistical tests indicate that the survival curves for the diabetic and nondiabetic groups do not differ significantly. Generally, these three test results will lead to the same conclusions, but the test you choose should depend on how you expect the survival distributions to differ to make best use of the different weightings that each test assigns to the time-points.

Comments: Figure 8.4 displays the SPSS plot of the two survival curves for the diabetic (gray) and nondiabetic (black) groups. The two Kaplan Meier curves overlap and suggest that there is no significant difference in the time to event between the two groups.

8.3.4 Stata Syntax and Output for Kaplan Meier Analysis

The Stata syntax follows:

```
. LTABLE SURVIVAL_TIME DIED, SURVIVAL HAZARD
```

STATA OUTPUT

Interval		Total	Deaths	Lost	Survival		std Error	[95% Conf. Int.]	
2	3		16539	0	1	1.0000	0.0000	.	.
3	4		16538	0	1	1.0000	0.0000	.	.
6	7		16537	0	3	1.0000	0.0000	.	.
7	8		16534	0	11	1.0000	0.0000	.	.
8	9		16523	0	15	1.0000	0.0000	.	.
9	10		16508	0	42	1.0000	0.0000	.	.
10	11	16466	0	84	1.0000	0.0000	.	.
11	12	16382	2	289	0.9999	0.0001	0.9995	1.0000
12	13	16091	4	1010	0.9996	0.0002	0.9992	0.9998
13	14	15077	7	662	0.9991	0.0002	0.9985	0.9995
14	15	14408	18	418	0.9979	0.0004	0.9970	0.9985
15	16	13972	17	310	0.9967	0.0005	0.9956	0.9975
16	17	13645	19	208	0.9953	0.0006	0.9940	0.9963

INTERVAL		BEG. TOTAL	CUM. FAILURE	STD. ERROR	HAZARD	STD. ERROR	[95% CONF. INT.]		
2	3	16539	0.0000	0.0000	0.0000	.	.	.	
3	4	16538	0.0000	0.0000	0.0000	.	.	.	
6	7	16537	0.0000	0.0000	0.0000	.	.	.	
7	8	16534	0.0000	0.0000	0.0000	.	.	.	
8	9	16523	0.0000	0.0000	0.0000	.	.	.	
9	10	16508	0.0000	0.0000	0.0000	.	.	.	
10	11	16466	0.0000	0.0000	0.0000	.	.	.	
11	12	16382	0.0001	0.0001	0.0001	0.0001	0.0000	0.0003	
12	13	16091	0.0004	0.0002	0.0003	0.0001	0.0000	0.0005	
13	14	15077	0.0009	0.0002	0.0005	0.0002	0.0001	0.0008	
14	15	14408	0.0021	0.0004	0.0013	0.0003	0.0007	0.0019	
15	16	13972	0.0033	0.0005	0.0012	0.0003	0.0006	0.0018	
16	17	13645	0.0047	0.0006	0.0014	0.0003	0.0008	0.0020	

Comments: For each time period (SURVIVAL_TIME), the table reports the Kaplan Meier estimates of the survival function used in plotting the survival curves (Survival). This is a measure of the probability of surviving a certain number of months.

The Stata syntax follows:

```
STS TEST DIABETES, LOGRANK
```

STATA OUTPUT

```
        FAILURE _D:     DIED
        ANALYSIS TIME _T:  SURVIVAL_TIME
Log-Rank   Test for Equality   of Survivor   Functions
           Events                Events
Diabetes   Observed              Expected
0          2254                  2261.24
1           233                   225.76
TOTAL      248 /                 2487.00
```

$$chi2(1) = 0.26$$
$$Pr>chi2 = 0.612$$

Comments: We also consider the tests of equality across strata to explore whether the survival curves vary across the groups. The log-rank test of equality is a nonparametric test for testing group differences. For our example of evaluating time to death for diabetic versus non-diabetic subjects, we obtain a p-value of 0.612, which suggests that the survival curves are not significantly different between the two groups.

The Stata syntax follows:

```
. STS GRAPH, BY (DIABETES)
```

STATA OUTPUT

Comments: The plot of the survival functions for each stratum is displayed in figure 8.5. The x-axis is the time to event (analysis time),

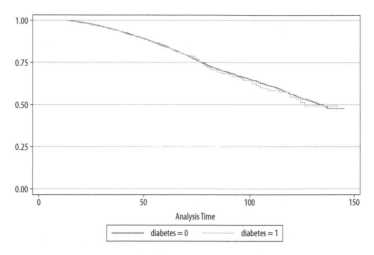

Figure 8.5 Survival plot for time to death by diabetes status.

while the y-axis is the probability of survival. The survival curves plotted for the recent/active diabetes (gray) and inactive/remote/absent diabetes (black) groups are not different.

8.4 Cox Proportional Hazards Regression Model

While we used the Kaplan Meier analysis, a nonparametric technique, to compare survival curves across groups, we cannot use the Kaplan Meier estimator to evaluate the impact of certain covariates. A popular regression model used in survival analysis is the Cox proportional hazards model (Cox 1972). This method is a semiparametric approach that allows us to model the time to event through the hazard function while adjusting for the impact of covariates. The Cox regression model is considered semiparametric, as it does not assume the distribution of the baseline hazard function but does require an assumption about the effect of the predictors on the hazard function.

We parameterize the hazard rate in terms of the predictors to describe the relationship between the covariates and the time to event. For example, the hazard function is:

$$h(t|X) = \exp\,(\beta_0 + \beta_1 X),$$

where the covariate of interest is X and the regression parameters are β_0 and β_1. In the Cox regression, we assume that a ratio of hazard rates $\dfrac{h(t|x_2)}{h(t|x_1)}$ is constant; hence the reason we refer to the model as the proportional hazards model. Our goal is to address the impact of the regression parameters (β) in determining the relationship between the covariates and the relative risk of death. This form allows the regression parameters to be any value (negative or positive), although the hazard function will always be positive. Because time t is not in the hazard function, we can focus on the impact of covariates (such as the presence of diabetes or an APOE 4 allele) on the hazard rate rather than evaluating time dependence. The Cox proportional hazards model parameters estimates are obtained using maximum likelihood methods.

PROPORTIONAL HAZARDS ASSUMPTION

A key assumption of the Cox proportional hazards regression model is the proportional hazards assumption. The model assumes that the ratio of hazards is constant over time. For example, if diabetic patients who are 60 years old have a hazard that is 1.1 times that of nondiabetic patients who are 60 years old, then we assume that diabetic patients who are 70 years old have a hazard that is 1.1 times that of nondiabetic patients who are 70 years old. While this assumption is often reasonable, in some cases it is not. For example, when predicting dementia on the basis of age, the hazard increases as age increases, and so this may not be an appropriate model.

Table 8.3 reports the Cox proportional hazards regression estimates. The Cox proportional hazards regression model identifies age, years smoking, diastolic blood pressure, and MMSE as statistically significantly associated with the time to death. Although body mass index (BMI) has a p-value of 0.049, which is less than

Table 8.3 Cox Proportional Hazards Regression Results

Parameter	Estimate	e^{estimate}	p-Value
Age	0.037	1.038	<0.0001
Years smoking	0.012	1.012	<0.0001
Systolic blood pressure	0.000	1.000	0.808
Diastolic blood pressure	−0.007	0.993	0.012
Heart rate	0.001	1.001	0.837
BMI	−0.011	0.990	0.049
MMSE	−0.121	0.886	<0.0001
Diabetes	−0.094	0.910	0.280
Hypertension	−0.019	0.981	0.712
Hypercholesterolemia	0.002	1.002	0.968

the cutoff of 0.05, we are cautious about stating that it is statistically significant. This variable should be further evaluated in other studies to determine the impact on time to death. The hazard ratio, which is also known as the relative risk, is calculated using the exp(estimate). This shows the relative risk of a certain covariate assuming that all other factors are held constant. For example, if a subject smokes one additional year, the rate of death increases by 1.012, or 101.2%. Alternatively, if a patient's hypertension status switches to inactive (from recent/active), the rate of death decreases by $1/0.981 = 1.019$, or 101.9%.

8.4.1 SAS Syntax and Output for the Cox Regression Model

The SAS syntax follows:

```
¹PROC PHREG DATA=CHAP8 PLOT(OVERLAY)=SURVIVAL;
²MODEL SURVIVAL_TIME*DIED(0)=AGE SMOKYRS BPSYS BPDIAS HRATE BMI
MMSE DIABETES HYPERTEN HYPERCHO;
RUN;
```

[1]PROC PHREG fits Cox regression models; we add PLOT=SURVIVAL to obtain the curves.
[2]Specify the outcome and the covariates of interest. Outcome is the time to event variable and the censoring variable.

SAS OUTPUT

The PHREG Procedure

Model Information	
Data Set	WORK.CHAP8
Dependent Variable	SURVIVAL_TIME
Censoring Variable	DIED
Censoring Value(s)	0
Ties Handling	BRESLOW

Number of Observations Read	16539
Number of Observations Used	12573

Summary of the Number of Event and Censored Values

Total	Event	Censored	Percent Censored
12573	1812	10761	85.59

Comments: We have descriptive information. There are 16,539 records in the data. Of the 12,573 records evaluated, 1,812 subjects had an event (died), while 10,761 did not. Thus 85.59% of subjects did not die as of the end of the study (percentage censored).

Convergence Status
Convergence criterion (GCONV=1E-8) satisfied.

Comments: We check that the model has converged before drawing any conclusions about the model results.

Model Fit Statistics

Criterion	Without Covariates	With Covariates
-2 LOG L	30044.592	28362.934
AIC	30044.592	28382.934
SBC	30044.592	28437.955

Testing Global Null Hypothesis: BETA=0			
Test	Chi-Square	DF	Pr > ChiSq
Likelihood Ratio	1681.6586	10	<.0001
Score	2518.7659	10	<.0001
Wald	2115.9868	10	<.0001

Comments: The Testing Global Null Hypothesis statistical test checks whether all of the covariates are significant in modeling time to death. From the likelihood ratio test (p-value < 0.0001), we see that at least one of the covariates evaluated statistical impacts at the time to death.

Analysis of Maximum Likelihood Estimates							
Parameter	DF	Parameter Estimate	Standard Error	Chi-Square	Pr > ChiSq	Hazard Ratio	Label
AGE	1	0.037	0.003	184.716	<.0001	1.038	AGE
SMOKYRS	1	0.011	0.001	64.953	<.0001	1.012	SMOKYRS
BPSYS	1	0.000	0.002	0.059	0.808	1.000	BPSYS
BPDIAS	1	−0.007	0.003	6.354	0.012	0.993	BPDIAS
HRATE	1	0.000	0.002	0.043	0.837	1.000	HRATE
BMI	1	−0.010	0.005	3.883	0.049	0.990	
MMSE	1	−0.121	0.003	1764.518	<.0001	0.886	MMSE
DIABETES	1	−0.094	0.087	1.169	0.280	0.910	
HYPERTEN	1	−0.019	0.052	0.137	0.712	0.981	
HYPERCHO	1	0.002	0.049	0.002	0.968	1.002	

Comments: We find that age (AGE), years smoking (SMOKYRS), diastolic blood pressure (BPDIAS), and MMSE significantly drive the time to death for subjects in our cohort. Systolic blood pressure (BPSYS), heart rate (HRATE), diabetes (DIABETES), hypertension (HYPERTEN), and hypercholesterolemia (HYPERCHO) are not found to significantly affect the time to death. Although BMI has a p-value that is less than the cutoff of 0.05 (p-value = 0.0488), this is very close to the cutoff and should be further evaluated; see http://www.amstat.org/asa/files/pdfs/P-ValueStatement.pdf.

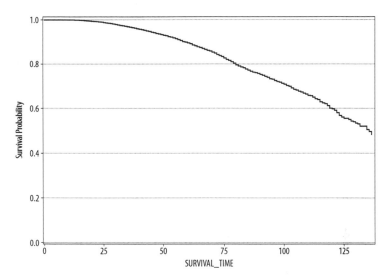

Figure 8.6 Survival plot at reference setting (mean of covariates).

Reference Set of Covariates for Plotting									
AGE	SMOKYRS	BPSYS	BPDIAS	HRATE	BMI	MMSE	DIABETES	HYPERTEN	HYPERCHO
71.613	10.000	134.000	75.000	68.000	26.900	25.586	0.106	0.456	0.474

Comments: A plot of the survival probability versus time is provided (fig. 8.6). Also, one has the reference set if one wants to compute the survival function.

8.4.2 R Syntax and Output for the Cox Regression Model

The R syntax follows:

```
1library(survival)
2y <- Surv(chap8$SURVIVAL_TIME,chap8$DIED)
3coxfit <- coxph(y~AGE+SMOKYRS+BPSYS+BPDIAS+HRATE+BMI+MMSE+DIABE
TES+HYPERTEN+HYPERCHO,data=chap8)
4summary(coxfit)
```

[1]This library contains functions including Kaplan Meier and Cox proportional hazards.

[2]The outcome is specified using the Surv() function, time to event (SURVIVAL_TIME), and the censoring variable (DIED).

[3]The coxph() function is used for performing Cox regression. The outcome (created by the Surv() function) is specified.

[4]The summary() function allows prints of the model characteristic.

R OUTPUT

```
summary(coxfit)
## Call:
## coxph(formula = y ~ AGE + SMOKYRS + BPSYS + BPDIAS + HRATE +
##     BMI + MMSE + DIABETES + HYPERTEN + HYPERCHO, data = chap8)
##
##   n= 12573, number of events= 1812
##    (3966 observations deleted due to missingness)
##
##                   coef   exp(coef)   se(coef)        z Pr(>|z|)
## AGE         0.0374180   1.0381268   0.0027446   13.633  < 2e-16 ***
## SMOKYRS     0.0115464   1.0116133   0.0014257    8.099 5.56e-16 ***
## BPSYS       0.0003575   1.0003576   0.0015252    0.234   0.8147
## BPDIAS     -0.0069914   0.9930330   0.0027578   -2.535   0.0112 *
## HRATE       0.0004696   1.0004697   0.0023094    0.203   0.8389
## BMI        -0.0104951   0.9895597   0.0053131   -1.975   0.0482 *
## MMSE       -0.1216780   0.8854334   0.0028836  -42.197  < 2e-16 ***
## DIABETES   -0.0948981   0.9094656   0.0869028   -1.092   0.2748
## HYPERTEN   -0.0198960   0.9803006   0.0520734   -0.382   0.7024
## HYPERCHO    0.0019323   1.0019342   0.0492434    0.039   0.9687
## ---
## Signif. codes:  0 '***' 0.001 '**' 0.01 '*' 0.05 '.' 0.1 ' ' 1
##
##           exp(coef)   exp(-coef) lower .95 upper .95
## AGE          1.0381      0.9633     1.0326    1.0437
## SMOKYRS      1.0116      0.9885     1.0088    1.0144
## BPSYS        1.0004      0.9996     0.9974    1.0034
## BPDIAS       0.9930      1.0070     0.9877    0.9984
```

```
## HRATE        1.0005      0.9995      0.9960      1.0050

## BMI          0.9896      1.0106      0.9793      0.9999

## MMSE         0.8854      1.1294      0.8804      0.8905

## DIABETES     0.9095      1.0995      0.7670      1.0783

## HYPERTEN     0.9803      1.0201      0.8852      1.0856

## HYPERCHO     1.0019      0.9981      0.9098      1.1035

##

## Concordance= 0.775   (se = 0.008 )

## Rsquare= 0.126    (max possible= 0.908 )

## Likelihood ratio test= 1694   on 10 df,    p=<2e-16

## Wald test           = 2133   on 10 df,    p=<2e-16

## Score (logrank) test = 2543   on 10 df,    p=<2e-16
```

Comments: There are 12,573 records with 1,812 deaths. There are 3,966 observations removed in the analysis owing to missing values. For each covariate in the analysis, the regression coefficient (coef), the exponentiated regression coefficient (exp(coef)), standard error (se(coef)), z-value, p-value, and confidence intervals are reported. Age (AGE), years smoking (SMOKYRS), diastolic blood pressure (BP-DIAS), and MMSE are identified as statistically significant predictors of the time to death. The likelihood ratio, Wald, and Score tests check whether any covariates were statistically significant, since the p-value (<2e-16) is less than 0.05. It suggests that at least one covariate was statistically significant.

8.4.3 SPSS Syntax and Output for the Cox Regression Model

The SPSS syntax follows:

```
COXREG Survival time
  /STATUS=died(1)
  /METHOD=ENTER AGE SMOKYRS BPSYS BPDIAS HRATE BMI MMSE
DIABETES HYPERTEN HYPERCHO
  /PLOT SURVIVAL HAZARDS
  /CRITERIA=PIN(.05) POUT(.10) ITERATE(20).
```

SPSS OUTPUT

Cox Regression

Omnibus Tests of Model Coefficients

-2 Log Likelihood	Overall (score)			Change From Previous Step			Change From Previous Block		
	Chi-square	df	Sig.	Chi-square	df	Sig.	Chi-square	df	Sig.
28362.934	2518.766	10	.000	1681.659	10	.000	1681.659	10	.000

Comments: The Chi-square test identifies whether any of the model coefficients are statistically significant (improved prediction of the outcome with addition of the covariates). The Chi-square value for this model is statistically significant ($p < 0.05$). Thus the predictors in this Cox regression model improve the prediction of time to death.

Variables in the Equation

	B	SE	Wald	df	Sig.	Exp(B)
AGE	.037	.003	184.717	1	.000	1.038
SMOKYRS	.011	.001	64.952	1	.000	1.012
BPSYS	.000	.002	.059	1	.808	1.000
BPDIAS	-.007	.003	6.354	1	.012	.993
HRATE	.000	.002	.043	1	.837	1.000
BMI	-.010	.005	3.883	1	.049	.990
MMSE	-.121	.003	1764.515	1	.000	.886
DIABETES	-.094	.087	1.169	1	.280	.910
HYPERTEN	-.019	.052	.137	1	.712	.981
HYPERCHO	.002	.049	.002	1	.968	1.002

Comments: Note that e^β is the hazard ratio of the outcome. To obtain the risk ratio to describe the association between the outcome and the

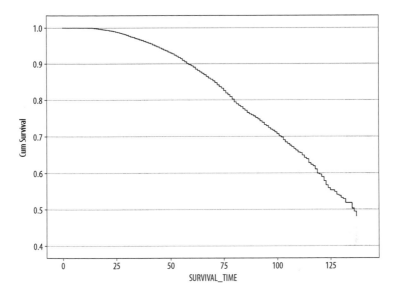

Figure 8.7 Survival plot at mean of covariates.

independent variables, we use the exponential of beta (Exp(B)) in SPSS. The beta values represent log of the hazard or risk for the outcome. There is a significant association between survival time and age (AGE), years smoking (SMOKYRS), diastolic blood pressure (BP-DIAS), and MMSE. We note that the p-value for BMI is 0.049, and so one should be cautious in evaluating the significance of this result. We find the risk ratios of death for these patients in 10 years are 10.38 for age and 10.12 for years smoking.

Comments: Plots of the survival function and hazard function are provided in the output, in figures 8.7 and 8.8, respectively.

8.4.4 Stata Syntax and Output for the Cox Regression Model

The STATA syntax follows:

```
STCOX AGE SMOKYRS BPSYS BPDIAS HRATE BMI MMSE DIABETES HYPERTEN HYPERCHO,        NOHR
```

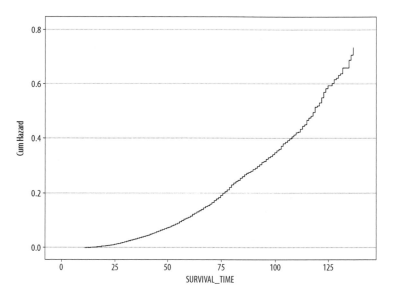

Figure 8.8 Hazard function at mean of covariates.

STATA OUTPUT

```
failure _d:    died
ANALYSIS TIME _T:      SURVIVAL_TIME
Iteration 0:   log likelihood = -15022.296
Iteration 1:   log likelihood = -14237.241
Iteration 2:   log likelihood = -14181.646
Iteration 3:   log likelihood = -14181.467
Iteration 4:   log likelihood = -14181.467
Refining estimates:
Iteration 0:   log likelihood = -14181.467
```

Comments: At each iteration, the log likelihood decreases.

```
Cox regression --      Breslow method for     ties
No. of subjects = 12,573       Number of obs    =    12,573
No. of failures = 1,812
Time at risk    = 641429
                               LR chi2(10)      =    1681.66
Log likelihood = -14181.467    Prob > chi2      =    0.0000
```

Comments: The likelihood for the remainder is $-1,4181.47$, and the likelihood for the fit is $1,681.66$ with a p-value of 0.0000.

_t	Coef.	Std. Err.	z	P>z	[95% Conf. Interval]	
AGE	0.037	0.003	13.590	0.000	0.032	0.043
SMOKYRS	0.011	0.001	8.060	0.000	0.009	0.014
BPSYS	0.000	0.002	0.240	0.808	-0.003	0.003
BPDIAS	-0.007	0.003	-2.520	0.012	-0.012	-0.002
HRATE	0.000	0.002	0.210	0.837	-0.004	0.005
BMI	-0.010	0.005	-1.970	0.049	-0.021	0.000
MMSE	-0.121	0.003	-42.010	0.000	-0.127	-0.115
DIABETES	-0.094	0.087	-1.080	0.280	-0.264	0.076
HYPERTEN	-0.019	0.052	-0.370	0.712	-0.121	0.083
HYPERCHO	0.002	0.049	0.040	0.968	-0.095	0.099

Comments: The regression parameter estimates (Coef.), standard errors (Std. Err.), z-values, p-values, and the 95% confidence intervals are reported in the output. We can calculate the hazard ratios (also called relative risks) by calculating e^{β}. For example, the model indicates that as the number of smoking years increases by one unit, and all other variables are held constant, the rate of death increases by $e^{0.037} = 1.038$, or 3.8%. Results such as this are determined by calculating the hazard ratio from the estimated regression coefficients.

The Stata syntax follows:

```
ESTAT PHTEST
```

STATA OUTPUT

```
        Test of Proportional Hazards      Assumption
        Time: Time
                          chi2          df          Prob>chi2
global test               35.71         10          0.0001
```

Comments: One of the primary assumptions of the Cox proportional hazards model is proportionality. This output reports the statistical test, checking the assumption of proportional hazards, where the null hypothesis is that the assumption was not violated. Because the p-value is $0.0001 < 0.05$, we find that there is evidence the proportional hazards assumption has been violated. This indicates that a time-dependent covariate in the model is significant.

8.5 Bayesian Survival Analysis Models

The use of Bayesian methods (see chap. 6) has become increasingly popular in modern statistical analysis, with applications in numerous scientific fields. In recent releases of SAS and Stata, there are numerous tools for Bayesian analysis with convenient access through several popular procedures. We perform Cox proportional hazards regression using Bayesian estimation. We implement prior information to estimate the posterior distributions for each covariate to understand the impact on the time to event.

Problem: Do covariates including age, years smoking, blood pressure, heart rate, BMI, MMSE score, hypertension, and hypercholesterolemia affect the time to death?

Solution: Table 8.4 reports the mean of the posterior distribution, the relative risk (exp(mean)), and the 95% highest posterior density (HPD) intervals. Intervals that include 0 indicate that the covariate was not found to statistically significantly affect the time to death.

From the Bayesian Cox regression analysis, we identify age, years smoking, diastolic blood pressure, heart rate, and MMSE as statistically significant drivers of the time to death. While the 95% HPD interval for BMI does not include 0, the upper bound of the interval is close to 0. These results are consistent with the frequentist Cox proportional hazards model result. We fit the Cox regression model using a Bayesian approach in SAS, R, and Stata.

Table 8.4 Bayesian Cox Proportional Hazards Regression Posterior Summary

Parameter	Mean	e^{mean}	95% HPD Interval Lower Bound	Upper Bound
Age	0.037	1.038	0.032	0.043
Years smoking	0.012	1.012	0.009	0.014
Systolic blood pressure	0.000	1.000	−0.003	0.003
Diastolic blood pressure	−0.007	0.993	−0.012	−0.001
Heart rate	0.000	1.000	−0.004	0.005
BMI	−0.011	0.990	−0.021	−0.001
MMSE	−0.121	0.886	−0.127	−0.115
Diabetes	−0.097	0.907	−0.265	0.069
Hypertension	−0.021	0.979	−0.124	0.077
Hypercholesterolemia	0.003	1.003	−0.093	0.102

8.5.1 SAS Syntax and Output for the Bayesian Cox Regression Model

The SAS syntax follows:

```
¹PROC PHREG DATA=CHAP8;

²MODEL SURVIVAL_TIME*DIED(0)=AGE SMOKYRS BPSYS BPDIAS HRATE BMI
MMSE DIABETES HYPERTEN HYPERCHO;

³BAYES SEED=1 OUTPOST=POST;

RUN;
```

[1]The PHREG procedure is used to evaluate Cox regression models.
[2]The time to event (SURVIVAL_TIME) and the censoring variable (DIED).
[3]The BAYES statement invokes the Bayesian analysis. The SEED= option is used to select a random seed so that the results are replicated. The OUTPOST= option saves the posterior distribution samples in an SAS dataset (POST). A prior was not specified, so the uniform prior is utilized by default.

SAS OUTPUT

```
                        The PHREG Procedure
                        Bayesian Analysis
```

Model Information	
Data Set	WORK.CHAP8
Dependent Variable	SURVIVAL_TIME
Censoring Variable	DIED
Censoring Value(s)	0
Model	Cox
Ties Handling	BRESLOW
Sampling Algorithm	ARMS
Burn-In Size	2000
MC Sample Size	10000
Thinning	1

Number of Observations Read	16539
Number of Observations Used	12573

Summary of the Number of Event and Censored Values

Total	Event	Censored	Percent Censored
12573	1812	10761	85.59

Comments: The PHREG Procedure table reports information about
the dataset used (dataset name, outcome variable, censoring variable) and about the Bayesian estimation method. The Adaptive Re-
jection Metropolis Sampling (ARMS) algorithm is utilized. There
are 2,000 burn-in iterations, and 10,000 Markov Chain iterations
(MC Sample Size) are used for the analysis. There are 16,539 observations in the dataset; 12,573 are utilized in the analysis owing to
missing values. There are 85.59% of these records that are censored
(DIED = 0).

Maximum Likelihood Estimates					
Parameter	DF	Estimate	Standard Error	95% Confidence Limits	
AGE	1	0.037	0.003	0.032	0.043
SMOKYRS	1	0.012	0.001	0.009	0.014
BPSYS	1	0.000	0.002	-0.003	0.003
BPDIAS	1	-0.007	0.003	-0.012	-0.002
HRATE	1	0.000	0.002	-0.004	0.005
BMI	1	-0.011	0.005	-0.021	0.000
MMSE	1	-0.121	0.003	-0.127	-0.115
DIABETES	1	-0.094	0.087	-0.264	0.076
HYPERTEN	1	-0.019	0.052	-0.121	0.083
HYPERCHO	1	0.002	0.049	-0.095	0.099

Comments: The Maximum Likelihood Estimates table reports the estimates, standard errors, and confidence limits for the frequentist (maximum likelihood) estimation approach discussed in section 8.4.

Uniform Prior for Regression Coefficients	
Parameter	Prior
AGE	Constant
SMOKYRS	Constant
BPSYS	Constant
BPDIAS	Constant
HRATE	Constant
BMI	Constant
MMSE	Constant
DIABETES	Constant
HYPERTEN	Constant
HYPERCHO	Constant

Comments: The prior distribution assumes that for each regression the coefficient is uniform. Because no prior distributions were specified, by default the uniform prior is utilized for each covariate.

				Initial Values of the Chain					
Chain	Seed	AGE	SMOKYRS	BPSYS	BPDIAS	HRATE	BMI	MMSE	DIABETES	HYPERTEN
1	1	0.037	0.012	0.0004	-0.007	0.001	-0.011	-0.121	-0.094	-0.019

Initial Values of the Chain	
Chain	HYPERCHO
1	0.002

Fit Statistics	
DIC (smaller is better)	28382.86
pD (Effective Number of Parameters)	9.959

Comments: The initial estimates and fit statistics, posterior summary statistics, and HPD intervals are reported. The initial estimates are the initial parameter values used in the sampling approach. The Fit Statistics report the fit of the model. The fit statistics reported include the Deviance Information Criterion (DIC), a Bayesian version of the Akaike Information Criterion, and the pD, which is the effective number of parameters. The DIC can be used to compare the fit of two models, where a smaller DIC value indicates a better fit.

Posterior Summaries and Intervals					
Parameter	N	Mean	Standard Deviation	95% HPD	Interval
AGE	10000	0.037	0.003	0.032	0.043
SMOKYRS	10000	0.012	0.001	0.009	0.014
BPSYS	10000	0.000	0.002	-0.003	0.003
BPDIAS	10000	-0.007	0.003	-0.012	-0.001
HRATE	10000	0.000	0.002	-0.004	0.005
BMI	10000	-0.011	0.005	-0.021	-0.001
MMSE	10000	-0.121	0.003	-0.127	-0.115
DIABETES	10000	-0.097	0.086	-0.265	0.069
HYPERTEN	10000	-0.021	0.052	-0.124	0.077
HYPERCHO	10000	0.003	0.050	-0.093	0.102

Comments: The Posterior Summaries and Intervals table reports the model parameter estimates (mean), the standard deviation, and the 95% HPD intervals. Because the prior distribution is noninformative, the results are similar to those obtained with the standard PROC PHREG analysis in section 8.4.

Parameter	ESS	Autocorrelation Time	Efficiency
AGE	7971.7	1.254	0.797
SMOKYRS	8779.4	1.139	0.878
BPSYS	5027.9	1.989	0.503
BPDIAS	5121.2	1.953	0.512
HRATE	9537.5	1.049	0.954
BMI	8251.8	1.212	0.825
MMSE	9713.1	1.030	0.971
DIABETES	8554.3	1.169	0.855
HYPERTEN	7362.6	1.358	0.736
HYPERCHO	8660.4	1.155	0.866

Comments: The effective sample size for each parameter is reported. This is used as an indicator of autocorrelation if the effective sample size is much lower than the actual data sample size.

Comments: The trace plot for the covariate age (AGE) is given in figure 8.9. While the SAS output prints trace plots for each covariate, we include one trace plot for reference. Trace plots are used to assess the convergence of the Markov chains. The trace plot centers at the mean value is 0.037 for age. There are only small fluctuations in the trace plot (top plot), the autocorrelations are small (bottom left plot), and the posterior density plot appears to be bell shaped (bottom right plot). These are all indicators that the Markov chain converged, and so it is appropriate to interpret the posterior results.

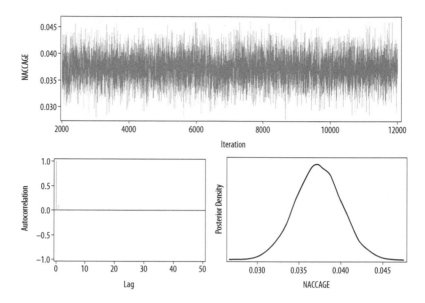

Figure 8.9 Diagnostics for age.

8.5.2 R Syntax and Output for the Bayesian Cox Regression Model

The R syntax follows:

```
1 library(survival)
2 library(spBayesSurv)
3 y <- Surv(chap8$SURVIVAL_TIME,chap8$DIED)
4 mcmc=list(nburn=2000,nsave=500,nskip=0,ndisplay=100)
5 bayescoxfit <- indeptCoxph(y~AGE+SMOKYRS+BPSYS+BPDIAS+HRATE+BMI
  +MMSE+DIABETES+HYPERTEN+HYPERCHO,data=chap8,mcmc=mcmc)
6 summary(bayescoxfit)

7 library(coda)
8 traceplot(mcmc(bayescoxfit$beta[1,]),main="AGE")
```

[1] The spBayesSurv library is used for the Bayesian Cox regression model fit. The survival library is needed to create the output variable using the Surv() function.

[2]The spBayesSurv library contains the indeptCoxph() function used for fitting Cox regression models using a Bayesian approach.

[3]The outcome for the analysis, y, requires time to event and the censoring variable.

[4]The indeptCoxph() function requires information for Markov Chain Monte Carlo (MCMC). We define the MCMC parameters using a list, and save it into the object mcmc. The list includes the number of burn in iterations (nburn=), the number of iterations to save (nsave=), a number related to the thinning interval (nskip=), and the frequency to display the current number of saved iterations number in the console (ndisplay=).

[5]We fit a Bayesian Cox proportional hazards regression model using the indeptCoxph() function. We specify the outcome (y, a function of the time to event and the censoring variable) and the predictors $(AGE + SMOKYRS + \cdots + HYPERCHO)$. The dataset is specified using data= statement. The MCMC settings are specified using mcmc=, and we set the settings to our list of saved settings (mcmc).

[6]Used to summarize the model parameter estimates (from the posterior distributions) after performing Cox regression using Bayesian estimation.

[7]The coda library is used to summarize and plot output from MCMC simulations. We load this library to produce trace plots for each of the covariates evaluated in Cox regression.

[8]The traceplot() function is used to generate trace plots. It produces a trace plot for the variable age (AGE), which is the first covariate listed in the analysis. To produce a trace plot for heart rate (HRATE, the fifth variable listed in the covariates), the code `traceplot(mcmc (bayescoxfit$beta[5],]),main="HRATE")` is used (the variable reference number in the model output and the variable name in the title were updated).

R OUTPUT

```
summary(bayescoxfit)
## Cox PH model with piecewise constant baseline hazards
## Call:
## indeptCoxph(formula = y ~ AGE + SMOKYRS + BPSYS + BPDIAS +
##     HRATE + BMI + MMSE + DIABETES + HYPERTEN + HYPERCHO,
##     data = chap8, mcmc = mcmc)
##
## Posterior inference of regression coefficients
## (Adaptive M-H acceptance rate: 0.104):
##                Mean       Median     Std. Dev.    95%CI-Low    95%CI-Upp
## AGE          0.0387116   0.0384343  0.0011105    0.0368475    0.0409512
## SMOKYRS      0.0102537   0.0102225  0.0003549    0.0096641    0.0108128
## BPSYS        0.0002411   0.0002278  0.0006322   -0.0010356    0.0013201
## BPDIAS      -0.0084329  -0.0083877  0.0008018   -0.0098212   -0.0068266
## HRATE        0.0008886   0.0009200  0.0002185    0.0004144    0.0011979
## BMI         -0.0110987  -0.0109108  0.0008560   -0.0127934   -0.0097646
## MMSE        -0.1184175  -0.1182942  0.0026587   -0.1238547   -0.1119211
## DIABETES    -0.1955612  -0.1906972  0.0302313   -0.2377181   -0.1350707
## HYPERTEN    -0.0289778  -0.0307356  0.0372677   -0.0956181    0.0395940
## HYPERCHO     0.0102557   0.0098375  0.0238408   -0.0331445    0.0467827
##
## Log pseudo marginal likelihood: LPML=-10884.65
## Number of subjects: n=12573
```

Comments: The R output for a Bayesian Cox proportional hazards model reports the mean, median, and standard deviation of each posterior distribution. The 95% HPD interval is used to determine statistical significance of each covariate. Using these results, we obtain similar conclusions to the previous frequentist Cox model fit.

8.5.3 Stata Syntax and Output for the Bayesian Cox Regression Model

The Stata syntax follows:

```
BAYES : STREG AGE SMOKYRS BPSYS BPDIAS HRATE BMI MMSE DIABETES
HYPERTEN HYPERCHO, DISTRIBUTION(WEIBULL)
```

STATA OUTPUT

```
(3,966 missing values generated)
        failure _d:  died
     analysis time _t:      survival_time
Burn-in . . .
Simulation . . .
```

Comments: The model details are given below.

```
                        Model summary
Likelihood:
_t ~ streg_weibull(xb__t,{ln_p})


Priors:
{_t:age} ~ normal(0,10000)                              (1)
{_t:smokyrs} ~ normal(0,10000)                          (1)
{_t:bpsys} ~ normal(0,10000)                            (1)
{_t:bpdias} ~ normal(0,10000)                           (1)
{_t:hrate} ~ normal(0,10000)                            (1)
{_t:bmi} ~ normal(0,10000)                              (1)
{_t:mmse} ~ normal(0,10000)                             (1)
{_t:diabetes} ~ normal(0,10000)                         (1)
{_t:hyperten} ~ normal(0,10000)                         (1)
{_t:hypercho} ~ normal(0,10000)                         (1)
{_t:_cons} ~ normal(0,10000)                            (1)
{ln_p} ~ normal(0,10000)
```

Comments: The prior probabilities are given for the parameters. We use a noninformative prior as normal with mean zero and variance 100^2.

```
(1) Parameters are elements of the          linear form xb__t.
Bayesian Weibull PH regression         MCMC iterations = 12,500
Random-walk Metropolis-Hastings sampling       Burn-in =  2,500
                                        MCMC sample size = 10,000
No. of subjects =   12573              Number of obs = 12,573
No. of failures =   1812
No. at risk      =  641429

                                        Acceptance rate = .3073
                                        Efficiency: min = .001776
                                                    avg = .005389
Log marginal likelihood = -3842.1231            max = .01224
```

Comments: MCMC settings are reported in the output (iterations = 12,500, burn-in = 2,500, sample size = 10,000) for the Bayesian Weibull proportional hazard (PH) regression. The output table reports the hazard ratios (exp(estimate), estimates are not reported), standard deviations, MCMC standard errors (MCSE), the median, and the 95% credible interval (lower and upper bounds).

	Haz. Ratio	Std. Dev.	MCSE	Median	[95% Cred. Interval]	
AGE	1.038	0.002	0.000	1.038	1.034	1.042
SMOKYRS	1.012	0.001	0.000	1.012	1.009	1.015
BPSYS	1.000	0.001	0.000	1.000	.998	1.003
BPDIAS	0.993	0.002	0.000	0.993	.988	0.998
HRATE	1.000	0.002	0.000	1.000	.996	1.004
BMI	0.990	0.004	0.001	0.990	.981	0.998
MMSE	0.884	0.002	0.000	0.884	.881	0.888
DIABETES	0.922	0.006	0.001	0.922	.911	0.933
HYPERTEN	0.981	0.006	0.001	0.981	.968	0.993

	Haz. Ratio	Std. Dev.	MCSE	Median	[95% Cred. Interval]	
HYPERCHO	0.997	0.003	0.001	0.997	.991	1.002
_CONS	0.000	0.000	0.000	0.000	.000	0.000
LN_P	0.899	0.012	0.003	0.900	.873	0.922

Comments: The output table reports the hazard ratios, which are exp(estimate) (estimates are not reported), standard deviations, MCMC standard errors (MCSE), the median, and the 95% credible interval (lower and upper bounds).

Note: _CONS estimates baseline hazard. Default priors are used for model parameters. There is a high autocorrelation after 500 lags.

8.6 Discussions and Conclusions

We fit survival analysis models to evaluate the time to an event. We reviewed methods to assess the time to event, as it is affected by several covariates. We use the semiparametric Cox regression models with the proportional hazard assumption. We also discussed the use of the Kaplan Meier method, a nonparametric approach to compare the survival time between two groups.

We used these survival models to analyze time to dementia diagnosis, concentrating on age, years of smoking, systolic blood pressure, diastolic, blood pressure, heart rate, BMI, MMSE, diabetes, hypertension, and hypercholesterolemia. We found that age, years of smoking, diastolic, and MMSE are significant predictors.

8.7 Exercises

Consider the time to death for patients in this chapter dataset (available at http://www.public.asu.edu/~jeffreyw/). The variable SURVIVAL_TIME is the time to event (death or censoring), and the variable DIED is the censoring variable (1 = death, 2 = censored).

1. Does the time to death differ among diagnosis groups (AD, DLB, FTD, VaD, and normal)? Which diagnosis groups have a significant impact on time to death?

2. Does the survival time differ significantly between men and women in this cohort? If so, which group has the longer estimated survival time?

3. Evaluate the impact of covariates including gender, race, diagnosis, and CDR-SUM score on time to death.

   a. Which covariates are statistically significant in affecting the time to death?

   b. Interpret the hazard ratios for each covariate. Which groups/values have an increased risk of death?

Chapter 9

Modeling Responses with Time-Dependent Covariates

9.1 Motivating Example

The regression models discussed thus far have been appropriate for the analysis of data with independent observations, or for data in which there is correlation on account of the repeated measurements. But it is common in longitudinal study data to have time-dependent covariates, or covariates that change values over time. As the covariate changes, one may be interested in understanding how the covariate values in a previous time affect the responses in a later time. Ignoring this relation affects the estimates of the standard errors, which in turn affects the test statistic and thus the conclusions regarding the significance of the covariate (Lai and Small 2007; Lalonde et al. 2014).

In this chapter, we fit two models to address such relations. We introduce the generalized method of moments (GMM) models to account for time-dependent covariates and revisit the generalized estimating equation (GEE) model (also discussed in chaps. 4 and 5). We also discuss the partitioned GMM model for addressing time-dependent covariates (Irimata et al. 2019).

We evaluate a subset of data from the National Alzheimer's Coordinating Center (NACC), which is the result of a longitudinal study of patients obtained across the United States. We consider a subset of 1,818 patients, each of which had four visits to one of 32 Alzheimer's Disease Centers (7,272 records). The patients have a mix of primary diagnoses, including 768 patients with Alzheimer's disease (AD), 24 patients with dementia with Lewy bodies (DLB), 14 patients with frontotemporal dementia (FTD), 74 patients with vascular dementia (VaD), and 938 nondemented (normal) patients. These data contain time-independent covariates such as age and time-dependent covariates

Table 9.1 Subset of Data

ID	ADC	Visit	Age	BMI	DIABETES	HYPERTEN	HYPERCHO	CDRSUM	DX_AD
000385	289	1	82	29.0	0	1	1	7.0	1
000385	289	2	83	29.0	0	0	1	5.0	1
000385	289	3	84	26.4	0	0	0	5.0	1
000385	289	4	84	29.0	0	0	0	7.0	1
000920	6061	1	64	25.8	0	0	1	0.0	0
000920	6061	2	65	25.8	0	0	1	0.0	0
000920	6061	3	67	26.3	1	0	1	0.0	0
000920	6061	4	68	25.7	0	0	0	0.0	0

such as BMI, diabetes, hypertension, and hypercholesterolemia (see section 9.2). The collection of responses over time introduces certain relations between covariate vales at present and those responses in the future.

In the NACC study data, we use models to estimate the Clinical Dementia Rating Scale Sum of Boxes (CDR-SUM) and the probability of an AD diagnosis while accounting for time-dependent and time-independent covariates. A subset of the data used in this chapter is provided (table 9.1), where DB = diabetic status, HT = hypertensive status, and HC = hypercholesterolemia status for 1= recent/active and 0 = remote/inactive/absent.

9.2 Background

The regression models used to analyze data in chapters 2 and 3 are appropriate for analyzing data with independent observations and time-independent covariates. By time-independent covariates, we mean that the relationship between the covariates and the outcome remains the same over the period of the study. Although the value of a variable such as age clearly increases as time increases, we do not expect that the impact of age will change as time increases, as age increases linearly with time. In chapters 4 and 5, we observed events repeatedly over time but concentrated on the inherent correlation among the responses and not among the covariate values and the future responses.

In this chapter, the GEE and GMM models address the changing values of the covariates. Time-dependent covariates are commonly encountered in longitudinal data and can have a significant impact on the results; hence these impacts should be accounted for in the model.

Initially, researchers addressed time-dependent covariates using GEE models with an independent working correlation structure (Pepe and Anderson 1994), as discussed in chapters 4 and 5. Lai and Small (2007) provided an alternative approach by using a GMM method to include the valid equations to estimate the regression parameters. The GMM approach relies on the identification of a set of valid moments conditions that are brought together to estimate the regression coefficients. One does not have to worry about the valid equations when fitting cross-sectional data, as all equations are valid (response in time t with covariate values in time t). It is the use of moments obtained on account of responses and covariates in different time periods that one needs to determine. Lai and Small (2007) developed a scheme to identify such valid moments by classifying each time-dependent covariate as belonging to one of three types. These types are distinguished on the basis of the type of correlation between the covariate and outcome across time. Lalonde et al. (2014) gave a method that allows one to question each component of the covariate with a later response rather than assume that the entire covariate is of a certain type. The method provided a test for identifying valid moment conditions. Both sets of researchers grouped all the valid moments equations into one, thereby obtaining a single coefficient for that covariate. Irimata et al. (2019) expanded on these methods to include a partitioning of the data matrix, which results in additional parameters to reflect the impact as the predictor changes over time.

While these methods have been readily accepted, they have not yet been fully implemented in common statistical software. In this chapter, we discuss the methods available at this time to address time-dependent covariates and discuss the available programs. The GMM model (Lalonde et al. 2014) is fit using R code (https://github.com /lalondetl/GMM) or through an SAS macro developed by Cai and Wilson (2015, 2016). The partitioned GMM model is available in an SAS macro (Irimata et al. 2019). These programs are designed to fit time-dependent covariates using balanced data, in which each patient has the same number of visits or measurements.

In this chapter, we demonstrate the fit of GMM and partitioned GMM regression models to evaluate CDR-SUM score and the probability of an AD diagnosis. In particular, we use GEE methods in section 9.3, GMM methods in section 9.4, and partitioned GMM methods in section 9.5.

9.3 GEE Model for Time-Dependent Covariates

We introduced GEE models for continuous data in chapter 4 and for binary data in chapter 5. These methods utilize a working correlation structure to account for the correlation between the repeated observations on the response. When longitudinal data include time-dependent covariates, however, Pepe and Anderson (1994) showed that the independent (IN) working correlation structure must be utilized to ensure statistical consistency. Although this correlation structure is obviously assumed when all observations on a given subject or unit are independent, the use of the IN structure provides a safe choice to ensure that certain assumptions are not violated. The fit of these models is similar to work demonstrated in chapters 4 and 5.

We consider a continuous response in this section and the binary response in the next. We model each patient's CDR-SUM score, a continuous response. We estimate this model using GEE with independent working correlation matrix to understand the impact of each covariate on the outcome with the use of SAS syntax (section 9.3.1).

Problem: How is a patient's CDR-SUM score affected by age, BMI, diabetes, and hypertension? The variables BMI, diabetes, hypertension, and hypercholesterolemia are time-dependent covariates.

Table 9.2 GEE Model Results

Parameter	Estimate	Std Err	p-Value
Intercept	−1.330	0.928	0.152
AGE	0.083	0.010	<0.0001
BMI	−0.056	0.018	0.002
DIABETES	0.487	0.330	0.141
HYPERTEN	−0.210	0.198	0.290
HYPERCHO	−0.060	0.184	0.743

Solution: We evaluate this question using a GEE model with an independent working correlation structure. The GEE model results are reported in table 9.2.

The GEE model indicates that age and BMI are statistically significant predictors of the CDR-SUM score. We find that diabetes, hypertension, and hypercholesterolemia are not significantly associated with the CDR-SUM score.

9.3.1 SAS Syntax and Output for GEE Model with Continuous Response

We use SAS PROC GENMOD to fit the GEE model to the continuous CDR-SUM score. We investigate predictors that are associated with cognitive and functioning ability. The SAS syntax and output follow:

```
¹PROC GENMOD DATA=LONGITUDINAL;
²CLASS ID VISITNUM(REF="1");
³MODEL CDRSUM = AGE BMI DIABETES HYPERTEN HYPERCHO;
⁴REPEATED SUBJECT = ID / WITHIN=VISITNUM CORR=IND CORRW;
RUN;
```

¹PROC GENMOD fits GEE models. The DATA= option is the dataset to evaluate.

²The CLASS statement specifies categorical variables, and the REF statement on the time variable changes the reference category to the first measurement instead of the fourth measurement (thus we compare all future visits to the first visit), which is automatically selected.

[3]The MODEL statement specifies the outcome and covariates (outcome = covariates).

[4]Measurement structure is within the time (VISITNUM) by subject (identified by ID). Select independent working correlation matrix (CORR=IND). CORRW prints the matrix.

SAS OUTPUT

Model Information	
Data Set	WORK.LONGITUDINAL
Distribution	Normal
Link Function	Identity
Dependent Variable	CDRSUM CDRSUM

Comments: The Model Information table summarizes the dataset being evaluated, the dependent variable (the outcome, CDR-SUM), as well as the assumed distribution and link function of the outcome (the default values are normal and identity, respectively).

Number of Observations Read	7272
Number of Observations Used	7272

Comments: We see that our dataset contains 7,272 observations, and because there are no missing values, all the observations are used in the model fit.

Class Level Information		
Class	Levels	Values
ID	1818	000385 000920 000959 001075 002171 002720
		002855 002865 004056 004683 005458 006029
		006035 007784 007824 007939 007962 008694
		008802 010063 010228 010492 010645 . . .
VISITNUM	4	2 3 4 1

Comments: The Class-Level Information table addresses the categorical variables and the number of levels or possible values in each.

Parameter Information	
Parameter	Effect
Prm1	Intercept
Prm2	AGE
Prm3	BMI
Prm4	DIABETES
Prm5	HYPERTEN
Prm6	HYPERCHO

Algorithm converged.

Comments: The Parameter Information table contains the names of the variables in the model and which parameters will be estimated. We obtained confirmation that the model converged, which means we can interpret the model results.

GEE Model Information	
Correlation Structure	Independent
Within-Subject Effect	VISITNUM (4 levels)
Subject Effect	ID (1818 levels)
Number of Clusters	1818
Correlation Matrix Dimension	4
Maximum Cluster Size	4
Minimum Cluster Size	4

Algorithm converged

Comments: The GEE Model Information table lists information about the correlation structure and repeated measurements. We evaluate 1,818 patients with multiple visits. We see that the minimum number of visits per patient is 4, and the maximum number of visits per patient is 4 (all patients have 4 visits).

	Working Correlation Matrix			
	Col1	Col2	Col3	Col4
Row1	1.000	0.000	0.000	0.000
Row2	0.000	1.000	0.000	0.000
Row3	0.000	0.000	1.000	0.000
Row4	0.000	0.000	0.000	1.000

GEE Fit Criteria	
QIC	7304.562
QICu	7278.000

Comments: The Working Correlation Matrix is printed with the CORRW option. Because we selected an independent correlation structure, the working correlation matrix is an identity matrix. The fit statistics Quasilikelihood under the Independence model Criterion (QIC) and the simplified QIC (QICu) are measures of the model fit and are used to compare multiple models.

			Analysis of GEE Parameter Estimates			
			Empirical Standard Error Estimates			
Parameter	Estimate	Standard Error	95% Confidence Limits		Z	Pr > |Z|
Intercept	-1.330	0.928	-3.148	0.489	-1.43	0.152
AGE	0.083	0.010	0.064	0.103	8.25	<.0001
BMI	-0.056	0.018	-0.092	-0.021	-3.09	0.002
DIABETES	0.487	0.330	-0.161	1.134	1.47	0.141
HYPERTEN	-0.210	0.198	-0.598	0.179	-1.06	0.290
HYPERCHO	-0.060	0.184	-0.420	0.300	-0.33	0.743

Comments: The Analysis of GEE Parameter Estimates table contains the regression parameter estimate, standard error, confidence inter-

Table 9.3 GEE Model Results

Parameter	Estimate	Std Err	p-Value
Intercept	−3.299	0.515	<0.0001
AGE	0.056	0.006	<0.0001
BMI	−0.046	0.010	<0.0001
DIABETES	0.103	0.156	0.510
HYPERTEN	−0.086	0.103	0.405
HYPERCHO	0.148	0.096	0.123

val, Z-value, and p-value for each parameter. We find that diabetes ($p = 0.141$), hypertension (0.290), and hypercholesterolemia (0.7433) are not significantly associated with the CDR-SUM score.

9.3.2 GEE Model for Time-Dependent Covariates
Binary Responses

In the previous section, we analyzed continuous responses. In this section, we use a similar approach but for binary responses. We consider each patient's probability of an AD diagnosis; a binary response is affected by the predictors.

Problem: How is a patient's probability of an AD diagnosis affected by age, BMI, diabetes, hypertension, and hypertension?

Solution: Since we recognize that the variables BMI, diabetes, hypertension, and hypercholesterolemia are time-dependent covariates, we use a GEE model (with an independent working correlation structure) to identify the factors associated with an AD diagnosis. The GEE model results are reported in table 9.3.

We find that the covariates age and BMI are significant drivers. Older patients are more likely to be diagnosed as AD. Patients with lower BMIs are more likely to be diagnosed with AD in this dataset.

9.3.3 SAS Syntax and Output for GEE Model with Binary Response

The GEE model is fit to predict the probability of an AD diagnosis using SAS. The SAS syntax follows:

```
¹PROC GENMOD DATA=LONGITUDINAL DESCENDING;
²CLASS ID VISITNUM(REF="1");
³MODEL DX_AD = AGE BMI DIABETES HYPERTEN HYPERCHO/DIST=BIN;
⁴REPEATED SUBJECT = ID / WITHIN=VISITNUM CORR=IND CORRW;
run;
```

[1]Using GEE, the DESCENDING option models the probability that
the outcome = 1.
[2]Specify the categorical variables ID and the visit number (VISIT-
NUM) using (REF="1").
[3]The outcome (DX_AD) and covariates (AGE BMI DIABETES HY-
PERTEN HYPERCHO). Outcome distribution is binomial (DIST=BIN).
[4]Subjects identify the cluster (ID). Repeated visits on each subject
(VISITNUM). Specify working correlation matrix (CORR=IND), the
identity matrix.

SAS OUTPUT

Model Information	
Data Set	WORK.LONGITUDINAL
Distribution	Binomial
Link Function	Logit
Dependent Variable	DX_AD

Number of Observations Read	7272
Number of Observations Used	7272
Number of Events	3072
Number of Trials	7272

Class Level Information		
Class	Levels	Values
ID	1818	000385 000920 000959 001075 002171 002720 002855 002865 004056 004683 005458 006029 006035 007784 007824 007939 007962 008694 008802 010063 010228 010492 010645
VISITNUM		4 2 3 4 1

	Response Profile	
Ordered Value	DX_AD	Total Frequency
1	1	3072
2	0	4200

PROC GENMOD is modelling the probability that DX_AD='1'.

Comments: The Model Information table indicates that we are evaluating a binary outcome variable with a logit link (logistic regression using GEE). There are no missing observations, so all 7,272 records are used in the analysis. There are 768 patients with an AD diagnosis (DX_AD = 1). There are 1,050 patients that do not have an AD diagnosis.

	Parameter Information	
Parameter		Effect
Prm1		Intercept
Prm2		AGE
Prm3		BMI
Prm4		DIABETES
Prm5		HYPERTEN
Prm6		HYPERCHO

	GEE Model Information
Correlation Structure	Independent
Within-Subject Effect	VISITNUM (4 levels)
Subject Effect	ID (1818 levels)
Number of Clusters	1818
Correlation Matrix Dimension	4
Maximum Cluster Size	4
Minimum Cluster Size	4

Comments: The Parameter Information and GEE Model Information tables summarize information about the model. We see that we are estimating six regression parameters for our covariates (Intercept, AGE, BMI, DIABETES, HYPERTEN, HYPERCHO). There are 1,818 patients, and each has four visits. We assume an independent working correlation structure, which is indicated by the identity matrix for the working correlation matrix.

| | | | Analysis of GEE Parameter Estimates | | | |
| | | | Empirical Standard Error Estimates | | | |
Parameter	Estimate	Standard Error	95% Confidence Limits		Z	Pr > |Z|
Intercept	-3.299	0.515	-4.308	-2.291	-6.410	<.0001
AGE	0.056	0.006	0.045	0.068	9.950	<.0001
BMI	-0.046	0.010	-0.066	-0.026	-4.480	<.0001
DIABETES	0.103	0.156	-0.203	0.409	0.660	0.510
HYPERTEN	-0.086	0.103	-0.288	0.116	-0.830	0.405
HYPERCHO	0.148	0.096	-0.040	0.335	1.540	0.123

Comments: The GEE output provides the parameter estimates, standard errors, confidence intervals, test statistics (Z), and p-values (Pr > $|Z|$) for each covariate. Age and BMI are identified as statistically significant predictors of an AD diagnosis.

9.4 GMM Model for Time-Dependent Covariates

While the GEE model with an independent working correlation structure (section 9.3) is a method for modeling time-dependent covariates in longitudinal data, it does not consider whether the moment conditions used to obtain estimates of the regression coefficients are valid.

When we deal with time-dependent covariates, there are certain relationships between the different time periods in the data that cannot be. There may be responses in one time period associated with predictors in an earlier time period. As such, not all the moment conditions are valid. This phenomenon, if not addressed, can produce inefficient estimates and less-than-desirable results. Lai and Small

(2007) addressed this issue with GMM estimation for continuous data. They utilized a three-type classification scheme, based on a relation between the predictor and the residual. But it is based on a group identification of the covariate's moments. Though this method was an improvement over GEE with an independent working correlation, the restriction to only three types of time-dependent covariates is at times too rigid and requires the user to identify the covariate type.

Lalonde et al. (2014) improved upon this approach of identifying valid moment conditions. Their approach does not require a grouping of time-dependent covariate's moments. Instead, they utilized a method based on bivariate correlations between the response and the covariate in each of different time periods. This allows one to evaluate each moment condition for validity. This approach eliminates the need for the researcher to identify which covariate type was most appropriate. This approach is suitable for both continuous and binary outcome data.

The GMM SAS macro is described in section 9.4.1 to fit the Lalonde et al. (2014) model. We apply the macro %GMM to evaluate the relationship between time-dependent covariates and the outcomes CDR-SUM and AD diagnosis.

Problem: What is the association between CDR-SUM and age, BMI, diabetes, hypertension, and hypercholesterolemia? How can we appropriately account for the time-dependent covariates BMI, diabetes, hypertension, and hypercholesterolemia?

Solution: The GMM model results indicate that all of the covariates evaluated are highly significant predictors of the CDR-SUM score (table 9.4). These results differ from the GEE results (table 9.3) that diabetes, hypertension, and hypercholesterolemia were not statistically significant. We find that incorporating the appropriate moment conditions accounts for the time-varying relationship of the predictors measures the varying impact of a particular covariates over time. The GMM approach examines the impact of different visits (evaluate

Table 9.4 GMM Model Results

Parameter	Estimate	Std Err	p-Value
Intercept	−0.875	0.021	0.000
AGE	0.064	0.001	0.000
BMI	−0.067	0.002	0.000
DIABETES	0.372	0.031	0.000
HYPERTEN	0.221	0.008	0.000
HYPERCHO	0.072	0.005	0.000
Visit = 2	0.570	0.013	0.000
Visit = 3	1.199	0.042	0.000
Visit = 4	2.070	0.164	0.000

effect of time) and finds that each time-point is statistically significant (table 9.4). We use the %GMM macro in SAS to fit a GMM regression models with time-dependent covariates to evaluate the CDR-SUM, a continuous score.

9.4.1 GMM SAS Macro

An SAS macro making use of PROC IML to perform GMM regression is presented (Cai and Wilson 2015, 2016). The macro facilitates the analysis of longitudinal data for both continuous and binary responses. It implements GMM linear regression and GMM logistic regression to appropriately account for time-dependent covariates (Lalonde et al. 2014). The macro is available at https://github.com /katherineirimata/TimeDependentGMM. The SAS macro is a flexible programming tool. Macros, such as the %GMM macro, allow statistical methods that have not yet been incorporated as official SAS procedures to be widely available to SAS users. It must be opened and loaded into each SAS session before it is called from the editor window. Carpenter (2016) gives a more in-depth discussion of the SAS macro language on this topic.

Our %GMM SAS macro is used to fit models with time-dependent covariates using a GMM estimation approach. It supports continuous and binary responses. The %GMM macro requires the macro %MVINTEGRATION (Cai and Wilson 2015), which calculates multivariate normal probabilities, to first be initialized (run in SAS). The

%MVINTEGRATION macro was adapted from an SAS/IML program by Alan Genz and Frank Bretz (Genz 1992, 1993). The macro runs using the SAS code:

```
%MVINTEGRATION(reflib=);
```

The macro option reflib is used to specify the file path at which to save a file (SAS Catalog of IML Modules). After the macro is called, the catalog will be saved in the specified file location (e.g., reflib="C:\User\Documents"). The GMM macro is called to load in the data and perform GMM regression for time-dependent covariates:

```
%GMM(DS=,
        FILE=,
        REFLIB=,
        TIMEVAR=,
        OUTVAR-,
        PREDVAR=,
        IDVAR=,
        ALPHA=0.05,
        DISTR=);
```

The option DS specifies the file location of the SAS dataset, listed in quotation marks (the SAS data file must be saved in a folder on the user's computer). FILE specifies the name of the SAS dataset saved in the folder in the DS location. The variables are specified using TIMEVAR (variable measuring time or visits), OUTVAR (outcome variable), and PREDVAR (predictor variables). The option IDVAR is used to specify the identifiers for the subjects (such as a name or ID number), which is numeric or characters. The significance level for the correlation test is given by ALPHA (typically we use 0.05). DISTR is used to specify the distribution of the outcome variable, and it has the options NORMAL (for continuous normally distributed variables) or BIN (for binary variables).

The %GMM macro produces output containing the regression parameter estimates (Estimate), standard deviations (StdDev), test statistics (Zvalue), and *p*-values (Pvalue). The macro output also includes the correlation tests between the residuals and the covariate(s) and identifies the valid moment conditions.

9.4.2 SAS Syntax and Output for GMM Model with Continuous Response

The syntax for fitting the GMM model to continuous CDR-SUM data in the SAS macro follows:

```
¹%MVINTEGRATION(REFLIB="C:\USER\DOCUMENTS\CHAPTER 9")
²%GMM(DS="C:\USER\DOCUMENTS\CHAPTER 9\DATA",
       FILE=CH5DATA_LONGITUDINAL_4VISITS,
       REFLIB=" C:\USER\DOCUMENTS\CHAPTER 9",
       TIMEVAR=VISITNUM,
       OUTVAR=CDRSUM,
       PREDVAR=AGE BMI DIABETES HYPERTEN HYPERCHO,
       IDVAR=ID,
       ALPHA=0.05,
       DISTR=NORMAL);
```

[1]MVINTEGRATION saves the catalog to the folder "CHAPTER 9" (using the specified path).
[2]The call to the macro GMM performs GMM linear regression for time-dependent variables, as the distribution is specified as normal (DISTR=NORMAL). The reference library for the catalog of IML modules is specified using REFLIB= (note that it is the same path as is specified in the %MVINTEGRATION call above). We are evaluating the impact of age (AGE), BMI, diabetes (DIABETES), hypertension (HYPERTEN), and hypercholesterolemia (HYPERCHO) on the outcome CDR-SUM (CDRSUM). We have repeated visit measurements (TIMEVAR=VISITNUM) on the patients who are identified by their ID numbers (IDVAR=ID).

SAS OUTPUT

		Outmtx		
	Estimate	StdDev	Zvalue	Pvalue
Intercept	-0.875	0.021	-42.235	0.000
AGE	0.064	0.001	44.475	0.000
BMI	-0.067	0.002	-43.401	0.000
DIABETES	0.371	0.031	11.847	0.000
HYPERTEN	0.221	0.008	26.815	0.000
HYPERCHO	0.072	0.005	13.862	0.000
t2	0.570	0.013	44.999	0.000
t3	1.198	0.042	28.747	0.000
t4	2.070	0.164	12.641	0.000

betavec								
-0.875	0.064	-0.067	0.371	0.221	0.072	0.570	1.198	2.070

Comments: For brevity, the integration, correlation test, and optimization output are excluded. We report the Outmtx and betavec tables. Outmtx contains the parameter estimates, standard errors, test statistics (Zvalue), and the p-values (Pvalue) for all covariates, including indicator variables for time. Betavec contains a summary of the regression parameters in a vector. Each column of betavec corresponds to the variables in the Outmtx table (i.e., Intercept, AGE, BMI, DIABETES, HYPERTEN, HYPERCHO, t2, t3, t4).

9.4.3 GMM Model with Binary Response

Problem: What is the association between the probability of an AD diagnosis and the covariates previously discussed? How can we appropriately account for the time-dependent covariates BMI, diabetes, hypertension, and hypercholesterolemia?

Solution: We fit the GMM logistic regression model to evaluate the probability of an AD diagnosis with time-dependent covariates (BMI,

Table 9.5 GMM Model Results

Parameter	Estimate	Std Err	p-Value
Intercept	−6.047	0.398	0.000
AGE	0.082	0.006	0.000
BMI	−0.009	0.001	0.000
DIABETES	0.007	0.005	0.215
HYPERTEN	−0.004	0.003	0.223
HYPERCHO	0.001	0.003	0.652
Visit = 2	−0.101	0.007	0.000
Visit = 3	−0.196	0.014	0.000
Visit = 4	−0.293	0.020	0.000

diabetes, hypertension, hypercholesterolemia) and time-independent covariates (age and visit) (table 9.5).

The GMM model to evaluate the probability of an AD diagnosis identifies age, BMI, and the three visit indicators (visit 2, visit 3, and visit 4) as statistically significant. Similar to the GEE results, GMM does not identify diabetes, hypertension, or hypercholesterolemia as having a significant impact on AD diagnosis over time.

9.4.4 SAS Syntax and Output for GMM Model with Binary Response

The syntax for fitting the GMM model to the probability of AD diagnosis data in the SAS macro follows:

```
1%GMM(DS="C:\USER\DOCUMENTS\CHAPTER 9\DATA",
        FILE=CHAP9,
        REFLIB="C:\USER\DOCUMENTS\CHAPTER 9",
        TIMEVAR=VISITNUM,
        OUTVAR=DX_AD,
        PREDVAR=AGE BMI DIABETES HYPERTEN HYPERCHO,
        IDVAR=ID,
        ALPHA=0.05,
        DISTR=BIN);
```

[1]We use the %GMM macro to perform GMM logistic regression. The outcome AD diagnosis (OUTVAR=DX_AD) is a binary variable

(DISTR=BIN). The SAS dataset chap9.sas7bdat is saved in the DATA folder (path specified using DS=). We evaluate the predictors age, BMI, diabetes, hypertension (HYPERTEN), and hypercholesterolemia (HYPERCHO).

SAS OUTPUT

	Outmtx			
	Estimate	StdDev	Zvalue	Pvalue
Intercept	-6.047	0.398	-15.205	0.000
AGE	0.082	0.006	14.430	0.000
BMI	-0.009	0.001	-8.204	0.000
DIABETES	0.007	0.005	1.241	0.215
HYPERTEN	-0.004	0.003	-1.218	0.223
HYPERCHO	0.001	0.003	0.452	0.652
t2	-0.101	0.007	-14.322	0.000
t3	-0.196	0.014	-14.483	0.000
t4	-0.293	0.020	-14.596	0.000

betavec								
-6.047	0.082	-0.009	0.007	-0.004	0.0012	-0.101	-0.196	-0.293

Comments: The %GMM output reports the estimated regression coefficients (Estimate), as well as the standard errors, Z-values, and p-values. We estimate the parameters for each covariate and three indicators for time (indicators for visits t2, t3, and t4).

9.5 Partitioned GMM Model for Time-Dependent Covariates

The partitioned GMM model assumes the relationship between each time-dependent covariate, and the outcome is not necessarily constant over time. In longitudinal studies with time-dependent covariates, this is a natural assumption, especially with regard to health. For instance, BMI may have a weak immediate impact on diabetes, but over time the impact may increase. The partitioned GMM model allows one to model the variation in the relation over time. It uses the methods of Lalonde et al. (2014) and Lai and Small (2007) to identify the valid moments. Each covariate yields more than one regression coefficient, based on the number of times the subject was surveyed.

The partitioned GMM model depends on T time periods (for our data, $T = 4$, as there are four visits) Each time-dependent covariate produces at most $T - 1$ regression coefficients of the general form:

$$g(\mu_{it}) = \beta_0 + \beta^{tt} X_i^{[0]} + \beta^{[1]} X_i^{[1]} + \beta^{[2]} X_i^{[2]} \cdots + \beta^{[T-1]} X_i^{[T-1]},$$

where β^{tt} denotes the effect of the covariate on the outcome when observed during the same time period, and $\beta^{[1]}$, $\beta^{[2]}$, ..., $\beta^{[T-1]}$ denote the lagged effects of the covariate on the outcome. For instance, $\beta^{[1]}$ represents the effect of the predictor on the outcome across a one time period lag, or equivalently when X is observed one time period before Y. The GMM method is used to obtain the regression coefficients.

Problem: Does the impact of covariate relationships on CDR-SUM change over time?

Solution: We evaluate the partitioned GMM model for the evaluation of CDR-SUM in terms of the time-independent variable age and the time-dependent variables BMI, diabetes, hypertension, and hypercholesterolemia. We use the Lalonde, Wilson, Yin (LWY) partitioned GMM approach. The parameter estimates, standard errors, and p-values are reported in table 9.6.

The model reveals regression parameter estimates and p-values for each covariate at the current time-point [0], one time lag [1], two time lags [2] and three time lags [3]. Age was considered a time-independent variable; therefore there is only one parameter estimate. BMI is found to statistically affect the CDR-SUM score for the current time period as well as for all three time lags. We also found that recent/active dia-

Table 9.6 Partitioned GMM Model Results

Parameter	Estimate	Std Err	p-Value
Intercept	−0.599	0.021	0.000
AGE	0.069	0.003	0.000
BMI [0]	−0.090	0.004	0.000
BMI [1]	0.015	0.001	0.000
BMI [2]	0.024	0.005	0.000
BMI [3]	0.027	0.007	0.000
DIABETES [0]	0.555	0.030	0.000
DIABETES [1]	0.083	0.008	0.000
DIABETES [2]	−0.161	0.008	0.000
DIABETES [3]	−0.423	0.005	0.000
HYPERTEN [0]	−0.242	0.038	0.000
HYPERTEN [1]	0.035	0.067	0.604
HYPERTEN [2]	−0.024	0.079	0.761
HYPERTEN [3]	0.121	0.042	0.004
HYPERCHO [0]	−0.162	0.030	0.000
HYPERCHO [1]	0.105	0.031	0.001
HYPERCHO [2]	−0.058	0.112	0.603
HYPERCHO [3]	0.132	0.046	0.004

betes is highly statistically significantly associated with the CDR-SUM score at all points. But we find that recent/active diabetes at two and three visits prior is associated with decreased CDR-SUM scores (toward normal cognition). Alternatively, recent/active diabetes in the current or previous time period is associated with increased CDR-SUM scores (indicator of dementia). This changing of relationship over time may have been the reason a relationship between diabetes and CDR-SUM could not be identified using the GEE model. The partitioned GMM model finds that recent/active hypertension in the current time period is associated with lower CDR-SUM scores, while recent/active hypertension three visits prior is associated with higher CDR-SUM scores. Recent/active hypercholesterolemia in the current time period, one visit prior, and three visits prior is also found to be a significant driver of CDR-SUM score. The GMM model provides a refined understanding of the impact of covariates on the outcome by identifying differential relationships at various time periods.

Problem: How do different factors affect the probability of an AD diagnosis over time? Does a low BMI at the first visit affect the probability of an AD diagnosis after four visits (approximately four years)? Is the impact limited to shorter time periods?

Solution: We used the partitioned GMM model to address the probability of an AD diagnosis and with predictors (age, BMI, diabetes, hypertension, and hypercholesterolemia) over time (table 9.7).

In the partitioned GMM model, age remains a significant predictor. We find that BMI is a statistically significant driver of the probability of AD diagnosis at all time periods. As BMI increases in our dataset, we find that the probability of AD decreases and continues to influence the probability of an AD diagnosis over time. The partitioned GMM model also identifies diabetes as a significant predictor at one and two time lags. Diabetes at one time period prior is associated with a lower probability of an AD diagnosis, while diabetes two time periods prior is associated with an increased likelihood of an AD diagnosis. Neither hypertension nor hypercholesterolemia

Table 9.7 Partitioned GMM Logistic Regression Model Results

Parameter	Estimate	Std Err	p-Value
Intercept	−3.389	0.373	0.000
Age	0.069	0.006	0.000
BMI [0]	−0.070	0.006	0.000
BMI [1]	−0.003	0.000	0.000
BMI [2]	−0.003	0.000	0.000
BMI [3]	−0.003	0.000	0.000
DIABETES [0]	0.102	0.096	0.287
DIABETES [1]	−0.043	0.017	0.011
DIABETES [2]	0.033	0.013	0.013
DIABETES [3]	−0.012	0.016	0.457
HYPERTEN [0]	−0.115	0.061	0.061
HYPERTEN [1]	−0.011	0.013	0.379
HYPERTEN [2]	−0.009	0.009	0.334
HYPERTEN [3]	−0.011	0.011	0.307
HYPERCHO [0]	0.091	0.055	0.099
HYPERCHO [1]	0.026	0.015	0.070
HYPERCHO [2]	0.012	0.012	0.319
HYPERCHO [3]	0.020	0.010	0.048

is identified as a statistically significant predictor for any of the time periods.

9.5.1 Partitioned GMM SAS Macro

The partitioned GMM approach is available in SAS through the %PARTITIONEDGMM macro produced by Irimata and Wilson (2018). The macro is available at https://github.com/kirimata /Partitioned-GMM. This SAS macro is suited to the analysis of either binary or continuous outcome longitudinal datasets, with equal numbers of visits for each subject. The macro allows for the use of either the partitioned LWY or partitioned Lai Small (LS) approaches for identifying valid moment conditions. The macro produces an estimate of the lagged regression parameters, as well as the standard errors, test statistics, and p-values. The %MVINTEGRATION macro must be initialized when the partitioned LWY model is fitted. The %PARTITIONEDGMM macro must also be loaded into the current SAS session before the partitioned GMM macro is used.

The %PARTITIONEDGMM macro has a number of options and defaults, which are adjusted to accommodate different data types. The macro takes the general format:

```
%PARTITIONEDGMM(
        DS=.,
        FILE=,
        TIMEVAR=,
        OUTVAR=,
        PREDVARTD=,
        IDVAR=,
        ALPHA=0.05,
        PREDVARTI=,
        DISTR=BIN,
        OPTIM=NLPCG,
        MC=LWY);
```

Many of the arguments in this macro are similar to those used in section 9.4.1. The DS argument is optional and is used to specify the folder of the SAS dataset to be analyzed. The FILE argument specifies either the SAS file within the DS folder or the dataset loaded in the SAS session to be analyzed. The argument TIMEVAR denotes the variable, which contains the time periods in the dataset. This variable must be numeric and contain sequential time periods. The next two arguments, OUTVAR and PREDVARTD, are used to specify the outcome variable and one or more time-dependent variables. The variable type for OUTVAR must be either binary or continuous, matching the argument for DISTR, which is either "bin" or "normal," respectively. Multiple time-dependent covariates are listed in PREDVARTD, separated by a space. The IDVAR argument is used to specify which variable contains the patient identifiers, which must be numeric and unique for each patient, while ALPHA is used to specify the significance level at which the moment conditions should be evaluated. By default, ALPHA is set to 0.05, and in most applications it need not be adjusted. The optional argument PREDVARTI is used to identify time-independent covariates, if any. The OPTIM argument specifies the optimization algorithm to be utilized and can take as arguments any of the optimization algorithms included in SAS IML. The last argument, MC, is used to select which moment condition check will be used. By default this is set to the Lalonde et al. (2014) approach, denoted by LWY, though the Lai and Small (2007) approach may also be used by changing this argument to LS. Irimata and Wilson (2018) provide a more in-depth discussion of the macro, as well as an additional example.

Once the %PARTITIONEDGMM macro is run, it produces as output estimates of the intercept, regression parameters for the time-independent covariates, and regression coefficients for the lagged time-dependent covariates. In addition to parameter estimates, the macro also produces estimates of the standard deviation, the Z-value for the test statistic, and a p-value, which is used to evaluate the significance of the predictor.

9.5.2 SAS Syntax and Output for the Partitioned GMM Model with Continuous Outcome

The SAS syntax for the continuous outcome in CDR-SUM follows:

```
¹%PARTITIONEDGMM(FILE=LONGITUDINAL2,
                TIMEVAR=VISITNUM,
                OUTVAR=CDRSUM,
                PREDVARTD=BMI DIABETES HYPERTEN HYPERCHO,
                IDVAR=ID,
                ALPHA=0.05,
                PREDVARTI=AGE,
                DISTR=NORMAL,
                OPTIM=NLPNRR,
                MC=LWY);
```

¹We perform a partitioned LWY approach using the %PARTITION-EDGMM macro. We evaluate the outcome CDR-SUM (OUTVAR= CDRSUM), which is a continuous variable (DISTR=NORMAL). Patients are identified by the variable ID (IDVAR=ID). The %PARTI-TIONEDGMM macro requires a numeric identification number for subjects. We consider the predictors age, BMI, diabetes, hypertension, and hypercholesterolemia, where age is assumed to be time independent (PREDVARTI=AGE) and BMI, diabetes, hypertension, and hypercho-lesterolemia are assumed to be time dependent (PREDVARTD=BMI DIABETES HYPERTEN HYPERCHO). We use the Newton Raphson ridge optimization method (OPTIM=NLPNRR).

SAS OUTPUT

Analysis of Partitioned GMM Estimates				
	Estimate	StdDev	Zvalue	Pvalue
Intercept	−0.599	0.021	−28.801	0.0000
AGE	0.069	0.003	22.249	0.000
BMI_0	−0.090	0.004	−21.134	0.000

	Estimate	StdDev	Zvalue	Pvalue
	Analysis of Partitioned GMM Estimates			
DIABETES_0	0.554	0.030	18.677	0.000
HYPERTEN_0	-0.242	0.038	-6.392	0.000
HYPERCHO_0	-0.161	0.030	-5.316	0.000
BMI_1	0.015	0.001	13.533	0.000
DIABETES_1	0.083	0.008	10.422	0.000
HYPERTEN_1	0.035	0.067	0.519	0.604
HYPERCHO_1	0.105	0.031	3.413	0.001
BMI_2	0.024	0.005	4.541	0.000
DIABETES_2	-0.161	0.008	-20.933	0.000
HYPERTEN_2	-0.024	0.079	-0.304	0.761
HYPERCHO_2	-0.058	0.112	-0.521	0.603
BMI_3	0.027	0.007	4.111	0.000
DIABETES_3	-0.423	0.005	-78.839	0.000
HYPERTEN_3	0.121	0.042	2.878	0.004
HYPERCHO_3	0.132	0.046	2.860	0.004

Comments: We exclude output related to the covariate types, optimization iterations, and moment conditions. We focus on the Analysis of Partitioned GMM Estimates table. This table reports the estimates (Estimate), standard errors (StdDev), test statistics (Zvalue), and *p*-values (Pvalue) for each covariate over time. The underscore followed by a number for each covariate indicates the time/visit lag. For example, BMI_3 is the parameter for BMI three visits prior.

9.5.3 SAS Syntax and Output for the Partitioned GMM Model with Binary Outcome

The SAS syntax for fitting the logistic regression model for AD diagnosis follows:

```
1%PARTITIONEDGMM(FILE=LONGITUDINAL2,
                TIMEVAR=VISITNUM,
```

```
OUTVAR=DX_AD,

PREDVARTD=BMI DIABETES HYPERTEN HYPERCHO,

IDVAR=NEWID,

ALPHA=0.05,

PREDVARTI=AGE,

DISTR=BIN,

OPTIM=NLPNRR,

MC=LWY);
```

[1]We use the dataset LONGITUDINAL2, which contains the numeric identification numbers (NEWID). We evaluate the probability of an AD diagnosis (OUTVAR=DX_AD), a binary outcome (DISTR=BIN), using the time-independent variable age (PREDVARTI=AGE) and the time-dependent variables BMI, diabetes, hypertension, and hypercholesterolemia (PREDVARTD=BMI DIABETES HYPERTEN HYPERCHO). We perform the partitioned LWY approach.

SAS OUTPUT

	Estimate	StdDev	ZValue	PValue
Intercept	−3.389	0.373	−9.098	0.000
AGE	0.069	0.006	12.326	0.000
BMI_0	−0.070	0.006	−11.466	0.000
DIABETES_0	0.102	0.096	1.066	0.287
HYPERTEN_0	−0.115	0.061	−1.878	0.060
HYPERCHO_0	0.091	0.055	1.649	0.099
BMI_1	−0.003	0.000	−8.051	0.000
DIABETES_1	−0.043	0.017	−2.553	0.011
HYPERTEN_1	−0.011	0.013	−0.879	0.379
HYPERCHO_1	0.026	0.015	1.813	0.070
BMI_2	−0.003	0.000	−8.566	0.000
DIABETES_2	0.033	0.013	2.474	0.013
HYPERTEN_2	−0.009	0.009	−0.967	0.334
HYPERCHO_2	0.012	0.012	0.996	0.319

	Estimate	StdDev	ZValue	PValue
BMI_3	-0.003	0.000	-8.107	0.000
DIABETES_3	-0.012	0.016	-0.743	0.457
HYPERTEN_3	-0.011	0.011	-1.022	0.307
HYPERCHO_3	0.020	0.010	1.975	0.048

Comments: The output reports the estimates, standard errors, test statistics, and p-values for each of the parameters. Because we are evaluating four time periods per patient, each covariate has estimates for the current time period and estimates for the three prior time lags. Age (AGE) is the only variable without lagged estimates, as it was assumed to be a time-independent covariate.

9.6 Summary and Discussions

In this chapter, we discuss the issue of time-dependent covariates in longitudinal studies. We present appropriate models for the analysis of such data. While a GEE model with an independent working correlation structure offers the most convenient approach for time-dependent covariates, it relies on all moment conditions to be valid.

The GMM models, Lai and Small (2007) and Lalonde et al. (2014), provided a means of identifying valid moment conditions but amalgamated the equations to produce one coefficient estimate for each covariate across time. The partitioned GMM model identifies valid moment conditions, partitions the coefficients, and provides differential interpretation across time. These models allow us to consider the complex relationships that arise in longitudinal data with time-dependent covariates. We apply these methods to dementia data by modeling the CDR-SUM score and the probability of an AD diagnosis.

9.7 Exercises

Using the data from this chapter, we are interested in identifying factors that are associated with recent/active diabetes. The dataset is located at http://www.public.asu.edu/~jeffreyw/.

1. Use time-dependent models to determine the impact of diagnosis (DX), BMI, systolic blood pressure (BPSYS), diastolic blood pressure (BPDIAS), and heart rate (HR) for patients with four ADC visits.

    a. Fit a time-dependent GEE logistic regression model.

    b. Fit a time-dependent GMM logistic regression model.

    c. Fit a partitioned GMM logistic regression model.

2. How do the model results in 1(a)–1(c) vary? Do any of the factors have a differential effect on diabetes over time?

Chapter 10

Joint Modeling of Mean and Dispersion

10.1 Motivating Example

Until now, we have concentrated on modeling the mean parameter of the distribution. This was the case when we fitted generalized linear models (GLMs) in chapter 3 and generalized linear mixed models in chapters 4 and 5, among others. In this chapter, we discuss modeling the mean and the variance simultaneously as functions of covariates. Previously, we either relied on the fact that the variance was constant or that the variance changed as a function of the mean. In this chapter, we address how nonconstant variance or how the violation of a variance assumption may affect the results of an analysis. We fit two submodels, one for the mean and one for the variance. We treat each of these submodels as a generalized linear model.

In chapter 3, we discussed GLMs where the mean of the distribution is explained through a systematic set of covariates with an appropriate link function. For example, we considered multiple linear regression models (a type of GLM with a normally distributed outcome and an identity link function) to address how a patient's age at death may be influenced by cardiovascular risk factors. We apply this technique to address the impact of cardiovascular risk factors on mean age at death (continuous response) and probability of an Alzheimer's disease (AD) diagnosis (binary response). We make some basic assumptions about the variance. In particular, we assume either that the variance was constant or that the distribution came from the exponential family. The former left no chance that the variance can change from subpopulation to subpopulation. The latter implies that the variance must change in accordance with the mean. In practice, however, these assumptions may not hold, and the variance needs special modeling. We discuss this phenomenon in this chapter.

Table 10.1 Subset of Data

ADC	ID	SEX	AGE	BMI	DX	DIABETES	HYPERTEN	HYPERCHO	AGEDEATH
8646	000731	2	82	33.80	1	0	1	1	84
1416	004864	1	80	33.50	1	0	0	0	81
8658	005734	1	76	24.90	8	1	1	0	77
6713	006109	1	73	27.20	8	0	1	1	75
4967	006556	1	60	25.60	1	0	0	1	63
8658	007556	2	74	25.50	8	0	1	1	76
490	007791	2	83	25.90	1	0	1	0	84
289	009523	1	83	22.20	1	1	1	0	86
6518	012692	2	89	24.80	1	0	1	1	91
4967	014469	1	68	27.10	1	0	0	0	77
8658	017390	2	85	21.30	8	0	0	1	87
289	018152	1	76	20.80	8	0	1	1	77

We demonstrate a fit of this joint modeling using data pertaining to 2,031 patients representing 33 Alzheimer Disease Centers (ADCs) from the National Alzheimer's Coordinating Center (NACC). For each patient, we have information on their baseline visit, which occurred between September 2005 and November 2016. A GLM fitted to these data for AD patients and normal subjects determined that body mass index (BMI), diagnosis, and hypertension were statistically significant predictors of age at death, while hypercholesterolemia and diabetes were not. While these results seem reasonable, a key assumption made in fitting the model is homoscedasticity (constant variance) across each subpopulation of the covariates (X). We found evidence that this key assumption may no longer be satisfied. We discuss how to address overdispersion or extra variation in the data by modeling both the mean and the dispersion. This method, the joint modeling of mean and dispersion, is one approach of modeling the extra variation. A subset of the data used in chapter 10 is displayed in table 10.1.

10.2 Overdispersion

Overdispersion is a term that describes excess variation in the data. Under a specified distribution, we expect a certain amount of variation in any statistical model. When there is greater variability in the data than expected, however, we refer to the data as being overdispersed.

Overdispersion is common in survey data and hierarchical data, where the data are not perfectly described by any particular known statistical distribution. Alternatively, underdispersion describes the case in which there is less variation in the data than expected. This is not frequently seen in practice, however.

Consider obtaining 100 observations from the subpopulations of X (ranging from 0 to 10) and the continuous response Y. A plot of the data, Y versus X, is given in figure 10.1a. It is clear that the variable Y has a linear relationship with the covariate X. This is an example of simple linear regression, as Y is assumed to be normally distributed, and there is homoscedasticity (constant variance) across all values of X. But if we repeat the exercise and obtain the graph in figure 10.1b, we see a deviation from the center as X increases. We refer to this as overdispersion. In these 100 observations, we notice that the observed values of Y are tightly clustered for small values of X, while there is a large variation in the values of Y for large values of X. This is a case of a heteroscedastic normal distribution, which violates the assumption of constant variance.

Figure 10.1 displays the same variance among the mean of the subpopulation. Figure 10.1b displays variance changing among the mean. Because the variance is not related to the mean in normal data, we

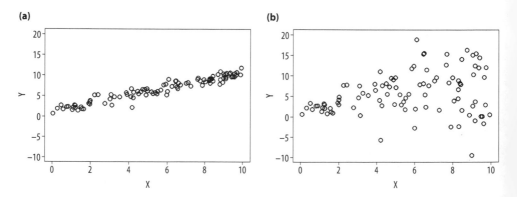

Figure 10.1 Plots of normal data (*a*) with constant variance and (*b*) with nonconstant variance.

usually encounter overdispersion in count and binary data. The Poisson distribution, which is used to model count data, is a member of the one-parameter exponential family. This distribution assumes that the mean and variance of the data are equal. When the variance is greater than the mean, we often refer to this as an overdispersed Poisson. In such cases, it is customary for researchers to utilize an alternative distribution for the data analysis. The negative binomial distribution is often used as an alternative to the Poisson distribution.

Similarly, for data following the binomial distribution, the mean and variance are related, as the mean is np and the variance is $np(1-p)$ where n is the sample size and p is the proportion, or the probability of the event of interest. When this relation does not hold, the overdispersed binomial is approximated using a beta-binomial distribution. The beta-binomial distribution relies on an additional free parameter that is used to address the overdispersion. We do not look at modified distributions to address the overdispersion; instead, we model the dispersion in the same light as we model the mean in a generalized linear model context.

10.3 Joint Modeling of Mean and Dispersion

In the regression models discussed in chapter 3, the focus is on modeling the mean. This is not uncommon, as researchers are often interested in understanding how the mean of the outcome is affected by one or more covariates. When the variance assumption is violated, however, the regression coefficients obtained are not efficient. Thus one must address the overdispersion. One approach is to model both the mean and dispersion. The joint modeling of the mean and dispersion, which is also referred to as a double generalized linear model (DGLM), simultaneously models the mean and the variance through the covariates using two GLMs (Smyth 1989).

10.3.1 Development of Joint Modeling

Pregibon (1984) introduced the possibility of jointly modeling the mean and dispersion through two GLMs. This was further explored through Efron's (1986) introduction of the double exponential family. One-parameter exponential family members, such as the Poisson and Bernoulli (described in section 10.2), require the variance to be a function of the mean. This is often violated in practice. Through double exponential families, Efron (1986) presented a second parameter to independently control the variance. This parameterization extended the use of regression to jointly model the variance dependent on observed covariates. Smyth (1989) also contributed to the development of joint modeling by parameterizing the dispersion submodel in terms of the deviance, a measure of dispersion in the data, and extending the technique to a class of generalized linear models.

Methods for accounting for heteroscedasticity and modeling dispersion have been explored extensively (Carroll and Ruppert 1982; Aitkin 1987; Davidian and Carroll 1987). Quasi-likelihood has been proposed as a method of modeling overdispersion in non-normal data (Lee and Nelder 2000). The quasi-likelihood model is an extension of the GLM, which relies on the specification of the mean-variance relationship (McCullagh and Nelder 1989). The flexible variance specification accounts for the dispersion in the model.

Researchers have also expanded the joint modeling method. Alternative estimation methods, such as trimmed likelihood estimation or maximum extended trimmed quasi-likelihood, have been implemented as an alternative to the maximum likelihood estimation to robustly estimate the model parameters and reduce the impact of outliers (Neykov et al. 2012). In addition, joint modeling has been applied to hierarchical settings (Lee and Nelder 2006). This extension, hierarchical double generalized linear models, allows random effects to be specified in the mean and dispersion submodels.

10.3.2 Joint Modeling Submodels

Joint modeling of mean and dispersion fits two interlinked submodels, one for the mean and one for the dispersion. Each submodel is a generalized linear model (chap. 3), and thus each model has random, systematic, and link components on independent observations.

Table 10.2, adapted from a table reported in a letter to the editor by Nelder et al. (1998), displays the components of the mean and dispersion submodels.

Table 10.2 summarizes joint GLMs for the mean and dispersion submodels. Each submodel shows the three components of a GLM (random, systematic, and link). We account for the variance through modeling the deviance d_i of the mean submodel. In the mean submodel, the three components are defined as summarized in table 10.2. The random component of the mean model is the outcome of interest Y, where $\mu = E(Y)$. This depends on the systematic component, which contains the set of covariates X and the mean regression coefficients β, and both the mean and systematic are connected by the link function $g(\cdot)$. The selection of the random component and the link function reflects the underlying distribution of the outcomes. The systematic component comprises covariates believed to have some impact on the mean response. For example, we may be interested in modeling an AD diagnosis in terms of age, BMI, diabetes (DB), hypertension (HT), and hypercholesterolemia (HC). The components of the mean model are defined in table 10.3.

In the dispersion submodel, the random component is determined using the deviances, d_i from the mean submodel, which has mean ϕ and variance $V(\phi)$. The deviances are modeled in terms of the covariates Z. The systematic component is flexible and can contain no covariates (intercept only), the same covariates as the mean model, a subset of the covariates from the mean model, or other covariates that

Table 10.2 Jointly Linked Mean and Dispersion Submodels

Component	Mean	Dispersion
Response	y_i	d_i
Mean	μ_i	ϕ_i
Variance	$\phi V(\mu_i)$	$2\phi_i^2$
Link	$\eta_i = g(\mu_i)$	$\eta_{d_i} = \log(\phi_i)$
Systematic	$\eta_i = \beta_0 + \beta_1 x_1 + \cdots + \beta_p x_p$	$\eta_{d_i} = \gamma_0 + \gamma_1 z_1 + \cdots + \gamma_k x_k$
Deviance	deviance, d_i	$2\{-\log(d/\phi) + (d-\phi)/\phi\}$
Weight	$1/\phi$	1

Table 10.3 Example of Mean Submodel

Component	Example Setup
Random	$DX\_AD_i \sim Bernoulli\ (p_i, p_i\ (1-p_i))$
Systematic	$\eta_i = \beta_0 + \beta_1 age + \beta_2 BMI + \beta_3 DB + \beta_4 HT + \beta_5 HC$
Link function	$\eta_i = logit\ (p_i)$

Table 10.4 Example of Dispersion Submodel

Component	Example Setup
Random	$d_i \sim \mathcal{D}_d\ (\phi_i, V_{di}\ (\phi_i))$
Systematic	$\eta_{di} = \gamma_0 + \gamma_1 age + \gamma_2 BMI + \gamma_3 DB + \gamma_4 HT + \gamma_5 HC$
Link function	$\eta_{di} = log(\phi_i)$

were not used in the mean model. Typically, a log link function is selected for the dispersion submodel (Nelder et al. 1998). For the example discussed above, we may be interested in investigating the impact of all of the covariates (age, BMI, diabetes, hypertension, and hypercholesterolemia) on the dispersion. Then, the dispersion submodel setup is presented as shown in table 10.4.

Each submodel is a GLM; thus the assumptions and model-checking methods apply to both the mean and dispersion submodel. The models are fit in an iterative process; hence the name joint modeling of the mean and dispersion. Joint modeling results in two sets of fitted equations with estimated regression parameters $\hat{\beta} = \beta_1, \ldots, \beta_p$ for the mean submodel and $\hat{\gamma} = \gamma_1, \ldots, \gamma_q$ for the dispersion submodel. This allows us to discuss the impact of covariates on both the mean and the variance of the data.

10.3.3 Advantages of Joint Modeling

In the analysis of correlated data, we focused on the modeling of the mean using appropriate techniques such as generalized estimation equations or random effects models, if the interest is only on modeling the mean. But one may use an alternative approach in the presence of significant clustering and a high intraclass correlation, the joint modeling of the mean and dispersion. Dispersion modeling has become increasingly common and may sometimes be the focus of the analysis in order to understand underlying factors that are associated with variation in the data as in reliability theory.

In addition to understanding the impact of covariates on the dispersion, an advantage of joint modeling includes efficient estimation. Correctly modeling the dispersion results in efficient estimation of the regression parameters for the mean submodel, while ignoring heterogeneity can result in a large loss of efficiency (Smyth and Verbyla 1999). Accounting for the dispersion through modeling also improves standard error estimates and confidence intervals (Smyth 1989).

10.4 Fitting Joint Modeling of Continuous Response

The two models (mean submodel and dispersion submodel) are interlinked, and thus the joint modeling of the mean and dispersion models are fit using an iterative procedure. The mean model is first fit using maximum likelihood. The deviance, a function of the residuals from the mean model, provides the outcome for the dispersion submodel. The dispersion submodel can similarly be estimated using a maximum likelihood approach through an iterative procedure. Successive iterations are used in the mean model, and weighted using the inverses of the fitted deviances. In each model estimation, the other submodel is fixed. Studies have suggested that two iterations are sufficient for fitting both GLMs, although this process is repeated until a specified convergence criterion is met.

Statistical software readily fits DGLMs and addresses the impact of many covariates on both the mean and variance. In SAS, PROC QLIM (qualitative and limited dependent variable model) fits models with heteroscedascity. The option HETERO within PROC QLIM is used to specify the covariates and the link function for the variance model. In R, the function DLGM (in the DGLM library) is used to jointly model the mean and variance, for specified systematic components and link functions for both submodels. The DGLM function in R is more flexible and is used in the analysis of a wider variety of statistical distributions.

We have information at baseline for 2,031 patients from 33 ADCs (1,681 patients clinically diagnosed with AD and 350 nondemented patients). We are interested in studying covariates that affect the age at death. We have evidence that there is overdispersion in the data, and so we use double generalized linear models to identify and address the excess variation.

Problem: Do BMI, diagnosis (AD or normal), diabetes, hypertension, and hypercholesterolemia explain the mean differences in age at death as well as the variance of age at death across subpopulations?

Solution: We begin joint modeling by fitting the mean and dispersion submodel with only an intercept term (no covariates) in the dispersion submodel. The mean submodel consists of covariates in BMI, diagnosis, diabetes, hypertension, and hypercholesterolemia. The "no covariate" approach addresses overdispersion. The parameter estimates for the mean and dispersion submodels are shown in table 10.5.

We find that BMI, diagnosis, and hypertension are significant predictors of the mean age at death. The intercept term for the disper-

Table 10.5 Joint Modeling of Continuous Response with No Covariates in Dispersion Submodel

Parameter	Mean		Dispersion	
	Estimate	p-Value	Estimate	p-Value
Intercept	92.07	0.000	4.63	0.0000
BMI	−0.30	0.000	—	—
DX = AD	−5.03	0.000	—	—
DIABETES	−1.01	0.211	—	—
HYPERTEN	3.89	0.000	—	—
HYPERCHO	0.01	0.991	—	—

Table 10.6 Joint Modeling of Continuous Response with Covariates in
Dispersion Submodel

Parameter	Mean		Dispersion	
	Estimate	p-Value	Estimate	p-Value
Intercept	91.89	0.0000	4.48	0.0000
BMI	−0.31	0.0000	0.01	0.0536
DX = AD	−4.45	0.0000	0.12	0.1377
DIABETES	−1.18	0.0750	−0.17	0.1262
HYPERTEN	3.85	0.0000	−0.49	0.0000
HYPERCHO	−0.18	0.6813	−0.29	0.0000

sion submodel is highly statistically significant, indicating that there is dispersion that must be modeled. Thus we fit a second joint model with the same covariates as in the mean submodel to determine whether any of the covariates contribute to the extravariation. The parameter estimates for adjustment to the dispersion submodel are reported in table 10.6.

We find that BMI, diagnosis, and hypertension are significant drivers of the mean age at death, although the parameter estimates now vary slightly after accounting for the dispersion through the covariates. In the dispersion submodel, hypertension and hypercholesterolemia are found to be significantly associated with the variance. Thus covariates affect the variance even if they do not significantly drive the mean (as is the case with hypercholesterolemia). One could further address these data by examining the impact of additional variables on the dispersion.

10.4.1 SAS Syntax and Output

Initially we fit mean submodels with covariates and the dispersion submodel with no covariate. The SAS syntax follows:

```
1PROC QLIM DATA=CHAP10;
2MODEL AGEDEATH=BMI DX_AD DIABETES HYPERTEN HYPERCHO;
3HETERO AGEDEATH~/LINK=EXP NOCONST;
RUN;
```

[1]PROC QLIM is used to model heteroscedasticity.

[2]The model statement is used to specify the mean model (random component = systematic component).

[3]The HETERO statement is used to specify the variance submodel (random component ~ systematic component). Because nothing is listed on the right-hand side of the equation, we are not considering any covariates for this model. The link function is specified as the exponential function, where it is defined as random component = EXP (systematic component). This is equivalent to the log link we use on the left-hand side. By default, the EXP link function is used in the HETERO statement. The NOCONST option specifies that there is no constant in the model.

SAS OUTPUT

The QLIM Procedure

Summary Statistics of Continuous Responses

Variable	Mean	Standard Error	Type	Lower Bound	Upper Bound	N Obs Lower Bound	N Obs Upper Bound
AGEDEATH	81.742	10.535	Regular				

Model Fit Summary

Number of Endogenous Variables	1
Endogenous Variable	AGEDEATH
Number of Observations	2031
Log Likelihood	−7579
Maximum Absolute Gradient	4.6731E-11
Number of Iterations	0
Optimization Method	Quasi-Newton
AIC	15172
Schwarz Criterion	15211

Algorithm converged.

| | | Parameter Estimates | | | |
Parameter	DF	Estimate	Standard Error	t Value	Approx Pr > |t|
Intercept	1	92.073	1.423	64.59	<.0001
BMI	1	-0.304	0.052	-5.90	<.0001
DX_AD	1	-5.025	0.598	-8.40	<.0001
DIABETES	1	-1.010	0.806	-1.25	0.211
HYPERTEN	1	3.892	0.482	8.08	<.0001
HYPERCHO	1	0.006	0.473	0.01	0.991
_Sigma	1	10.101	0.158	63.73	<.0001

Comments: PROC QLIM reports descriptive statistics for the outcome variable (age at death) as well as fit statistics for the joint model fit. The fit statistics include the log likelihood, Akaike Information Criterion (AIC), and Schwarz Criterion. We use the covariates BMI, diagnosis, diabetes, hypertension, and hypercholesterolemia to investigate the variance in age at death. The model reveals that BMI, diagnosis, and hypertension are significant covariates in explaining the variation in mean age at death. The model gives a constant variance of 10.10, which is statistically significant. We examine the impact of covariates on the variance as a further evaluation.

DISPERSION SUBMODEL CONTAINS COVARIATES IN THE MEAN SUBMODEL

We include covariates in the dispersion submodel. The SAS syntax follows:

```
PROC QLIM DATA=CHAP10;
 MODEL AGEDEATH=BMI DX_AD DIABETES HYPERTEN HYPERCHO;
¹HETERO AGEDEATH~BMI DX_AD DIABETES HYPERTEN HYPERCHO/LINK=EXP
NOCONST;
 RUN;
```

¹In this HETERO statement, we specify AGEDEATH ~ (covariates). This models the variance of age at death in terms of the specified covariates.

SAS OUTPUT

The QLIM Procedure

Summary Statistics of Continuous Responses

Variable	Mean	Standard Error	Type	Lower Bound	Upper Bound	N Obs Lower Bound	N Obs Upper Bound
AGEDEATH	81.742	10.535	Regular				

Model Fit Summary

Number of Endogenous Variables	1
Endogenous Variable	AGEDEATH
Number of Observations	2031
Log Likelihood	−7526
Maximum Absolute Gradient	0.018
Number of Iterations	53
Optimization Method	Quasi-Newton
AIC	15075
Schwarz Criterion	15143

Algorithm converged.

Parameter Estimates

Parameter	DF	Estimate	Standard Error	t Value	Approx Pr > |t|
Intercept	1	91.887	1.346	68.25	<.0001
BMI	1	−0.310	0.049	−6.29	**<.0001**
DX_AD	1	−4.454	0.538	−8.27	**<.0001**
DIABETES	1	−1.176	0.660	−1.78	0.075
HYPERTEN	1	3.849	0.466	8.26	**<.0001**
HYPERCHO	1	−0.185	0.450	−0.41	0.682
_Sigma	1	9.402	0.930	10.11	**<.0001**
_H.BMI	1	0.014	0.007	1.92	0.054
_H.DX_AD	1	0.124	0.085	1.47	0.142
_H.DIABETES	1	−0.173	0.113	−1.52	0.128
_H.HYPERTEN	1	−0.488	0.068	−7.18	**<.0001**
_ H.HYPERCHO	1	−0.294	0.067	−4.40	**<.0001**

Comments: We consider the impact of covariates in the dispersion submodel. The parameter estimates for the dispersion submodel are denoted with "_H." in front of the variable names. From the dispersion submodel, we identify hypertension and hypercholesterolemia as statistically significant predictors in modeling the variance of age at death. Thus there is significant dispersion in data unaccounted for through the mean model.

10.4.2 R Syntax and Output

Initially, we fit the mean submodels with covariates and the dispersion submodel with no covariate. The R syntax follows:

```
¹library(dglm)
²md <- dglm(AGEDEATH~BMI+DX+DIABETES+HYPERTEN+HYPERCHO,
           ~ 1, family = stats::gaussian, dlink =
"log",data=chap10)
³summary(md)
```

¹The DGLM library is used to fit double generalized linear models in R.
²The DGLM function in the DGLM library is used to perform joint modeling of the mean and variance. The first option specifies the mean submodel (random component ~ systematic component). The second option specifies the dispersion submodel (~systematic component). In this case, since the dispersion submodel is specified as ~1, we consider only an intercept term (no covariates). The FAMILY= option specifies the distribution of the outcome of interest (random component). The DLINK= option is used to specify the link function used in the dispersion submodel, and DATA= specifies the R data frame to access the data.
³The summary statement gives the joint modeling output (saved as "md").

R OUTPUT

summary(md)

```
##
## Call: dglm(formula = AGEDEATH ~ BMI + DX + DIABETES + HYPERTEN +
##      HYPERCHO, dformula = ~1, family = stats::gaussian, dlink = "log",
##      data = chap10)
##
## Mean Coefficients:
##                   Estimate Std. Error      t value      Pr(>|t|)
## (Intercept) 92.073450069 1.42766589 64.49229522 0.000000e+00
## BMI          -0.304408117 0.05167901 -5.89036313 4.501076e-09
## DX1          -5.025121204 0.59882945 -8.39157324 8.875454e-17
## DIABETES     -1.010090687 0.80707016 -1.25155252 2.108775e-01
## HYPERTEN      3.892100017 0.48268242  8.06347987 1.255659e-15
## HYPERCHO      0.005503452 0.47397147  0.01161136 9.907368e-01
## (Dispersion Parameters for gaussian family estimated as below )
##
##    Scaled Null Deviance: 2208.172 on 2030 degrees of freedom
## Scaled Residual Deviance: 2031 on 2025 degrees of freedom
##
## Dispersion Coefficients:
##                Estimate Std. Error z value Pr(>|z|)
## (Intercept) 4.625358 0.03138051 147.3959        0
## (Dispersion parameter for Gamma family taken to be 2 )
##
##    Scaled Null Deviance: 2682.845 on 2030 degrees of freedom
## Scaled Residual Deviance: 2682.845 on 2030 degrees of freedom
##
## Minus Twice the Log-Likelihood: 15157.83
## Number of Alternating Iterations: 3
```

Comments: In the DGLM output, the estimates, standard errors, test statistics, and p-values for the mean and dispersion submodels are reported (Mean Coefficients and Dispersion Coefficients, respectively).

These results indicate that the intercept term for the dispersion sub-model is highly statistically significant, and thus there is unexplained variation that needs to be accounted for. The model fit, including the deviance and −2*loglikelihood, are reported. We see that the joint models required three iterations to converge.

DISPERSION SUBMODEL CONTAINS COVARIATES IN THE MEAN SUBMODEL

We include covariates in the dispersion submodel. The R syntax follows:

```
[1]md2 <- dglm(AGEDEATH~BMI+DX+DIABETES+HYPERTEN+HYPERCHO,
            ~ BMI+DX+DIABETES+HYPERTEN+HYPERCHO,
            family = stats::gaussian, dlink = "log",data=chap10)
summary(md2)
```

[1]In this joint modeling fit, the dispersion submodel is specified in terms of the same covariates as the mean submodel.

R OUTPUT

```
summary(md2)
##
## Call: dglm(formula = AGEDEATH ~ BMI + DX + DIABETES + HYPERTEN +
##      HYPERCHO, dformula = ~BMI + DX + DIABETES + HYPERTEN +
##      HYPERCHO, family = stats::gaussian, dlink = "log", data = chap10)
##
## Mean Coefficients:
##                Estimate Std. Error      t value       Pr(>|t|)
## (Intercept)  91.8870944 1.34352915  68.3923341  0.000000e+00
## BMI          -0.3098851 0.04913776  -6.3064549  3.495410e-10
## DX1          -4.4543326 0.53597802  -8.3106628  1.721174e-16
## DIABETES     -1.1762419 0.66038910  -1.7811347  7.504031e-02
## HYPERTEN      3.8486723 0.46427441   8.2896500  2.042262e-16
## HYPERCHO     -0.1846590 0.44959831  -0.4107199  6.813214e-01
## (Dispersion Parameters for gaussian family estimated as below )
```

```
##
##     Scaled Null Deviance: 2215.435 on 2030 degrees of freedom
## Scaled Residual Deviance: 2031 on 2025 degrees of freedom
##
## Dispersion Coefficients:
##                Estimate    Std. Error    z value      Pr(>|z|)
## (Intercept)    4.4819005  0.199579236  22.456748  1.099475e-111
## BMI            0.0139443  0.007224419   1.930162   5.358677e-02
## DX1            0.1242639  0.083712811   1.484407   1.377010e-01
## DIABETES      -0.1725546  0.112823628  -1.529419   1.261606e-01
## HYPERTEN      -0.4882355  0.067476144  -7.235676   4.632168e-13
## HYPERCHO      -0.2935996  0.066258405  -4.431129   9.374089e-06
## (Dispersion parameter for Gamma family taken to be 2 )
##
##     Scaled Null Deviance: 2702.747 on 2030 degrees of freedom
## Scaled Residual Deviance: 2594.976 on 2025 degrees of freedom
##
## Minus Twice the Log-Likelihood: 15051.35
## Number of Alternating Iterations: 3
```

Comments: This second submodel, fitting covariates in the dispersion submodel, required three iterations to converge. We see that two covariates (hypertension and hypercholesterolemia) are found to statistically significantly affect the dispersion.

10.5 Fitting Joint Modeling of Binary Response

We consider joint modeling of the mean and dispersion models to model binary outcome data. We consider the 2,031 baseline visits for patients with AD diagnoses versus normal subjects. We wish to address covariates associated with an AD diagnosis.

Problem: Do age, BMI, diabetes, hypertension, and hypercholesterolemia explain the mean and the variation in the probability of an AD diagnosis?

Solution: We begin by first checking for overdispersion in the data. We fit the dispersion submodel with an intercept term. The parameter estimates for both submodels are shown in table 10.7.

The McKelvey-Zavoina (MZ) R^2 provides a measure of the fit of the data. It is computed as:

$$R_{MZ}^2 = \frac{\sum_{i=1}^{N}(\hat{y}_i - \overline{\hat{y}_i})^2}{N + \sum_{i=1}^{N}(\hat{y}_i - \overline{\hat{y}_i})^2}.$$

The covariate in the dispersion submodel has a value of -0.14.

The mean submodel results suggests that age, diabetes, hypertension, and hypercholesterolemia are significantly associated with the probability of an AD diagnosis. We find that hypercholesterolemia is associated with an increased probability of an AD diagnosis, while diabetes and hypertension are associated with a higher probability of a normal diagnosis. The intercept for the dispersion submodel is statistically significant, and we continue our analysis by finding informational covariates in the dispersion submodel (table 10.8).

We identify age, diabetes, and hypertension as significantly associated with the probability of an AD diagnosis, although hypercholesterolemia is no longer identified as significant (p-value = 0.05). In the dispersion submodel, we see that age and hypertension drive the variance of the outcome.

Table 10.7 Joint Modeling of Binary Response with No Covariates in Dispersion Submodel

Parameter	Mean		Dispersion	
	Estimate	p-Value	Estimate	p-Value
Intercept	6.46	0.000	−0.14	0.000
AGE	−0.05	0.000	—	—
BMI	−0.02	0.094	—	—
DIABETES	−0.44	0.014	—	—
HYPERTEN	−0.37	0.003	—	—
HYPERCHO	0.26	0.028	—	—

Table 10.8 Joint Modeling of Binary Response with Covariates in Dispersion Submodel

Parameter	Mean		Dispersion	
	Estimate	p-Value	Estimate	p-Value
Intercept	6.12	0.000	−2.30	0.000
AGE	−0.05	0.000	0.02	0.000
BMI	−0.02	0.098	0.01	0.104
DIABETES	−0.45	0.024	0.20	0.072
HYPERTEN	−0.38	0.002	0.20	0.003
HYPERCHO	0.24	0.050	−0.09	0.183

10.5.1 SAS Syntax and Output

Initially, we fit mean submodels with covariates and dispersion submodels with no covariate. The SAS syntax follows:

```
PROC QLIM DATA=CHAP10;
¹MODEL DX_AD=AGE BMI DIABETES HYPERTEN HYPERCHO/
DISCRETE(D=LOGIT);
²HETERO DX_AD~/LINK=EXP NOCONST;
RUN;
```

[1]As it is a binary outcome; we use the option DISCRETE in the model statement. Specify that we are using a logit link with D = LOGIT.
[2]We have heterogeneity, without considering the impact of specific covariates.

SAS OUTPUT

The QLIM Procedure

Discrete Response Profile of DX_AD

Index	Value	Total Frequency
1	0	350
2	1	1681

Model Fit Summary

Number of Endogenous Variables	1
Endogenous Variable	DX_AD

Model Fit Summary	
Number of Observations	2031
Log Likelihood	-885.970
Maximum Absolute Gradient	0.002
Number of Iterations	16
Optimization Method	Quasi-Newton
AIC	1784
Schwarz Criterion	1818

Goodness-of-Fit Measures		
Measure	Value	Formula
Likelihood Ratio (R)	94.792	2 * (LogL - LogL0)
Upper Bound of R (U)	1866.7	- 2 * LogL0
Aldrich-Nelson	0.0446	R / (R + N)
Cragg-Uhler 1	0.046	1 - exp(-R/N)
Cragg-Uhler 2	0.076	(1-exp(-R/N)) / (1-exp(-U/N))
Estrella	0.047	1 - (1-R/U)^(U/N)
Adjusted Estrella	0.041	1 - ((LogL-K)/LogL0)^(-2/N*LogL0)
McFadden's LRI	0.051	R / U
Veall-Zimmermann	0.093	(R * (U+N)) / (U * (R+N))
McKelvey-Zavoina	0.292	
N = # of observations, K = # of regressors		

Algorithm converged.

Parameter Estimates					
Parameter	DF	Estimate	Standard Error	t Value	Approx Pr > |t|
Intercept	1	6.463	0.716	9.020	<.0001
AGE	1	-0.054	0.007	-7.560	<.0001
BMI	1	-0.022	0.014	-1.560	0.118
DIABETES	1	-0.436	0.191	-2.290	0.022
HYPERTEN	1	-0.366	0.129	-2.830	0.005
HYPERCHO	1	0.263	0.128	2.060	0.040

Comments: The mean submodel suggests that age, diabetes, and hypertension are significant in modeling the mean. The goodness-of-fit measures give some idea of the model fit but must be compared to some distribution.

DISPERSION SUBMODEL CONTAINS COVARIATES IN THE MEAN SUBMODEL

We include covariates in the dispersion submodel. The SAS syntax follows:

```
PROC QLIM DATA=CHAP10;
MODEL DX_AD=AGE BMI DIABETES HYPERTEN HYPERCHO/
DISCRETE(D=LOGIT);
¹HETERO DX_AD~AGE BMI DIABETES HYPERTEN HYPERCHO/ LINK=EXP
NOCONST;
RUN;
```

[1]We address the heterogeneity for this binary outcome example in terms of the covariates used in the mean submodel.

SAS OUTPUT

The QLIM Procedure

Discrete Response Profile of DX_AD

Index	Value	Total Frequency
1	0	350
2	1	1681

Model Fit Summary

Number of Endogenous Variables	1
Endogenous Variable	DX_AD
Number of Observations	2031
Log Likelihood	−883.468
Maximum Absolute Gradient	0.001
Number of Iterations	140

Optimization Method	Quasi-Newton
AIC	1789
Schwarz Criterion	1851

Goodness-of-Fit Measures		
Measure	Value	Formula
Likelihood Ratio (R)	99.795	2 * (LogL - LogL0)
Upper Bound of R (U)	1866.700	-2 * LogL0
Aldrich-Nelson	0.047	R / (R + N)
Cragg-Uhler 1w	0.048	1 - exp(-R/N)
Cragg-Uhler 2	0.080	(1-exp(-R/N)) / (1-exp(-U/N))
Estrella	0.049	1 - (1-R/U)^(U/N)
Adjusted Estrella	0.038	1 - ((LogL-K)/LogL0)^(-2/N*LogL0)
McFadden's LRI	0.054	R / U
Veall-Zimmermann	0.098	(R * (U+N)) / (U * (R+N))
McKelvey-Zavoina	0.258	

N = # of observations, K = # of regressors

Algorithm converged

Parameter Estimates				
Parameter	DF	Estimate	Standard Error	t Value	Approx Pr > |t|
Intercept	1	5.130	2.532	2.030	0.043
AGE	1	-0.053	0.030	-1.780	0.075
BMI	1	0.009	0.029	0.320	0.749
DIABETES	1	-0.381	0.423	-0.900	0.368
HYPERTEN	1	-0.082	0.232	-0.350	0.723
HYPERCHO	1	0.214	0.294	0.730	0.467
_H.AGE	1	-0.025	0.011	-2.170	0.030
_H.BMI	1	0.041	0.039	1.050	0.294
_H.DIABETES	1	-0.111	0.735	-0.150	0.880
_H.HYPERTEN	1	0.359	0.441	0.810	0.415
_H.HYPERCHO	1	0.116	0.478	0.240	0.808

Comments: The joint modeling model estimates are reported in the Parameter Estimates table. From the heteroscedasticity model parameters (_H.), we see that age is significantly associated with the variance of the probability of an AD diagnosis.

10.5.2 R Syntax and Output

Initially, we fit mean submodels with covariates and dispersion submodels with no covariate. The R syntax follows:

```
library(dglm)
```

```
¹md3 <- dglm(DX_AD~AGE+BMI+DIABETES+HYPERTEN+HYPERCHO,
            ~ 1, family = stats::binomial, dlink =
"log",data=chap10)
summary(md3)
```

[1]We specify the DGLM options as usual. For binary outcome data, we specify that the statistical distribution is binomial using the family= option.

R OUTPUT

```
summary(md3)
##
## Call: dglm(formula = DX_AD ~ AGE + BMI + DIABETES + HYPERTEN +
##      HYPERCHO, dformula = ~1, family = stats::binomial, dlink = "log",
##      data = chap10)
##
## Mean Coefficients:
##                   Estimate   Std. Error     z value      Pr(>|z|)
## (Intercept)     6.46322039  0.669082972    9.659819  4.466525e-22
## AGE            -0.05358013  0.006618273   -8.095786  5.689577e-16
## BMI            -0.02169973  0.012965198   -1.673690  9.419149e-02
## DIABETES       -0.43590417  0.178077787   -2.447830  1.437194e-02
## HYPERTEN       -0.36574409  0.120918173   -3.024724  2.488602e-03
## HYPERCHO        0.26263556  0.119360645    2.200353  2.778186e-02
```

```
## (Dispersion Parameters for binomial family estimated as below )
##
##    Scaled Null Deviance: 2139.651 on 2030 degrees of freedom
## Scaled Residual Deviance: 2031 on 2025 degrees of freedom
##
## Dispersion Coefficients:
##               Estimate Std. Error    z value     Pr(>|z|)
## (Intercept) -0.1364533 0.03138051  -4.348346 1.371678e-05
## (Dispersion parameter for Gamma family taken to be 2 )
##
##    Scaled Null Deviance: 1259.64 on 2030 degrees of freedom
## Scaled Residual Deviance: 1259.64 on 2030 degrees of freedom
##
## Minus Twice the Log-Likelihood: 1753.863
## Number of Alternating Iterations: 5
```

Comments: The joint modeling parameter estimates for the mean and dispersion submodels are reported. We have evidence of significant overdispersion in the data owing to the statistically significant intercept in the dispersion submodel. We find that the binary outcome model requires five iterations to converge.

DISPERSION SUBMODEL CONTAINS COVARIATES

We include covariates in the dispersion submodel. The R syntax follows:

```
[1]md4 <- dglm(DX_AD~AGE+BMI+DIABETES+HYPERTEN+HYPERCHO,
            ~ AGE+BMI+DIABETES+HYPERTEN+HYPERCHO,
            family = stats::binomial, dlink =
"log",data=chap10)
summary(md4)
```

[1]We address joint modeling of the mean and dispersion using the DGLM function. We consider a binary outcome, and we model the variance in terms of the specified set of covariates.

R OUTPUT

summary(md4)

```
##
## Call: dglm(formula = DX_AD ~ AGE + BMI + DIABETES + HYPERTEN +
##      HYPERCHO, dformula = ~AGE + BMI + DIABETES +
##      HYPERTEN + HYPERCHO, family = stats::binomial, dlink = "log",
##      data = chap10)
##
## Mean Coefficients:
##                 Estimate  Std. Error   z value    Pr(>|z|)
## (Intercept)    6.12016828 0.615822819  9.938197 2.839203e-23
## AGE           -0.04891478 0.006028615 -8.113769 4.907353e-16
## BMI           -0.02193412 0.013251095 -1.655269 9.787000e-02
## DIABETES      -0.44647570 0.198154301 -2.253172 2.424831e-02
## HYPERTEN      -0.37990137 0.123128346 -3.085410 2.032721e-03
## HYPERCHO       0.23603151 0.120459130  1.959432 5.006218e-02
## (Dispersion Parameters for binomial family estimated as below )
##
##      Scaled Null Deviance: 2141.607 on 2030 degrees of freedom
## Scaled Residual Deviance: 2031 on 2025 degrees of freedom
##
## Dispersion Coefficients:
##                 Estimate  Std. Error   z value    Pr(>|z|)
## (Intercept)   -2.30198361 0.319500868 -7.204937 5.807071e-13
## AGE            0.02271774 0.003094511  7.341302 2.115267e-13
## BMI            0.01187978 0.007301892  1.626946 1.037486e-01
## DIABETES       0.20293576 0.112689657  1.800838 7.172849e-02
## HYPERTEN       0.20162040 0.068593076  2.939370 3.288807e-03
## HYPERCHO      -0.08810591 0.066175761 -1.331392 1.830599e-01
## (Dispersion parameter for Gamma family taken to be 2 )
##
##      Scaled Null Deviance: 1234.482 on 2030 degrees of freedom
## Scaled Residual Deviance: 1151.197 on 2025 degrees of freedom
```

```
##
## Minus Twice the Log-Likelihood: 1671.227
## Number of Alternating Iterations: 5
```

Comments: The dispersion submodel with covariates requires five iterations to converge. We find that age and hypertension are significantly associated with increased variation in the data.

10.6 Summary and Discussions

In this chapter, we introduce the concept of joint models to model overdispersion. While a key assumption in linear regression is homoscedasticity, it is possible for heteroscedascity to be present in the data. The joint modeling of the mean and the dispersion is one approach to address extra variation through covariates to model the dispersion submodel. We address a subset of data obtained from NACC and identify factors that contributed to modeling the dispersion in the age at death and also the probability of AD diagnosis.

The joint modeling of the mean and the dispersion has an added benefit. It reduces the amount of unexplained variation by modeling first the mean and then the dispersion. We conclude that the joint model of the mean and the dispersion (Smyth 1989) was a much better fit for the data compared to the logistic regression model (Agresti 1990).

10.7 Exercises

Consider the data modeled using a logistic regression model in chapter 2 (http://www.public.asu.edu/~jeffreyw/). There are 2,031 AD patients and normal subjects used in identifying covariates associated with diabetes. We considered the predictors diagnosis (DX), BMI, systolic blood pressure (BPSYS), diastolic blood pressure (BPDIAS), and heart rate (HR) and obtained the following model fit:

$$\log\left(\frac{\hat{p}_{DB}}{1-\hat{p}_{DB}}\right) = -5.73 - 0.34\text{DX} + 0.12\text{BMI} + 0.02\text{BPSYS}$$
$$- 0.05\text{BPDIAS} + 0.02\text{HR},$$

where BMI, BPSYS, BPDIAS, and HR were identified as statistically significant.

1. Model the probability of diabetes using logistic regression with the covariates above, and verify that you obtain the same parameter estimates.
2. Use joint modeling of the mean and dispersion with an intercept term for the dispersion submodel (no covariates), and identify if there is constant excess variation present in the data. Interpret the findings.
3. Use joint modeling of the mean and dispersion, and address the dispersion submodel with the same covariates used in the mean submodel. Which covariates, if any, contribute to excess variation?
4. Select additional covariates from the dataset that were not addressed in the mean model. Are any of these statistically significant drivers of the dispersion?
5. In the DGLMs fit in exercises 3 and 4, does the significance of any of the covariates in the mean submodel vary compared to exercise 1?

Chapter 11

Neural Networks and Other Machine Learning Techniques for Big Data

11.1 Motivating Example

Artificial neural networks (ANNs), as well as regression and other machine learning methods, are often the models of choice in health and health-related research. A neural network is a method used to identify relationships between connected input and output variables. Neural networks (NNs) use nonlinear functions to connect each layer, and each connection has a corresponding weight. This method of analysis is particularly effective for prediction when interpretation is not necessary, and it is currently one of the most popular data mining tools available (Zhao 2012).

In health and health-related studies, decision-making processes often require reliable statistical models. Health management specialists need simple and accurate estimation techniques to predict patient outcomes in the hospital planning process. Traditionally, logistic regression and ANNs have been used for predictions and classifications.

In chapters 2, 3, and 4, we employed regression models for the prediction of dementia subtypes. Because of the linear relationship in the parameters, however, regression models may not provide accurate predictions in complex situations, including cases of nonlinear outcomes and extreme values. In the use of regression models, there are certain distributional assumptions, such as no multicollinearity among the covariates. Violation of model assumptions and of certain model characteristics often leads to inefficient estimates (Neter and Wasserman 1974). In the study of many diseases, the presence of the disease is influenced by many interrelated factors, and it is sometimes difficult to describe their relationships using conventional methods. Thus artificial neural networks are highly recommended to identify the complicated relations and strong nonlinearity between different parameters and diseases. Many researchers consider ANN to be one of the best techniques for extracting information from nonlinear data. But the use of neural network methods is an important tool for a wide variety of applications across many disciplines, including prediction of dementia diseases where traditional statistical techniques are used.

In this chapter, we revisit the dataset consisting of baseline visits for patients in Alzheimer's Disease Center (ADC) 4967 that was previously assessed in chapter 3. These data contain 761 records for patients with visits between October 2005 and April 2014. While these data contain only 761 records, which is relatively small, we use this as a starting point to introduce the following concepts, which can be applied to much larger data.

11.2 Neural Network Models

Neural networks have become increasingly popular. NNs can be supervised models and are used to determine an outcome of interest given a specified number of inputs (covariates of interest). The number of outputs is based on the number of values we are seeking to predict or classify. A single output corresponds to regression, in which we use specified covariates of interest to predict one outcome of interest (Hastie et al. 2009).

The idea was inspired by biological neural networks in which neurons in the brain are connected by synapses and can process signals. Similarly, artificial neurons in a neural network are connected by some number of connections, referred to as edges. Weights are used in the calculation, and they are adjusted during the fitting of the neural network. There are one or more hidden layers between the inputs and outputs, which contain the artificial neurons. The user selects the number of hidden layers. Increasing the number of hidden layers increases the complexity of the neural network. In addition, the user specifies the number of neurons within each hidden layer. Figure 11.1 shows an example of a neural network structure. There is one hidden layer with four neurons. The arrows on the edges indicate the flow

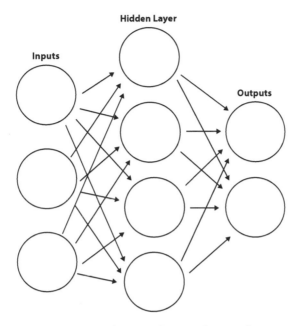

Figure 11.1 Diagram of a neural network.

of the data from the three inputs, to the hidden layer, to the two outputs.

The use of regression and neural network methods has been seen as competing with model-building methods (Eftekhar et al. 2005). Neural network methods have largely been used in the areas of prediction and classification (Warner and Misra 1996). Neural network models are also preferred in the area of pattern recognition (Setyawati et al. 2002). Many papers have been written about the relationship between NNs and statistical models (Ripley 1994). Cheng and Titterington (1994) provided a complete analysis and comparison of different network techniques with traditional statistical techniques and showed the strong association between NNs and discriminant analysis. Schumacher et al. (1996) compared NNs and logistic regression and analyzed the similarities and dissimilarities. Warner and Misra (1996) compared the performances of regression analysis and neural networks using simulated data from known functions and real-world problems.

Several authors presented cases where it would be advantageous to use neural network models in place of parametric regression models. Others have compared regression analysis with neural networks in terms of notation and implementation. Ripley (1994) presented the statistical aspects of NNs and classified them as one of the flexible nonlinear regression methods. In this chapter, we review and compare NNs with standard logistic regression techniques used for prediction of dementia diseases. When comparing methods, one should look at a number of factors, including size of the data, selection of model, validation methods, assumptions, and significant differences.

Section 11.3 provides a brief introduction to the terminologies used with neural networks, as well as a comparison of neural network and statistical model terminology. Section 11.4 presents analyses, and section 11.5 presents summary and findings in tabular form. Section 11.8 concludes the chapter with a brief discussion of some issues relating to neural networks and statistical techniques.

11.3 Terminologies in Neural Networks

Neural network models are similar to some statistical models; however, the terminology used in the NN literature is totally different from that used in statistics (Sarle 1994). These terminologies are shown in table 11.1 and reproduced from Paswan and Begum (2013).

A comparison of logistic regression models with neural network structures is well documented (Sarle 1994). A perceptron is a simple type of NN that obtains a linear combination of the inputs with a bias referred to as the net input. The output is obtained by applying an activation function to the net input. The activation functions are: linear (identity) function, hyperbolic tangent, logistic (sigmoidal), threshold, and Gaussian function. A perceptron consists of one or more outputs. Each output has a separate bias and a set of weights. It is usually the case that the same activation function is used for each output, though different activation functions are sometimes used. Perceptrons are trained through the least squares procedure, which is the minimization of the sum of squared errors over all outputs and over the training sets. As such, when a perceptron has a linear activation

Table 11.1 Terminology in Neural Networks versus Statistical Methods

Neural Network	Statistical Methods
Features	Variables
Inputs	Independent variables
Outputs	Predicted variables
Targets or training values	Dependent variables
Errors	Residuals
Training, learning, adaptation, or self-organization	Estimation
Error function, cost function, or Lyapunov function	Estimation criteria
Patterns or training pairs	Observations
Weights (synaptic)	Parameter estimate
Higher-order neurons	Interactions
Functional links	Transformations
Supervised learning or heteroassociation	Regression or discriminant analysis
Unsupervised learning, encoding, or autoassociation	Data reduction
Competitive learning or adaptive vector quantization	Cluster analysis
Generalization	Interpolation

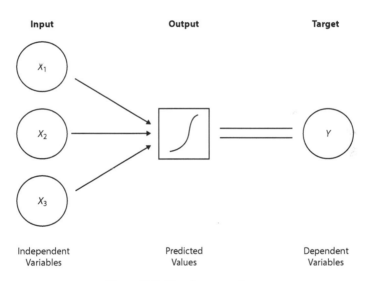

Figure 11.2 Simple perceptron.

function, it is the same as using a linear regression model (Weisberg 1985; Myers 1986). A perceptron with a logistic activation function is equivalent to a logistic regression model (Hosmer and Lemeshow 1989), which is depicted in figure 11.2 as simple nonlinear perceptron.

A model is nonlinear if it considers estimated weights between inputs and the hidden layer, and the hidden layer uses a nonlinear activation function like the logistic function. The resulting model is known as a multilayer perceptron (MLP). An MLP may have multiple inputs and outputs. The number of hidden neurons is less than the number of inputs and outputs. It can also have direct connection from the input layer to the output layer. In statistical terminology, these are known as main effects.

MLPs are universal approximators (White 1992); thus MLPs can be used when we know little about the relationship between the dependent and independent variables. The complexity of the MLP model differs by varying the number of hidden layers and the number of hidden neurons in each hidden layer. An MLP that contains a small number of hidden neurons is known as a parametric model, and it can be used as an alternative to polynomial regression. An MLP is considered a quasi-parametric model, similar to projection pursuit regression (Friedman and Stuetzle 1981), when it contains a moderate number of hidden neurons. Generally, an MLP with one hidden layer is the same as the projection pursuit regression model. The only difference is that an MLP uses a predetermined functional form for the activation function in the hidden layer, whereas a projection pursuit uses a flexible nonlinear smoother.

11.3.1 Measuring Model Performance

It is often of interest to measure the performance of a particular machine learning model. Many of the approaches discussed above are tuned or adjusted by the user, such as selecting the number of neighbors in k-neural network or the number of hidden layers and nodes in neural nets. Comparing the error for various parameterizations or for different approaches is often used to select the final model.

In order to measure the error of the approach, multiple datasets are used to build and examine the model performance. The training dataset is used to build the model and to determine the model parameters. This dataset "trains" the model using the data, and it is used for parameter estimation and variable selection. In some cases, a validation dataset is used to tune the parameters or to perform any adjusts to the model such as pruning with decision trees. The test dataset is used to examine the final model performance. The error rate determined from the test dataset is considered the error rate of the final model.

The multiple datasets are generated by randomly splitting the original data into unique subsets for training and testing (and, in some cases, validation). This allows us to measure the error and prevent overfitting to the data. For example, 80% of the data may be randomly selected for the training dataset, while the remaining 20% is used for testing.

We fit statistics such as the mean square error (MSE) to compare models. The MSE is calculated as: $\frac{1}{n} \sum_{i=1}^{n} (Y_i - \hat{Y}_i)^2$, where $\hat{Y}$ denotes model fit. This measures the average squared values of the error, where values closer to zero indicate smaller errors. The MSE is commonly used, although other fit statistics such as the mean absolute error or the mean absolute percentage error may also be considered. In classification applications, the percentage of records correctly categorized may be identified. To evaluate various approaches, the models should be used to fit the test dataset, and the fit statistic is calculated for both methods. For example, we may consider using regression and a neural network to fit a certain dataset. We can calculate the fit statistic (such as MSE) on both models to compare the performance of the two methods. The method with a lower MSE has smaller error and thus should be preferred.

11.4 Prediction of an Alzheimer's Disease Diagnosis Using Logistic Regression and Artificial Neural Networks

ANNs are often used as an alternative tool to logistic regression for the prediction of binary outcomes (Cheng and Titterington 1994; Sarle 1994). We apply both of these methods in the prediction of an Alzheimer's disease (AD) diagnosis.

Problem: How do we predict a diagnosis of AD given information about age, BMI, diabetes, hypertension, and hypercholesterolemia?

Solution: Previously, we addressed AD diagnosis with a logistic regression analysis using covariates such as age, BMI, diabetes, hypertension, and hypercholesterolemia. We now discuss predicting an AD diagnosis using a neural network. We use the data of 761 patients from ADC 4967, including information on the patient's age, BMI, the presence of diabetes, the presence of hypertension, and the presence of hypercholesterolemia. We conduct this analysis using the R and SPSS software programs. The results are reported below.

Classification

Sample	Observed	Predicted		Percent Correct
		0	1	
Training	0	12	122	9.0%
	1	14	408	96.7%
	Overall Percent	4.7%	95.3%	75.5%
Testing	0	9	39	18.8%
	1	5	152	96.8%
	Overall Percent	6.8%	93.2%	78.5%

Dependent Variable: DX_AD

The results are summarized in figure 11.3.

11.4.1 R Syntax and Output for Fitting Neural Networks

The R syntax follows:

```
#Split training/testing data
set.seed(38445)
1index <- sample(1:nrow(dta),round(0.8*nrow(dta)))
2train <- dta[index,]
3test <- dta[-index,]
#Fit Neural Net
4library(neuralnet)
5nn <- neuralnet(DX_AD~AGE+BMI+DIABETES+HYPERTEN+HYPERCHO,data=train,hidden=4,linear.output=T)
6plot(nn)
```

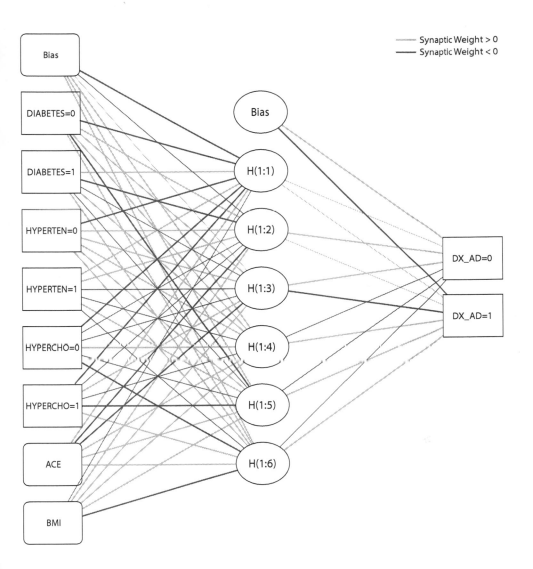

Hidden layer activation function: Hyperbolic tangent
Output layer activation function: Softmax

Figure 11.3 Neural network for Alzheimer's diagnosis.

```
#Calculate MSE
```

```
⁷test_ord <- data.frame(test$AGE,test$BMI,test$DIABETES,test$HYP
ERTEN,test$HYPERCHO,test$DX_AD)
⁸pr.nn <- compute(nn,test_ord[,1:5])
⁹MSE.nn <- sum((test_ord$test.DX_AD - pr.nn$net.result)^2)/
nrow(test_ord)
MSE.nn
```

[1]The sample() function randomly selects a specified number of values. The input variables are sample(x, size, replace=FALSE), where x is the values being sampled from, size is the number of values to select in the sample, and replace specifies whether the values should be sampled with replacement. By default, replace=FALSE. In this case, we are sampling 80% of the values from 1 to n (the size of the dataset) to randomly select observations to use in the training dataset (use 0.8*number of rows in dataset).

[2]The training dataset is created by subsetting the original dataset with the randomly selected indices.

[3]The testing dataset is created by selecting all the observations except the indices used in the training dataset (remaining 20% of observations).

[4]The neuralnet library contains the neuralnet() function for fitting neural networks.

[5]The neuralnet() function is used to fit neural networks where output ~ input. The option hidden= is used to specify the number of hidden layers. Hidden = n specifies one layer with n nodes. Specifying hidden = $c(n_1, n_2, \ldots, n_h)$ specifies h hidden layers with n_1 nodes in the first layer, n_2 nodes in the second layer, and so on. The option linear.output=TRUE specifies regression, while linear.output=FALSE is used for classification. Note that neuralnet() can only handle quantitative variables, so all factor variables must be converted to binary indicator variables. In addition, if there are issues with convergence, the user can adjust the number of hidden layers and nodes within each layer, or adjust the value of the option stepmax= (which has a default value of 1e+05).

[6]The plot() option produces the neural network plot, which is shown in the output below.

[7]We create a dataset that contains only the input and output variables of the test dataset, which are in order of the predictors listed in the neuralnet() function.

[8]The compute function is used to calculate the predictions of the specified dataset using the specified model. In this case, we apply the neural network model that has been previously fit (saved in nn) to the test dataset.

[9]We use the true values of the outcome in the test dataset, along with the predicted values, in the formula for MSE to measure the error of the model.

R OUTPUT

```
plot(nn)
MSE.nn
## [1] 0.1709164803
```

Comments: The plot() statement produces the plot of the neural network (displayed in fig. 11.4). The call to MSE.nn prints the value of the mean square error of the neural network, which is 0.17.

11.4.2 SPSS Syntax and Output for Fitting Neural Networks

The SPSS syntax follows:

```
*Multilayer Perceptron Network.
MLP DX_AD (MLEVEL=N) BY DIABETES HYPERTEN HYPERCHO WITH AGE BMI
 /RESCALE COVARIATE=STANDARDIZED
  /PARTITION TRAINING=7 TESTING=3 HOLDOUT=0
  /ARCHITECTURE  AUTOMATIC=YES (MINUNITS=1 MAXUNITS=50)
  /CRITERIA TRAINING=BATCH OPTIMIZATION=SCALEDCONJUGATE
LAMBDAINITIAL=0.0000005
    SIGMAINITIAL=0.00005 INTERVALCENTER=0 INTERVALOFFSET=0.5
MEMSIZE=1000
  /PRINT CPS NETWORKINFO SUMMARY CLASSIFICATION
```

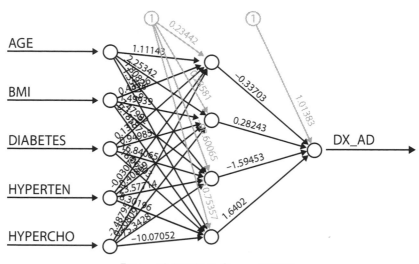

Error: 48.287313 Steps: 27271

Figure 11.4 Neural network for Alzheimer's diagnosis.

```
/PLOT NETWORK ROC GAIN LIFT PREDICTED
/SAVE PREDVAL
/STOPPINGRULES ERRORSTEPS= 1 (DATA=AUTO) TRAININGTIMER=ON
(MAXTIME=15) MAXEPOCHS=AUTO
    ERRORCHANGE=1.0E-4 ERRORRATIO=0.001
/MISSING USERMISSING=EXCLUDE.
```

SPSS OUTPUT

Multilayer Perceptron
Case Processing Summary

		N	Percent
Sample	Training	556	73.1%
	Testing	205	26.9%
Valid		761	100.0%
Excluded		0	
Total		761	

Comments: There are two sets. The training set has 73.1% of the data, and the testing set has 26.9% of the data.

Network Information

Input Layer	Factors	1	DIABETES
		2	HYPERTEN
		3	HYPERCHO
	Covariates	1	NACCAGE
		2	BMI
	Number of Units[a]		8
	Rescaling Method for Covariates		Standardized
Hidden Layer(s)	Number of Hidden Layers		1
	Number of Units in Hidden Layer 1[a]		6
	Activation Function		Hyperbolic tangent
Output Layer	Dependent Variables	1	DX_AD
	Number of Units		2
	Activation Function		Softmax
	Error Function		Cross-entropy

a. Excluding the bias unit

Comments: We fit the model with i hidden layers and one output layer.

Comments: Figure 11.5 displays the model fitted with the input and output layers.

Model Summary

Training	Cross Entropy Error	278.174
	Percent Incorrect Predictions	24.5%
	Stopping Rule Used	1 consecutive step(s) with no decrease in error[a]
	Training Time	0:00:00.13
Testing	Cross Entropy Error	99.589
	Percent Incorrect Predictions	21.5%

Dependent Variable: DX_AD
a. Error computations are based on the testing sample.

Comments: There are 21.5% of incorrect predictions for testing, as opposed to 24.5% for training.

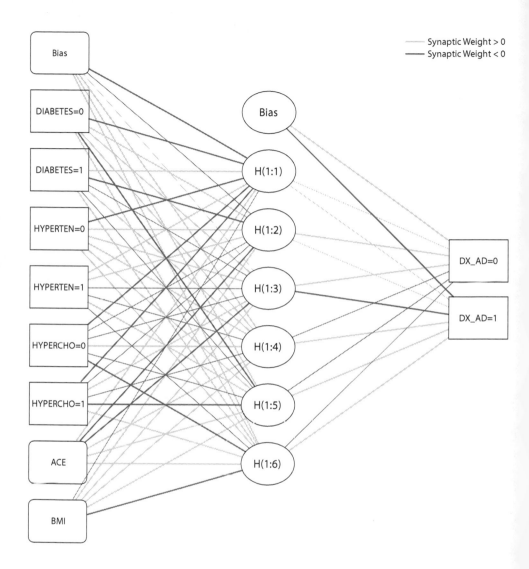

Synaptic Weight > 0
Synaptic Weight < 0

Hidden layer activation function: Hyperbolic tangent
Output layer activation function: Softmax

Figure 11.5 Neural network for Alzheimer's diagnosis.

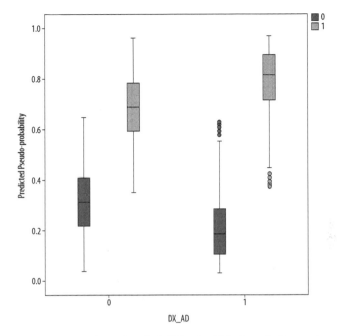

Figure 11.6 Predicted probabilities by Alzheimer's diagnosis.

Comments: The predicted probabilities are shown in figure 11.6 for the event and nonevent.

Classification

| Sample | Observed | Predicted | | |
		0	1	Percent Correct
Training	0	12	122	9.0%
	1	14	408	96.7%
	Overall Percent	4.7%	95.3%	75.5%
Testing	0	9	39	18.8%
	1	5	152	96.8%
	Overall Percent	6.8%	93.2%	78.5%

Dependent Variable: DX_AD

Comments: The receiver operating characteristic (ROC) curves for the fit models are given in figure 11.7.

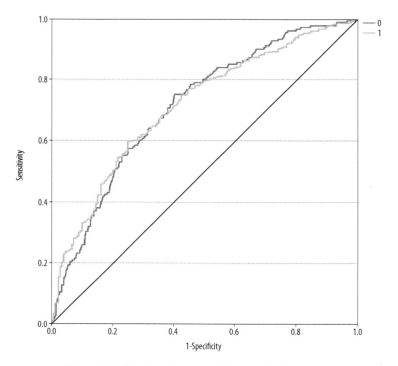

Figure 11.7 Receiver Operator Characteristic curves.

We use the remaining 152 observations as our training dataset. We apply the neural network to our training data to predict the probability of an AD diagnosis for each subject. We calculate the MSE using these predicted values and get a MSE of 7.15. This is compared to MSEs of other models to determine the performance of the model. Note that the results vary slightly across the programs as different observations are selected for the training and testing data (different randomizations selected using different seeds).

11.5 Conclusions

We consider a comparison of multilayered networks and traditional logistic regression for AD diagnosis prediction. It is clear from the literature that ANNs approximate any nonlinear mathematical function. This aspect of NNs is particularly useful when the relationship between the variables is not known or is complex, and hence it is difficult to handle statistically. The determination of various parameters associated with NNs, such as the number of hidden layers and the number of nodes in the hidden layer, however, is not straightforward, and finding the optimal configuration of neural networks is a time-consuming process. In this respect, a statistical model clearly stands out, as it allows interpretation of coefficients of the individual variables. In addition, the parametric assumptions of these models allow one to draw inferences regarding the significance of certain variables in prediction or classification problems. Neural networks and statistical models are not competing methodologies for data analysis. There is an overlap between the two fields. Neural networks include several models, such as MLPs that are useful for statistical applications. Statistical methodology is directly applicable to NNs in a variety of ways, including estimation criteria, optimization algorithms, confidence intervals, and graphical methods. Better communication between the fields of statistics and NNs would benefit both. Neural networks are flexible and allow the user to specify the number of hidden layers and the number of nodes. This popular technique has good model performance, and the interpretation, based on a biological neural system, is easy to understand.

11.6 Exercises

Using data from NACC (data link: http://www.public.asu.edu/~jeffreyw/), use a neural network to classify patients by diagnosis: AD, dementia with Lewy bodies (DLB), frontotemporal dementia (FTD), vascular dementia (VaD), and normal. The variables Diagnosis and DX are used to identify the true diagnosis (for training or for calculating the error rate in the test dataset), where DX = 1 is AD, DX = 2 is DLB, DX = 3 is FTD, DX = 4 is VaD, and DX = 8 is normal. Split the data so that 80% of the observations are used in the training dataset and 20% are used in the testing dataset.

1. Fit a neural network to predict the five diagnosis categories using the training data.
   a. Calculate the error rate of the classification using the test dataset.

    b. How does the error rate change as the number of hidden layers is adjusted?

2. Fit a second neural network that predicts whether a patient has dementia. This is a binary classification where a patient has dementia if DX = 1, 2, 3, or 4, and a patient does not have dementia if DX = 8.

    a. Calculate the error rate of the binary classification using the test dataset.

    b. How does the error rate change as the number of hidden layers is adjusted?

3. Fit a logistic regression model that predicts whether a patient has dementia.

    a. Calculate the error rate of the classification in the test dataset.

    b. How does the error rate of the logistic regression model compare to the error rate of the neural network?

Chapter 12

Case Study

12.1 Introduction

In this chapter, we present a case study that demonstrates the use of statistical methods discussed in this book. We are interested in understanding the impact of demographic and cardiovascular risk factors on cognitive change. In this case study, we investigate the association in patients Alzheimer's disease (AD), dementia with Lewy bodies (DLB), and frontotemporal dementia (FTD), as well as nondemented elderly individuals (normal). We evaluate two measures of cognition that have been utilized throughout this book, including the Mini-Mental State Examination (MMSE) and the Clinical Dementia Rating Scale Sum of Boxes (CDR-SUM). Using both measures of cognition allows us to verify the relationships we identify in the data. We provide a systematic approach of reviewing the data, evaluating associations, and building a final model. Of the four statistical programs used in this textbook, we choose SAS to demonstrate the analysis of these data. SAS does not suffer from the convergence issues we found with SPSS and STATA for some of the advanced models, and SAS outputs are easily reproduced with clarity and style. SAS will often produce additional graphs and output without extra syntax required, as compared to R. We provide supplementary code for R, SPSS, and Stata at http://www.public.asu.edu/~jeffreyw/.

In this analysis, we consider a subset of dementia patients clinically diagnosed with AD (5,077 patients), DLB (172 patients), FTD (488 patients), and 6,198 individuals lacking a dementia diagnosis (normal). Each individual has between 2 and 12 visits, for a total of 45,112 records. The individuals represent 35 ADCs. We present several statistical evaluations and models as we build up to the construction of a

Table 12.1 A Subset of Data Used in a Case Study

ADC	ID	MOFROMINDEX	MMSE	CDRSUM	AGE	BMI	HRATE	HYPERTEN	HYPERCHO
5452	271	0	29	0.5	81	21.5	72	0	1
5452	271	12	30	3.5	82	21.6	74	0	0
5452	271	23	25	6	83	20.2	68	0	1
5452	271	37	24	6	84	20.6	80	0	1
5452	271	64	16	12	86	20.2	72	0	0
354	287	0	26	1.5	79	32.6	70	1	0
354	287	14	29	1.5	80	31.4	64	1	0
289	385	16	22	7	82	29	68	1	1
289	385	28	21	5	83	29	72	0	1
289	385	41	20	5	84	26.4	86	0	0
289	385	50	16	7	84	29	74	0	0

generalized linear mixed model (discussed in chaps 4 and 5). We use random intercepts in the form of a generalized linear model (GLM) to account for the correlation at the patient level and the center levels for each dementia subtype. A subset of the data, showing three patients from three different ADCs, is shown in table 12.1.

12.2 Background

Dementia patients often experience cognitive decline, and many studies have been performed to understand factors that may affect the rate of decline. Recent investigations have identified differential associations between cardiovascular risk factors and changes in cognition (Bergland et al. 2017; Irimata et al. 2018). We wish to explore some of these relationships in our data.

RESEARCH QUESTION

In this case study, we investigate the impact of demographic and cardiovascular risk factors on the rate of cognitive decline. We consider three dementia subtypes—AD, DLB, and FTD—as well as a normal subgroup. The aim of this chapter is to walk the reader through the process of identifying associations and building statistical models in a multivariable setting.

On the basis of the analytical tools presented in this textbook, we conducted the following:

1. Data review and cleaning with well-defined exclusions.
   Items to consider in this process:
   - Missing data
   - Minimum and maximum values of each variable fall within a reasonable range
   - Exclusions (confounding diagnoses, specific subtypes, etc.)
   - In longitudinal analyses, the minimum number of visits per patient required to include in the analysis
2. Data description at the univariate stage (evaluate each covariate one at a time).
3. Data description and analysis for two variables at a time (i.e., looking at relationships between one covariate and the outcome).
4. Data analysis in the multivariable setting under independence (i.e., estimating the value of the outcome using all covariates such as cardiovascular risk factors, age, gender, and the like).
5. Data analysis in the multivariable setting using random effects for correlated observations (extending #4 to account for clustering such as the impact of visiting a particular center).

12.3 Study Data

We begin our analysis by reviewing the study data. Prior to starting any statistical analyses, we should understand the background of the study, including the samples being evaluated, time period of the study, as well as the data collection methods. As stated previously in chapter 1, when utilizing any dataset, one must understand the design of the study. It is highly recommended to work with the personnel of the particular study, as they understand the caveats and limitations of the data.

12.3.1 Data Origin

We obtain data with permission from the National Alzheimer's Coordinating Center (NACC) Uniform Data Set (UDS) for this analysis (https://www.alz.washington.edu) (Morris et al. 2006; Beekly et al. 2007; Weintraub et al. 2009). The UDS contains information on patients' demographic information and clinical evaluations (Morris et al. 2006; Beekly et al. 2007; Weintraub et al. 2009). Online, NACC provides the Researcher's Data Dictionary, which provides a description of all the data elements. In our study, the records contain visit information collected between August 2005 and November 2017.

12.3.2 Data Inclusion

We focus on the analysis of individuals with AD, DLB, and FTD, as well as normal individuals. In this evaluation, we exclude patients with VaD or mixed diagnoses. Because we are interested in the change in cognition over time, we are studying patients who have two or more visits to ADC over the course of the study. Each patient has one primary diagnosis throughout the study, and we do not consider cases with changing diagnoses. The Uniform Data Set (UDS; see https://www.alz.washington.edu/WEB/forms_uds.html) collects data on a variety of diagnoses. When working with large datasets, it is helpful to discuss how the specific cohort being evaluated was selected, as exclusion criteria could create potential biases in a study. In some instances, one may want to compare the demographics between cases within their study and cases they excluded.

12.3.3 Data Summary

We utilize a longitudinal dataset consisting of 45,112 observations for 11,935 individuals. We calculate the number of observations (NUM_OBS), the number of ADCs represented in the data (NUM_ADC), and the number of patients (NUM_SUBJ) using SAS PROC SQL:

```
PROC SQL;
        SELECT COUNT(ADC) AS NUM_OBS,
                     COUNT(DISTINCT ADC) AS NUM_ADC,
                     COUNT(DISTINCT ID) AS NUM_SUBJ
        FROM CHAP12;
QUIT;
```

Our focus is on individuals with diagnoses of AD, DLB, FTD, and normal. Although we have already selected these individuals for our

Table 12.2 Frequency of Dementia Subtypes

Diagnosis	DX	Frequency	Relative Frequency (%)
AD	1	5,077	42.54
DLB	2	172	1.44
FTD	3	488	4.09
Normal	8	6,198	51.93

analyses, we wish to examine the distribution of individuals by diagnosis at baseline (the first recorded visit). We create a first visit indicator (1 = first visit, 0 = follow-up visit) using the following SAS syntax:

```
PROC SORT DATA=CHAP12;

BY ADC ID;

RUN;

DATA CHAP12;

SET CHAP12;

IF FIRST.ID THEN FIRSTVISIT = 1;

ELSE FIRSTVISIT=0;

BY ADC ID;

RUN;
```

We use the first visit indicator (FIRSTVISIT) to evaluate the distribution of diagnoses at the baseline visit:

```
PROC FREQ DATA=CHAP12;

TABLES DIAGNOSIS/LIST MISSING;

WHERE FIRSTVISIT=1;

RUN;
```

The results are summarized in table 12.2.

12.4 Data Analysis: Descriptive Statistics

We use statistical measures (chapter 2) to provide information on the response (output) and predictors (input). It is important to summarize and examine the covariates within the dataset to understand the range of values represented in the data. A data dictionary or description of the variables is helpful for interpreting the meaning of codes for binary and categorical variables. Using frequency tables can also help identify missing or unusual values.

12.4.1 Data Description at the Univariate Stage

RESPONSE VARIABLES

In our study, we consider two continuous response variables (MMSE and CDR-SUM), which are used as measures of cognitive and functional abilities. The MMSE (Folstein et al. 1975) scores range between 0 and 30. Scores closer to 0 suggest severe cognitive impairment, while scores closer to 30 suggest no cognitive impairment. The CDR-SUM score is a total score for six domains measuring cognitive and functioning abilities (Hughes et al. 1982). The total score ranges between 0 and 18, where scores near 0 suggest no cognitive impairment, while scores near 18 suggest severe cognitive impairment. We use descriptive statistics for continuous variables to examine the distribution of the responses in our data. A summary of the responses was obtained by diagnosis through the following SAS syntax:

```
PROC SORT DATA=CHAP12;
BY DX;
RUN;
PROC MEANS DATA=CHAP12;
VAR MMSE CDRSUM;
BY DX;
WHERE FIRSTVISIT=1;
RUN;
```

Because the data contain multiple diagnoses and we would like to report summary statistics for each diagnosis, we must first sort the data by diagnosis (using PROC SORT). PROC MEANS reports the frequency (N), mean, standard deviation (Std Dev), minimum, and maximum for both responses by diagnosis group. We report the summary statistics for MMSE and CDR-SUM at baseline. The results are summarized in table 12.3.

Table 12.3 Descriptive Statistics for MMSE and CDR-SUM

Diagnosis	Response	Frequency	Mean	Std Dev	Min	Max
AD	MMSE	5,077	22.24	5.51	0	30
	CDR-SUM	5,077	4.82	3.42	0	18
DLB	MMSE	172	23.43	4.80	8	30
	CDR-SUM	172	4.77	2.96	1	18
FTD	MMSE	488	22.98	6.35	0	30
	CDR-SUM	488	4.82	3.71	0	18
Normal	MMSE	6,198	29.03	1.32	17	30
	CDR-SUM	6,198	0.06	0.27	0	8

From the descriptive statistics, there is a wide range of MMSE and CDR-SUM values for patients with AD, DLB, and FTD, while normal subjects tend to have mean scores closer to 30 for MMSE and 0 for CDR-SUM, suggesting little to no cognitive decline (as expected). The mean MMSE score for normal subjects is higher than the MMSE score for dementia patients (29.03), while the mean CDR-SUM score is lower than the CDR-SUM score for dementia patients (0.06), which is consistent with the scoring systems for both evaluations. Interestingly, we note that there are cases of dementia patients (diagnoses of AD, DLB, or FTD) in which the MMSE is close to 30 and the CDR-SUM is close to 0 (indicating no cognitive decline). These records are closely investigated to determine how many dementia patients have cognitive scores that indicate no cognitive decline.

COVARIATES

We wish to understand how a variety of demographic and cardiovascular risk factors are associated with cognitive change for normal subjects and patients with dementia. In this study, we evaluate the impact of six predictors, including gender, age, body mass index (BMI), heart rate, hypertension, and hypercholesterolemia. The factors age, BMI, and heart rate are continuous variables. Age of the patient is recorded in years, while BMI is calculated as a function of weight and height. We obtain descriptive statistics for the predictors at baseline using PROC MEANS. We use the following SAS syntax:

```
PROC MEANS DATA=CHAP12;

VAR AGE BMI HRATE;

BY DX;

WHERE FIRSTVISIT=1;

RUN;
```

The summary statistics (frequency, mean, standard deviation, minimum, and maximum) for the continuous variables are summarized in table 12.4 by diagnosis.

The information in table 12.4 provides a means to compare the covariate values across dementia subtypes and normal individuals. Normal individuals tend to be slightly younger (mean of 70.29 years). The FTD group has the highest average BMI of 27.80. The heart rates are fairly consistent between the four groups, although the DLB group had the lowest average recorded heart rate of 66.70 beats per minute. The descriptive statistics are used to check whether the minimum and maximum values of each variable fall within a reasonable range. For example, because most people who have dementia tend to develop it later in life, it is not surprising that the mean ages for dementia in our study (AD, DLB, or FTD) are all in the 70s. As the NACC primarily recruits elderly individuals, we see that this is also true for the mean age of the normal group.

Table 12.4　Descriptive Statistics for Covariates by Subtypes

Diagnosis	Covariate	Frequency	Mean	Std Dev	Min	Max
AD	AGE	5,077	74.83	9.13	35	101
	BMI	5,077	26.23	4.53	13.6	53.7
	HRATE	5,077	67.53	10.87	38	138
DLB	AGE	172	71.03	7.62	51	88
	BMI	172	26.35	4.28	18.0	51.4
	HRATE	172	66.70	10.52	41	100
FTD	AGE	488	64.64	8.93	30	92
	BMI	488	27.80	5.12	16.8	46.9
	HRATE	488	68.56	11.61	42	116
Normal	AGE	6,198	70.29	10.02	21	100
	BMI	6,198	27.48	5.32	14.1	60.9
	HRATE	6,198	68.17	10.60	36	159

The factors gender, hypertension, and hypercholesterolemia are binary. Gender (variable SEX) has two values, male (SEX=1) and female (SEX=2). Hypertension and hypercholesterolemia have the values recent/active (HYPERTEN=1 and HYPERCHO=1) and remove/inactive/absent (HYPERTEN=0 and HYPERCHO=0). We are interested in understanding how the presence or absence of these conditions affects cognitive changes. For binary and categorical variables, we use frequency tables. The SAS syntax follows:

```
PROC FREQ DATA= CHAP12;
TABLES SEX HYPERTEN HYPERCHO/LIST MISSING;
BY DX;
WHERE FIRSTVISIT=1;
RUN;
```

PROC FREQ produces frequency tables for the variables SEX, HYPERTEN, and HYPERCHO for the values at baseline. The option LIST MISSING reports whether any of these variables have missing values in the output. The binary covariates are summarized in table 12.5.

The DLB group had the highest percentage of males (79.65%), while the normal group had the lowest percentage of males (32.46%). Although hypertension and hypercholesterolemia statuses change

Table 12.5 Frequency Distribution of Binary Variables by Subtype

	AD		DLB		FTD		Normal	
	N	Percentage	N	Percentage	N	Percentage	N	Percentage
SEX								
Male	2,397	47.21	137	79.65	302	61.89	2,012	32.46
Female	2,680	52.79	35	20.35	186	38.11	4,186	67.54
HYPERTEN								
Absent	2,628	51.76	109	63.37	310	63.52	3,383	54.58
Present	2,449	48.24	63	36.63	178	36.48	2,815	45.42
HYPERCHO								
Absent	2,524	49.71	88	51.16	285	58.40	3,365	54.29
Present	2,553	50.29	84	48.84	203	41.60	2,833	45.71

during the study, at baseline the AD group had the highest percentage of patients with hypertension and hypercholesterolemia.

12.4.2 Data Description and Analysis for Two Variables at a Time

We begin with baseline data (FIRSTVISIT=1). For the continuous covariates, we use a one-way analysis of variance (ANOVA) for mean comparisons across the four diagnoses (AD, DLB, FTD, and normal). This is a two-variable-at-a-time approach, as we do not consider the impact of other covariates for each analysis. These bivariate analyses are a useful tool for understanding the data and identifying differences between groups. But this is by no means our final determination, as two-at-a-time analyses often give a different conclusion compared to the multivariable setting. At baseline, we assume we have independent observations, and as such we use the appropriate test (*F*-test) in the one-way ANOVA. For these tests, we check the *p*-value in the output. In the ANOVA, the null hypothesis is that the factor is not associated with the outcome.

We compare the response variable across the four groups. Because the response variables MMSE and CDR-SUM are continuous, we use one-way ANOVA to test for significant differences between the baseline cognitive scores across groups. The SAS syntax follows:

```
PROC GLM DATA=CHAP12;
CLASS DX;
MODEL MMSE=DX;
MEANS DX/BON;
WHERE FIRSTVISIT=1;
RUN;
PROC GLM DATA= CHAP12;
CLASS DX;
MODEL CDRSUM=DX;
MEANS DX/BON;
WHERE FIRSTVISIT=1;
RUN;
```

Table 12.6 Comparison of Significant Differences across Dementia Group

	Overall p-Value	AD vs. Normal	DLB vs. Normal	FTD vs. Normal	AD vs. DLB	AD vs. FTD	DLB vs. FTD
MMSE	<0.0001	*	*	*	*	*	
CDR-SUM	<0.0001	*	*	*			

Note: Asterisks indicate significant differences between the specified subgroups for the specified variables.

The p-values in the SAS output are summarized in table 12.6. The overall p-value for the ANOVA, testing for any differences in the variable value across groups, is reported in the first column. The following columns report differences between specific diagnoses. Asterisks indicate significant differences, while blank boxes indicate no significant difference.

From these analyses, there are statistically significant differences between the covariates and responses (overall p-value < 0.05). The average MMSE score differed significantly among all groups except the DLB and FTD groups. As for the average CDR-SUM scores, three groups differed, while no significant differences were detected between AD and DLB, AD and FTD, and DLB and FTD patients.

The differences for MMSE and CDR-SUM across dementia groups are displayed in figures 12.1 and 12.2, respectively. These plots are obtained as by-products from the PROC generalized linear model (GLM) SAS syntax provided above. In each plot, DX = 1 represents AD, DX = 2 represents DLB, DX = 3 represents FTD, and DX = 8 represents normal subjects. The numbers reported next to each box and whisker plot are observation numbers of the outliers in the data.

The boxplot of MMSE by diagnosis group provides a visual of the information provided in table 12.3. We can see that the MMSE scores for the normal group (DX = 8) ranges from 17 (last dot on plot) to 30, although most scores are centered around 30, which indicates no cognitive decline. The numbers listed below the box and whisker plot (9712, 9731, etc.) are the observation numbers of each outlier that are provided by default in PROC GLM. From the plot, the MMSE scores of patients with AD diagnoses (DX = 1) vary the most (largest spread),

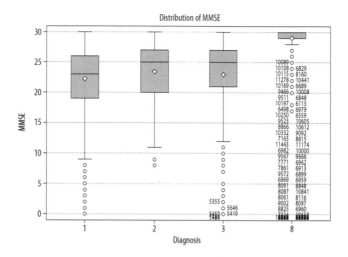

Figure 12.1 Boxplots of MMSE across diagnosis groups.

followed by MMSE scores for patients with DLB diagnoses (DX = 2), MMSE scores for patients with FTD diagnoses (DX = 3), and MMSE scores for normal subjects (DX = 8). Although the minimum scores for AD and FTD patients are 0, the values are outliers, and in fact most patients with these two diagnoses have higher MMSE scores (greater than 9 and 16, respectively).

From the boxplot of CDR-SUM scores across diagnosis groups, each of the dementia diagnoses (AD, DLB, and FTD) has an outlying value (high values of CDR-SUM), although most patients had CDR-SUM scores below 12. As expected, the normal subjects had CDR-SUM scores tightly centered around 0, although there are outliers with individuals having CDR-SUM scores as high as 8.

We examine the factors and the covariates, as they affect MMSE and CDR-SUM separately. We consider gender, hypertension, and hypercholesterolemia as factors and BMI, age, and heart rate as covariates in the bivariate analyses at baseline. We use the two-sample independent t-test for the factors and simple linear regression for the covariates. The following SAS syntax performs t-tests for the response variable MMSE:

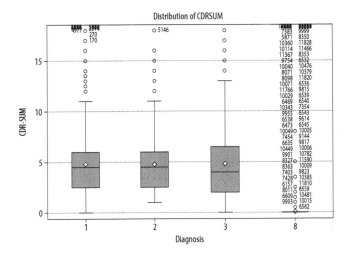

Figure 12.2 Boxplots of CDR-SUM across diagnosis groups.

```
PROC TTEST DATA=CHAP12;
CLASS SEX;
VAR MMSE;
BY DX;
WHERE FIRSTVISIT=1;
RUN;


PROC TTEST DATA=CHAP12;
CLASS HYPERTEN;
VAR MMSE;
BY DX;
WHERE FIRSTVISIT=1;
RUN;


PROC TTEST DATA=CHAP12;
CLASS HYPERCHO;
VAR MMSE;
BY DX;
WHERE FIRSTVISIT=1;
RUN;
```

Table 12.7 Bivariate Analysis for MMSE and Categorical Variables

Variable	AD			DLB		
	95% CI		p-Value	95% CI		p-Value
Sex (males-females)	0.504	1.111	<0.0001	1.687	5.132	0.0001
Hypertension	−0.444	0.162	0.3626	−1.924	1.078	0.5786
Hypercholesterolemia	−1.220	−0.614	<0.0001	−1.118	1.776	0.6542
Variable	FTD			Normal		
	95% CI		p-Value	95% CI		p-Value
Sex (males-females)	−0.589	1.820	0.3159	−0.336	−0.189	<0.0001
Hypertension	−1.798	0.347	0.1846	0.255	0.389	<0.0001
Hypercholesterolemia	−1.531	0.762	0.5104	0.025	0.157	0.0070

The information obtained from the SAS output is summarized in table 12.7.

MMSE significantly differs between males and females in the AD, DLB, and normal groups. Hypertension showed a difference in the normal group. MMSE scores greatly differed by hypercholesterolemia status for the AD group. Hypercholesterolemia also shows that it has an impact on MMSE score at baseline in the normal group.

The code to evaluate simple linear regression for each of the continuous covariates on MMSE is provided below:

```
PROC REG DATA=CHAP12;
MODEL MMSE=BMI;
BY DX;
WHERE FIRSTVISIT=1;
RUN;


PROC REG DATA=CHAP12;
MODEL MMSE=HRATE;
BY DX;
WHERE FIRSTVISIT=1;
RUN;


PROC REG DATA=CHAP12;
MODEL MMSE=AGE;
```

```
BY DX;
WHERE FIRSTVISIT=1;
RUN;
```

In table 12.8, we find that BMI has a significant impact on MMSE in the DLB and normal groups, but not for any other diagnoses. Since the parameter estimate for BMI is negative for the normal group, we conclude that higher BMIs are associated with lower MMSE scores. Alternatively, the parameter estimate for BMI is positive in the DLB group, which indicates that higher BMIs are associated with higher MMSE scores. In the AD group, we find that heart rate is significantly associated with the MMSE score, where heart rate is inversely related to cognitive score. The covariate age shows an impact on MMSE in the DLB, FTD, and normal groups.

We perform similar analyses for the CDR-SUM score. The SAS syntax for the two-sample t-test follows:

```
PROC TTEST DATA=CHAP12;
CLASS SEX;
VAR CDRSUM;
BY DX;
WHERE FIRSTVISIT=1;
RUN;
```

Table 12.8 Bivariate Analysis for MMSE and Continuous Variables

	AD		DLB		FTD		Normal	
Variable	Estimate	p-Value	Estimate	p-Value	Estimate	p-Value	Estimate	p-Value
BMI								
Intercept	21.72659	<0.0001	18.65855	<0.0001	22.70353	<0.0001	29.62727	<0.0001
BMI	0.01949	0.2535	0.18108	0.0343	0.00985	0.8610	−0.02170	<0.0001
Heart Rate								
Intercept	23.73700	<0.0001	23.99934	<0.0001	23.16845	<0.0001	28.95374	<0.0001
Heart Rate	−0.02220	0.0018	−0.00853	0.8074	−0.00279	0.9107	0.00113	0.4746
Age								
Intercept	22.96992	<0.0001	31.74784	<0.0001	27.39996	<0.0001	30.84469	<0.0001
Age	−0.00978	0.2487	−0.11710	0.0145	−0.06842	0.0336	−0.02580	<0.0001

```
PROC TTEST DATA=CHAP12;
CLASS HYPERTEN;
VAR CDRSUM;
BY DX;
WHERE FIRSTVISIT=1;
RUN;

PROC TTEST DATA=CHAP12;
CLASS HYPERCHO;
VAR CDRSUM;
BY DX;
WHERE FIRSTIVISIT=1;
RUN;
```

The information obtained from the SAS output is summarized in table 12.9.

We find that CDR-SUM differs significantly between males and females in all four groups (AD, DLB, FTD, and normal groups). Differences in the CDR-SUM score for subjects with recent/active hypertension versus a remote/inactive/absent status were detected in the normal group. Hypercholesterolemia has an impact on CDR-SUM in the AD and normal groups. The SAS code to evaluate simple linear regression of CDR-SUM with each of the continuous covariates follows:

Table 12.9 Bivariate Analysis for CDR-SUM and Categorical Variables

Variable	AD			DLB		
	95% CI		p-Value	95% CI		p-Value
Sex (males-females)	−0.6489	−0.2742	<0.0001	−2.9706	−0.1097	0.0355
Hypertension	−0.2760	0.1000	0.3587	−0.8841	0.9701	0.9272
Hypercholesterolemia	0.2732	0.6491	<0.0001	−0.8365	0.9506	0.8998

Variable	FTD			Normal		
	95% CI		p-Value	95% CI		p-Value
Sex (males-females)	0.2590	1.6073	0.0068	0.0150	0.0484	0.0002
Hypertension	−0.4257	0.9442	0.4574	−0.0443	−0.0164	<0.0001
Hypercholesterolemia	−0.0731	1.2613	0.0808	−0.0428	−0.0150	<0.0001

```
PROC REG DATA=CHAP12;
MODEL CDRSUM=BMI;
BY DX;
WHERE FIRSTVISIT=1;
RUN;


PROC REG DATA=CHAP12;
MODEL CDRSUM=HRATE;
BY DX;
WHERE FIRSTVISIT=1;
RUN;


PROC REG DATA=CHAP12;
MODEL CDRSUM=AGE;
BY DX;
WHERE FIRSTVISIT=1;
RUN;
```

We find that BMI has a significant impact on the CDR-SUM score for FTD and normal subjects (table 12.10). Heart rate is found to significantly affect CDR-SUM in the AD, DLB, and normal groups. Age showed an impact on CDR-SUM in the AD and DLB groups.

While these analyses (the two-sample t-test and simple linear regression) suggest some associations exist between the covariate and outcome across diagnosis groups, the tests consider only two variables at a time. It is an established fact that the behavior of variables in isolation with another variable is not the same in the presence of multivariable (Chen et al. 2017). We use generalized linear models to look at the combined effects of factors and covariates on MMSE and CDR-SUM.

12.5 Data Analysis: Modeling

Within each diagnosis, our variables of interest are MMSE and CDR-SUM. We wish to determine the simultaneous impact of the covariates

Table 12.10 Bivariate Analysis for CDR-SUM and Continuous Variables

Variable	AD		DLB		FTD		Normal	
	Estimate	p-Value	Estimate	p-Value	Estimate	p-Value	Estimate	p-Value
BMI								
Intercept	4.70603	<0.0001	7.05166	<0.0001	2.85113	0.0021	0.01853	0.3032
BMI	0.00421	0.6910	−0.08646	0.1024	0.07099	0.0302	0.00155	0.0161
Heart Rate								
Intercept	3.49110	<0.0001	0.90283	0.5271	3.39344	0.0008	0.00014492	0.9948
Heart rate	0.01963	<0.0001	0.05803	0.0066	0.02088	0.1490	0.00089366	0.0056
Age								
Intercept	2.07124	<0.0001	−1.54554	0.4564	3.36259	0.0063	0.05439	0.0248
Age	0.03669	<0.0001	0.08896	0.0025	0.02262	0.2292	0.00009508	0.7805

and factors for each diagnosis. As a starting point, we fit GLMs, evaluating the covariates at baseline to understand the impact of early measures.

12.5.1 Data Analysis of Multivariable Predictors under Independence

We fit GLMs for MMSE and CDR-SUM to understand how each outcome is affected by our covariates of interest. Using the sequence of covariates gives a better explanation of the variation in the responses. A GLM allows us to look at the simultaneous impact of several factors and covariates on the MMSE and CDR-SUM for each diagnosis. A model with multiple predictors is certain to give a better explanation of the variation in MMSE and CDR-SUM than the two-at-a-time approach we explored previously. The two-at-a-time approach assumes that no other covariates may affect the association. We fit GLMs for each diagnosis, including AD, DLB, FTD, and normal.

GENERALIZED LINEAR MODEL: MMSE

We investigate the impact of gender, age, BMI, heart rate, hypertension, and hyperglycosemia on MMSE. Four models are fitted for the mean of MMSE, one for each diagnosis group. We assume that MMSE is normally distributed. Because we are evaluating continuous data with a normal distribution as the random component, we use an identity link function (chap. 3). Thus one can write the model as:

$$E\,(\mathrm{MMSE}_i) = \beta_0 + \beta_1\mathrm{SEX}_i + \beta_2\mathrm{AGE}_i + \beta_3\mathrm{BMI}_i + \beta_4\mathrm{HRATE}_i$$
$$+ \beta_5\mathrm{HYPERTEN}_i + \beta_6\mathrm{HYPERCHO}_i.$$

We fit this model through SAS. The SAS syntax follows:

```
PROC GENMOD DATA=CHAP12;
        CLASS ADC ID SEX(REF="1");
        MODEL MMSE = SEX AGE BMI HRATE HYPERTEN HYPERCHO /
DIST=NORMAL
LINK=IDENTITY;
        WHERE FIRSTVISIT=1;
        BY DX;
RUN;
```

For the variable SEX, we specify male (SEX=1) as the reference group in the CLASS statement. The statement BY DX in the SAS code indicates that a model is fit for each value of the diagnosis.

The scaled deviance for each of the four models is close to 1 (table 12.11), which signifies that the model provides an adequate fit. If the scaled deviance is much greater than 1, it signifies that the model does not provide an adequate fit, and an alternative model should be investigated.

We fit four models for MMSE at baseline, one for each dementia group and for the normal group. We provide the parameter estimates and significance results in table 12.12. Significant covariates are listed in bold, where $\alpha = 0.05$.

For patients with AD, we find that gender, heart rate, and hypercholesterolemia are significantly associated with the MMSE score at baseline. For patients with DLB, gender and age are statistically

Table 12.11 Generalized Linear Models Fit Statistics for MMSE by Diagnosis

	AD	DLB	FTD	Normal
Criterion	Value/DF	Value/DF	Value/DF	Value/DF
Deviance	30.05	20.89	40.03	1.65
Scaled deviance	1.0014	1.0424	1.0146	1.0011

Table 12.12 Parameter Estimates and _p_-Values for MMSE by Diagnosis

	AD		DLB		FTD		Normal	
Parameter	Estimate	_p_-Value	Estimate	_p_-Value	Estimate	_p_-Value	Estimate	_p_-Value
Intercept	**23.943**	**<0.0001**	**28.077**	**<0.0001**	**29.789**	**<0.0001**	**31.220**	**<0.0001**
SEX = 2 (Female)	**−0.699**	**<0.0001**	**−3.313**	**0.0002**	−0.561	0.3474	**0.228**	**<0.0001**
AGE	−0.010	0.2619	**−0.097**	**0.0379**	**−0.091**	**0.0074**	**−0.025**	**<0.0001**
BMI	0.001	0.9672	0.067	0.4298	−0.036	0.5483	**−0.022**	**<0.0001**
HRATE	**−0.016**	**0.0308**	0.017	0.6153	−0.005	0.8493	0.001	0.6581
HYPERTEN	−0.062	0.7069	0.885	0.2676	1.123	0.0896	**−0.149**	**<0.0001**
HYPERCHO	**0.887**	**<0.0001**	−0.542	0.4863	0.445	0.4710	0.047	0.1651
Scale	5.478	—	4.476	—	6.282	—	1.283	—

Note: Boldface indicates significant covariates, where $\alpha = 0.05$.

significant predictors. In the FTD subgroup, age is found to significantly drive the baseline MMSE score. For normal subjects, gender, age, BMI, and hypertension are significant covariates.

GENERALIZED LINEAR MODEL: CDR-SUM

Similarly, we investigate the impact of gender, age, BMI, heart rate, hypertension, and hypercholesterolemia on CDR-SUM with similar assumptions to the evaluation of MMSE. The model for each diagnosis is expressed as:

$$E\,(\mathrm{CDRSUM}_i) = \beta_0 + \beta_1 \mathrm{SEX}_i + \beta_2 \mathrm{AGE}_i + \beta_3 \mathrm{BMI}_i + \beta_4 \mathrm{HRATE}_i \\ + \beta_5 \mathrm{HYPERTEN}_i + \beta_6 \mathrm{HYPERCHO}_i.$$

There are also four models fitted for the mean of CDR-SUM, one for each dementia group.

The SAS syntax follows:

```
PROC GENMOD DATA=CHAP12;
        CLASS ADC ID SEX(REF="1");
        MODEL CDRSUM = SEX AGE BMI HRATE HYPERTEN HYPERCHO /
DIST=NORMAL
LINK=IDENTITY;
        WHERE FIRSTVISIT=1;
        BY DX;
RUN;
```

The scaled deviance for each of these models is close to 1 (table 12.13).

The parameter estimates and p-values for the impact of the covariates on the CDR-SUM score for each subgroup are summarized in table 12.14.

For patients with AD, gender, age, heart rate, and hypercholesterolemia are significantly associated with the CDR-SUM score at baseline. For patients with DLB, gender, age and heart rate are statistically

Table 12.13 Generalized Linear Model Fit Statistics for CDR-SUM by Diagnosis

	AD	DLB	FTD	Normal
Criterion	Value/DF	Value/DF	Value/DF	Value/DF
Deviance	11.46	7.92	13.25	0.07
Scaled deviance	1.0014	1.0424	1.0146	1.0011

Table 12.14 Parameter Estimates and p-Values for CDR-SUM by Diagnosis

	AD		DLB		FTD		Normal	
Parameter	Estimate	p-Value	Estimate	p-Value	Estimate	p-Value	Estimate	p-Value
Intercept	0.613	0.2855	−4.152	0.1601	−0.940	0.6169	0.005	0.9011
SEX = 2 (Female)	0.401	<0.0001	1.175	0.0333	−0.949	0.0057	−0.033	<0.0001
AGE	0.037	<0.0001	0.086	0.0028	0.045	0.0210	−0.000	0.2878
BMI	0.019	0.0833	−0.027	0.6129	0.078	0.0237	0.001	0.4780
HRATE	0.014	0.0013	0.051	0.0128	0.023	0.1165	0.001	0.0012
HYPERTEN	0.068	0.5033	0.107	0.8281	−0.505	0.1849	0.025	0.0011
HYPERCHO	−0.486	<0.0001	−0.377	0.4319	−0.758	0.0330	0.021	0.0035
Scale	3.383	—	2.756	—	3.614	—	0.268	—

Note: Boldface indicates significant covariates, where $\alpha = 0.05$.

Table 12.15 Comparison of Predictors (*p*-Values) for MMSE versus CDR-SUM

Parameter	AD		DLB		FTD		Normal	
	MMSE	CDR-SUM	MMSE	CDR-SUM	MMSE	CDR-SUM	MMSE	CDR-SUM
Intercept	**<0.0001**	0.2855	**<0.0001**	0.1601	**<0.0001**	0.6169	**<0.0001**	0.9011
SEX = 2 (Female)	**<0.0001**	**<0.0001**	**0.0002**	**0.0333**	0.3474	**0.0057**	**<0.0001**	**<0.0001**
AGE	0.2619	**<0.0001**	**0.0379**	**0.0028**	**0.0074**	**0.0210**	**<0.0001**	0.2878
BMI	0.9672	0.0833	0.4298	0.6129	0.5483	**0.0237**	**<0.0001**	0.4780
HRATE	**0.0308**	**0.0013**	0.6153	**0.0128**	0.8493	0.1165	0.6581	**0.0012**
HYPERTEN	0.7069	0.5033	0.2676	0.8281	0.0896	0.1849	**<0.0001**	**0.0011**
HYPERCHO	**<0.0001**	**<0.0001**	0.4863	0.4319	0.4710	**0.0330**	0.1651	**0.0035**

Note: Boldface indicates significant covariates, where $\alpha = 0.05$.

significant predictors. In the FTD subgroup, gender, age, BMI and hypercholesterolemia are found to significantly drive the baseline CDR-SUM score. For normal subjects, gender, heart rate, hypertension, and hypercholesterolemia are significant covariates.

A comparison of the significant predictors for MMSE and CDR-SUM at baseline is summarized in table 12.15. The *p*-values from tables 12.12 and 12.14 are summarized below.

Some predictors are significant for both MMSE and CDR-SUM within diagnosis groups. For AD patients in our cohort, gender, heart rate, and hypercholesterolemia were significant predictors for both models. For DLB patients, gender and age were significant predictors for both models. For FTD patients, age was found to be significant for both MMSE and CDR-SUM scores at baseline. For normal subjects, gender and hypertension were statistically significant for both outcomes.

12.5.2 MMSE and CDR-SUM over Time

We have repeated observations of MMSE and CDR-SUM scores for patients. Two-dimensional plots for all patients over time based on their MMSE and CDR-SUM scores are given in figures 12.3 and 12.4, respectively. The upward and downward trends (not linear) on the graphs show the differences in patients over time. In other words, pa-

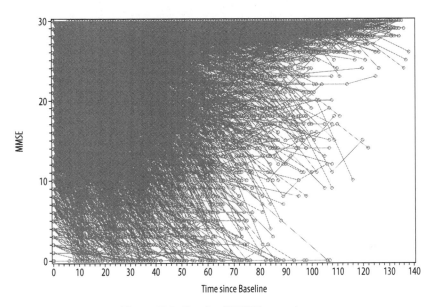

Figure 12.3 Graph of MMSE over time.

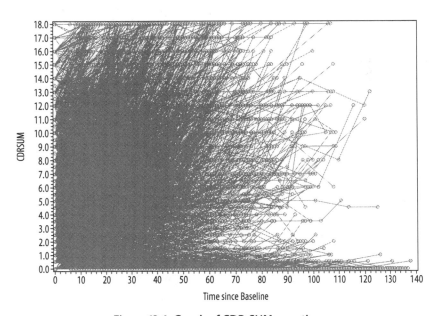

Figure 12.4 Graph of CDR-SUM over time.

tients are random effects. The SAS syntax that provides these graphs
follows:

```
PROC GPLOT DATA=CHAP12;
  PLOT MMSE*MOFROMINDEX = ID / NOLEGEND;
RUN;


PROC GPLOT DATA=CHAP12;
  PLOT CDRSUM*MOFROMINDEX = ID / NOLEGEND;
RUN;
```

While these GLMs help us to understand the relationship between
various factors and cognition at baseline, we cannot necessarily rely
on these model results to address questions beyond the baseline data,
as the observations are correlated (not independent). They are correlated because patients are repeatedly measured and also because they
belong to the same center. Thus we use tools from chapter 4 to address
random effects models for intraclass correlation (ICC). The GLM allows one to examine results at baseline or at any cross-sectional period
in the data, but it cannot assess the longitudinal nature of the data.
However, we are interested in factors and covariates affecting MMSE
and CDR-SUM over time. The fact that these patients are repeatedly
measured negates the assumption of independence. Moreover, the fact
that these patients are evaluated in a center with certain common policies negates any chances of independent observations. To account for
these aspects, we fit generalized linear mixed models.

We evaluate the effect of the covariates investigated previously (sex,
age, BMI, heart rate, hypertension, and hypercholesterolemia) on
MMSE and CDR-SUM by diagnosis using generalized linear mixed
models. On the basis of information provided in chapter 4, we use
three-level hierarchical models to account for the correlation from the
repeated measures on the patients (patient effect) and on the center
(center effect). We also include the number of months from the baseline

visit (MOFROMINDEX) and interactions between time and select variables (BMI, heart rate, hypertension, and hypercholesterolemia) to understand how these factors affect changes in MMSE or CDR-SUM over time. We fit models separately for each diagnosis. Nonsignificant interactions are eventually removed. Before one engages in the fit of generalized linear mixed models, however, it is helpful to explore the intraclass correlation present in the data due to the random effects.

We first estimate the intraclass correlation due to patients and due to center for each group (AD, DLB, FTD, and normal) based on the responses MMSE and CDR-SUM. We do this by fitting a mixed model with only random effects and no covariates.

INTRACLASS CORRELATION: MMSE

We examine the ICC to evaluate the strength of the clustering. The ICC is obtained for within patients and for within centers with the help of the following SAS syntax:

```
PROC GLIMMIX DATA=CHAP12 NOCLPRINT;
        CLASS ADC ID;
        MODEL MMSE = /DIST=NORMAL DDFM=RESIDUAL S;
        RANDOM INTERCEPT /SUBJECT=ID(ADC);
        RANDOM INTERCEPT/SUBJECT=ADC;
        BY DX;
RUN;
```

The SAS outputs led us to the following results for MMSE (table 12.16). We compute the intraclass correlation for patients and centers on MMSE scores.

The first three rows give the variance estimate for time within the patient (variance among the patient as random effects), patients within the ADC (variance among the center random effects), and the residual (the variance among the observations). The variance estimates for the subject level (ID) are larger than the variance estimates for ADC.

Table 12.16 Intraclass Correlation for MMSE

	AD	DLB	FTD	Normal
Variance Parameter Estimates				
ID (ADC) (SAS output)	26.2628	19.6257	35.8416	0.7948
ADC (SAS output)	3.9419	0.4107	4.6442	0.1486
Residual	16.3221	24.2294	29.9151	0.8936
Intraclass Correlation				
Patients	0.5645	0.4434	0.5091	0.4327
Center	0.0847	0.0093	0.0660	0.0809
Total explained	0.6492	0.4527	0.5751	0.5136

This is expected, as the subject level is the lower level of clustering and is expected to have a stronger effect. To quantify the percentage of variation explained by each level of clustering, we calculate the ICC. For example, for patients with an AD diagnosis, $(26.2628)/(26.2628 + 3.9419 + 16.3221) = 0.5645$; thus 56.45% of the variation in MMSE is accounted for by patient-level clustering. In addition, the center level accounts for 8.47% of the variation in the data. The random effects for ID and ADC are found to be significant, and so we fit a three-level hierarchical model with interactions.

HIERARCHICAL MODELS: MMSE

Initially, we present a three-level hierarchical model with interactions for MMSE on AD, DLB, FTD, and normal groups, while accounting for clustering at the patient and center levels (random statements). The necessary SAS syntax follows:

```
PROC GLIMMIX DATA=CHAP12 NOCLPRINT;
        CLASS ADC ID SEX(REF="1");
        MODEL MMSE = MOFROMINDEX SEX AGE BMI HRATE HYPERTEN
HYPERCHO
MOFROMINDEX*BMI MOFROMINDEX*HRATE
MOFROMINDEX*HYPERTEN MOFROMINDEX*HYPERCHO/DIST=NORMAL
DDFM=RESIDUAL S;
```

```
      RANDOM INTERCEPT /SUBJECT=ID(ADC);
      RANDOM INTERCEPT/SUBJECT=ADC;
      BY DX;
RUN;
```

We obtain the following results from the SAS outputs (table 12.17). The initial part of those outputs (not shown) tells us that the random component is Gaussian with an identity link, and the estimates were obtained through a process referred to as restricted maximum likelihood.

From the model output, we find that the covariates time since baseline (MOFROMINDEX), gender, age, heart rate, and the interaction between time and BMI are statistically significant predictors of MMSE for the AD subtype. In the DLB diagnosis group, we similarly found that time since baseline, gender, and age were statistically significant. We also found that the interaction between time and hypertension drives the MMSE score for this group. Time since baseline, hypertension, and two interaction terms (interaction between time and BMI and interaction between time and hypertension) are identified as significant predictors of MMSE in the FTD subgroup. For normal individuals, the MMSE score was found to be associated with gender, age, BMI, and the interaction term between time and hypertension.

We explore other models by refitting the models for each diagnosis using the significant covariates. We include time since baseline in all models as a measurement between visits. In the case of significant interaction terms, we include the corresponding covariate in the model (e.g., if MOFROMINDEX*BMI is significant, BMI must also be included in the model). We obtain parsimonious models with fewer parameters for interpretation purposes (table 12.18).

The significance of the random effects for each of the reduced models is reported (table 12.19).

The random intercepts at the subject level and at the patient level were statistically significant in four models (AD, DLB, FTD, and the normal diagnosis). This indicates significant correlation between the

Table 12.17 Generalized Linear Mixed Models for MMSE by Diagnosis

Parameter	AD		DLB		FTD		Normal	
	Estimate	p-Value	Estimate	p-Value	Estimate	p-Value	Estimate	p-Value
Intercept	20.413	<0.0001	29.740	<0.0001	28.425	<0.0001	31.540	<0.0001
MOFROMINDEX	-0.181	<0.0001	-0.257	0.008	-0.381	<0.0001	0.003	0.1375
Female	-0.627	0.0002	-3.456	0.001	-0.832	0.236	0.208	<0.0001
AGE	0.043	<0.0001	-0.112	0.037	-0.054	0.170	-0.031	<0.0001
BMI	-0.009	0.5789	0.092	0.361	-0.082	0.206	-0.018	<0.0001
HRATE	-0.013	0.0027	-0.014	0.663	-0.012	0.582	0.000	0.8862
HYPERTEN	-0.224	0.0897	1.618	0.062	1.586	0.017	0.011	0.6792
HYPERCHO	0.149	0.2261	0.079	0.921	-0.009	0.987	0.036	0.1479
MOFROMINDEX*BMI	0.002	<0.0001	0.004	0.148	0.008	<0.001	0.000	0.3993
MOFROMINDEX*HRATE	0.000	0.8559	0.000	0.970	-0.000	0.980	0.000	0.2183
MOFROMINDEX*HYPERTEN	0.006	0.0573	-0.058	0.027	-0.049	0.019	-0.001	0.0030
MOFROMINDEX*HYPERCHO	0.001	0.8119	0.038	0.100	0.009	0.604	0.000	0.5808

Note: Boldface indicates significant covariates, where $\alpha = 0.05$.

Table 12.18 Reduced Generalized Linear Mixed Models for MMSE by Diagnosis

AD		
Parameter	Estimate	p-Value
Intercept	20.586	<0.0001
MOFROMINDEX	−0.183	<0.0001
SEX = 2 (Female)	−0.636	0.0002
AGE	0.042	<0.0001
BMI	−0.012	0.4377
HRATE	−0.014	<0.0001
MOFROMINDEX*BMI	0.002	<0.0001

DLB		
Parameter	Estimate	p-Value
Intercept	32.416	<0.0001
MOFROMINDEX	−0.130	<0.0001
SEX = 2 (Female)	−4.028	<0.0001
AGE	−0.126	0.0163
HYPERTEN	1.672	0.0369
MOFROMINDEX*HYPERTEN	−0.036	0.1289

FTD		
Parameter	Estimate	p-Value
Intercept	23.584	<0.0001
MOFROMINDEX	−0.385	<0.0001
BMI	−0.073	0.2476
HYPERTEN	1.400	0.0258
MOFROMINDEX*BMI	0.008	<0.0001
MOFROMINDEX*HYPERTEN	−0.044	0.0266

Normal		
Parameter	Estimate	p-Value
Intercept	31.527	<0.0001
MOFROMINDEX	0.002	<0.0001
SEX = 2 (Female)	0.204	<0.0001
AGE	−0.031	<0.0001
BMI	−0.016	<0.0001
HYPERTEN	0.015	0.5491
MOFROMINDEX*HYPERTEN	−0.001	0.0069

measurements collected from the same patient. The random effect for ADC, accounting for similarities between MMSE measurements collected at the same clinic, was statistically significant in the models for patients with a diagnosis of AD and the normal group. We note that the

Table 12.19 Random Intercepts for MMSE by Diagnosis

	AD		DLB		FTD		Normal	
	ID (ADC)	ADC	ID (ADC)	ADC	ID (ADC)	ADC	ID (ADC)	ADC
Estimate	31.5015	2.9329	21.8917	0	45.6548	4.2151	0.7032	0.1221
Standard error	0.7036	0.8162	3.0387	—	3.5754	2.7646	0.0175	0.0321
Test statistic	44.7718	3.5934	7.2043	—	12.7691	1.5247	40.1829	3.8037

random effect for the center effect for the DLB subgroup could not be estimated.

HIERARCHICAL MODELS: CDR-SUM

Similar to the modeling of MMSE, we model the CDR-SUM score. The SAS syntax follows:

```
PROC GLIMMIX DATA=CHAP12 NOCLPRINT;
        CLASS ADC ID;
        MODEL CDRSUM = /DIST=NORMAL DDFM=RESIDUAL S;
        RANDOM INTERCEPT /SUBJECT=ID(ADC);
        RANDOM INTERCEPT/SUBJECT=ADC;
        BY DX;
RUN;
```

We obtain the intraclass correlation (table 12.20). We found that 60.35% of the variation in the CDR-SUM score was explained by patients (52.49%) and center (7.86%) within the AD group. The totals for the other subgroups were 43.20% for DLB, 55.69% for FTD, and 57.47% for normal. The center ICC for CDR-SUM is much higher than the ICC for MMSE for the DLB group (0.0766 vs. 0.0093). This indicates that the center tends to have a stronger impact on the CDR-SUM scores as compared to the MMSE scores for this diagnosis group.

We fit three-level hierarchical models to the CDR-SUM response data, as we did with the MMSE responses. The following SAS syntax gave our results:

Table 12.20 Intraclass Correlation for CDR-SUM

	AD	DLB	FTD	Normal
Variance parameter estimates				
ID (ADC)	9.8620	5.8753	10.6147	0.0312
ADC	1.4774	1.2666	1.6241	0.0065
Residual	7.4507	9.3886	9.7361	0.0279
Intraclass correlation				
Patients	0.5249	0.3554	0.4830	0.4756
Center	0.0786	0.0766	0.0739	0.0991
Total explained	0.6035	0.4320	0.5569	0.5747

```
PROC GLIMMIX DATA=CHAP12 NOCLPRINT;

        CLASS ADC ID SEX(REF="1");

        MODEL CDRSUM = MOFROMINDEX SEX AGE BMI HRATE HYPERTEN
HYPERCHO
MOFROMINDEX*BMI MOFROMINDEX*HRATE
                        MOFROMINDEX*HYPERTEN
MOFROMINDEX*HYPERCHO/DIST=NORMAL
DDFM=RESIDUAL S;

        RANDOM INTERCEPT /SUBJECT=ID(ADC);

        RANDOM INTERCEPT/SUBJECT=ADC;

        BY DX;

RUN;
```

The model results (parameter estimates and p-values) are reported in table 12.21.

From the model results, we find that the covariates associated with CDR-SUM vary by dementia subtype. We use these initial findings to obtain a more parsimonious model for each diagnosis. The model estimates from models fit with the significant parameters for each diagnosis are reported in table 12.22.

The variance estimates and standard errors of the random intercepts are reported in table 12.23. We calculate the test statistic to determine the significance of each random intercept. The test statistics for the subject level indicate that the clustering due to patient is

Table 12.21 Generalized Linear Mixed Models for CDR-SUM by Diagnosis

Parameter	AD		DLB		FTD		Normal	
	Estimate	p-Value	Estimate	p-Value	Estimate	p-Value	Estimate	p-Value
Intercept	1.383	0.0179	-2.657	0.4174	1.329	0.4854	0.003	0.9292
MOFROMINDEX	0.103	<0.0001	0.192	0.0007	0.162	<0.0001	0.000	0.9438
SEX=2	0.461	<0.0001	1.444	0.0223	-1.100	0.0034	-0.028	<0.0001
AGE	0.027	<0.0001	0.097	0.0030	0.026	0.2267	0.000	0.2502
BMI	0.024	0.0138	-0.003	0.9639	0.066	0.0640	0.001	0.0284
HRATE	0.009	0.0018	0.022	0.2673	0.021	0.0790	0.000	0.0170
HYPERTEN	0.048	0.5657	-0.711	0.1700	-0.891	0.0164	0.003	0.5789
HYPERCHO	-0.166	0.0342	-0.890	0.0619	-0.170	0.6024	0.009	0.0537
MOFROMINDEX*BMI	-0.001	<0.0001	-0.004	0.0378	-0.003	0.0024	0.000	0.0720
MOFROMINDEX*HRATE	0.000	0.0092	0.000	0.8062	0.000	0.4131	0.000	0.0797
MOFROMINDEX*HYPERTEN	-0.002	0.4521	0.033	0.0346	0.012	0.3053	0.000	0.0854
MOFROMINDEX*HYPERCHO	-0.001	0.6393	-0.008	0.5823	-0.003	0.7715	-0.000	0.0156

Note: Boldface indicates significant covariates, where $\alpha = 0.05$.

Table 12.22 Reduced Generalized Linear Mixed Models for CDR-SUM by Diagnosis

	AD	
Parameter	Estimate	p-Value
Intercept	1.364	0.019
MOFROMINDEX	0.102	<0.0001
SEX = 2 (female)	0.462	<0.0001
AGE	0.027	<0.0001
BMI	0.026	0.0088
HRATE	0.009	0.0017
HYPERCHO	−0.186	0.0033
MOFROMINDEX*BMI	−0.001	<0.0001
MOFROMINDEX*HRATE	0.000	0.0091

	DLB	
Parameter	Estimate	p-Value
Intercept	−1.137	0.7040
MOFROMINDEX	0.176	0.0001
SEX = 2 (female)	1.640	0.0096
AGE	0.090	0.0059
BMI	0.000	1.0000
HYPERTEN	−1.083	0.0273
MOFROMINDEX*BMI	−0.004	0.0451
MOFROMINDEX*HYPERTEN	0.032	0.0319

	FTD	
Parameter	Estimate	p-Value
Intercept	4.187	<0.0001
MOFROMINDEX	0.182	<0.0001
SEX = 2 (female)	−0.988	0.0085
BMI	0.070	0.0434
HYPERTEN	−0.711	0.0187
MOFROMINDEX*BMI	−0.003	0.0030

	Normal	
Parameter	Estimate	p-Value
Intercept	0.031	0.1358
MOFROMINDEX	0.000	0.8087
SEX = 2 (female)	−0.029	<0.0001
BMI	0.002	0.0004
HRATE	0.000	0.1135
HYPERCHO	0.008	0.0611
MOFROMINDEX*HYPERCHO	−0.000	0.1544

Table 12.23 Random Intercepts for CDR-SUM by Diagnosis

	AD		DLB		FTD		Normal	
	ID (ADC)	ADC	ID (ADC)	ADC	ID (ADC)	ADC	ID (ADC)	ADC
Estimate	12.1013	1.0934	7.9568	1.2703	12.7853	1.2917	0.0309	0.0063
Std err	0.2719	0.3036	1.1563	0.7582	1.0228	0.6652	0.0007	0.0018
Test statistic	44.5064	3.6014	6.8813	1.6754	12.5003	1.9418	44.1729	3.5000

statistically significant for all four models split by diagnosis (as the test statistic is greater than 1.96). The random effects at the center level are significant in the AD group and the normal group.

12.6 Discussion and Conclusions

Our study of cognitive scores by diagnosis required the use of generalized mixed models to account for the repeated measurements on the patients. For the AD diagnosis, we identified time since baseline, gender, age, heart rate, and the interaction term between time since baseline and BMI as significant predictors of MMSE. For the analysis of CDR-SUM scores for AD patients, we identified the same covariates as statistically significant, as well as BMI, hypercholesterolemia, and the interaction term between time since baseline and heart rate. In the evaluation of DLB patients, we find that the covariates time since baseline, gender, age, and hypertension are statistically significant predictors of MMSE. We found that time since baseline, gender, age, hypertension, the interaction between time since baseline and BMI, and the interaction time since baseline and hypertension are statistically significant predictors of the CDR-SUM scores. For FTD patients, we found that time since baseline, hypertension, the interaction term between time since baseline and BMI, and the interaction term between time since baseline and hypertension were significant covariates affecting MMSE. For the analysis of CDR-SUM scores in the FTD subgroup, time since baseline, gender, BMI, hypertension, and the interaction between time since baseline and BMI were significant predictors. For normal subjects, time since baseline, gender, age, BMI, and the interaction between time since baseline and hypertension were statistically significantly associated with MMSE. Alternatively, in the analysis of CDR-SUM, we found that only gender and BMI significantly affected the outcome. Through a comparison of both outcomes, we see that the covariates show varying impacts on MMSE and CDR-SUM scores.

While the study reveals differential associations across diagnosis groups and identifies covariates with a significant impact on cognition, we found the change in cognition over time to be important. The significant interaction terms between time since baseline and certain covariates indicate that the cardiovascular risk factor affects the rate of change on the cognitive score over time.

The case study in this chapter walked the reader through various considerations in the data analysis process. We began with an examination of the single variable, then two-at-a-time, then GLMs with several predictors assuming independent observation. We addressed the failure of the independence of observations assumptions and modeled the correlation through the fit of a generalized linear mixed model. We examined covariate relationships and differences that exist across dementia subtypes. While we selected a subset of covariates to focus on in this analysis, one may find that they have many more covariates to examine before determining a final model. We did not focus on covariate selection, other than the data processing and fitting of a parsimonious model.

Acknowledgments

JRW received funding support from the National Institutes of Health (NIH) Alzheimer's Consortium Fellowship Grant NHS0007.

The National Alzheimer's Coordinating Center (NACC) database is funded by National Institute on Aging (NIA) / NIH Grant U01 AG016976. NACC data are contributed by the NIA-funded Alzheimer's Disease Centers: P30 AG019610 (PI Eric Reiman, MD), P30 AG013846 (PI Neil Kowall, MD), P50 AG008702 (PI Scott Small, MD), P50 AG025688 (PI Allan Levey, MD, PhD), P50 AG047266 (PI Todd Golde, MD, PhD), P30 AG010133 (PI Andrew Saykin, PsyD), P50 AG005146 (PI Marilyn Albert, PhD), P50 AG005134 (PI Bradley Hyman, MD, PhD), P50 AG016574 (PI Ronald Petersen, MD, PhD), P50 AG005138 (PI Mary Sano, PhD), P30 AG008051 (PI Thomas Wisniewski, MD), P30 AG013854 (PI M. Marsel Mesulam, MD), P30 AG008017 (PI Jeffrey Kaye, MD), P30 AG010161 (PI David Bennett, MD), P50 AG047366 (PI Victor Henderson, MD, MS), P30 AG010129 (PI Charles DeCarli, MD), P50 AG016573 (PI Frank LaFerla, PhD), P50 AG005131 (PI James Brewer, MD, PhD), P50 AG023501 (PI Bruce Miller, MD), P30 AG035982 (PI Russell Swerdlow, MD), P30 AG028383 (PI Linda Van Eldik, PhD), P30 AG053760 (PI Henry Paulson, MD, PhD), P30 AG010124 (PI John Trojanowski, MD, PhD), P50 AG005133 (PI Oscar Lopez, MD), P50 AG005142 (PI Helena Chui, MD), P30 AG012300 (PI Roger Rosenberg, MD), P30 AG049638 (PI Suzanne Craft, PhD), P50 AG005136 (PI Thomas Grabowski, MD), P50 AG033514 (PI Sanjay Asthana, MD, FRCP), P50 AG005681 (PI John Morris, MD), and P50 AG047270 (PI Stephen Strittmatter, MD, PhD).

References

Chapter 1. Introduction to Statistical Software and Alzheimer's Data

Beekly, D. L., E. M. Ramos, W. W. Lee, W. D. Deitrich, M. E. Jacka, J. Wu, J. L. Hubbard, T. D. Koepsell, J. C. Morris and W. A. Kukull (2007). "The National Alzheimer's Coordinating Center (NACC) database: The Uniform Data Set." *Alzheimer Disease and Associated Disorders* 21(3): 249–258.

Bell, J. F., A. L. Fitzpatrick, C. Copeland, G. Chi, L. Steinman, R. L. Whitney, D. C. Atkins, L. L. Bryant, F. Grodstein, E. Larson et al. (2015). "Existing data sets to support studies of dementia or significant cognitive impairment and comorbid chronic conditions." *Alzheimer's and Dementia* 11(6): 622–638.

Braak, H., and E. Braak (1991). "Neuropathological stageing of Alzheimer-related changes." *Acta Neuropathologica* 82(4): 239–259.

Chadwick, C. (1992). "The MRC Multicentre Study of Cognitive Function and Ageing: A EURODEM incidence study in progress." *Neuroepidemiology* 11: 37–43.

Collett, D. (2003). *Modelling binary data*. Boca Raton, FL: Chapman & Hall / CRC.

Daniel, W. W., and C. L. Cross (2013). *Biostatistics: A foundation for analysis in the health sciences*. Hoboken, NJ: Wiley.

Dawber, T. R., W. B. Kannel and L. P. Lyell (1963). "An approach to longitudinal studies in a community: The Framingham Study." *Annals of the New York Academy of Sciences* 107: 539–556.

Hauser, R. M., and R. J. Willis (2004). "Survey design and methodology in the health and retirement study and the Wisconsin longitudinal study." *Population and Development Review* 30: 209–235.

Hofman, A., D. E. Grobbee, P. T. de Jong and F. A. van den Ouweland (1991a). "Determinants of disease and disability in the elderly: The Rotterdam Elderly Study." *European Journal of Epidemiology* 7(4): 403–422.

Hofman, A., W. A. Rocca, C. Brayne, M. M. Breteler, M. Clarke, B. Cooper, J. R. Copeland, J. F. Dartigues, A. da Silva Droux, O. Hagnell et al. (1991b). "The prevalence of dementia in Europe: A collaborative study of 1980–1990 findings. Eurodem Prevalence Research Group." *International Journal of Epidemiology* 20(3): 736–748.

Ikram, M. A., A. van der Lugt, W. J. Niessen, G. P. Krestin, P. J. Koudstaal, A. Hofman, M. M. Breteler and M. W. Vernooij (2011). "The Rotterdam Scan Study: Design and update up to 2012." *European Journal of Epidemiology* 26(10): 811–824.

Marek, K., D. Jennings, S. Lasch, A. Siderowf, C. Tanner, T. Simuni, C. Coffey, K. Kieburtz, E. Flagg, S. Chowdhury et al. (2011). "The Parkinson Progression Marker Initiative (PPMI)." *Progress in Neurobiology* **95**(4): 629–635.

Mirra, S., A. Heyman, D. McKeel, S. Sumi, B. Crain, L. Brownlee, F. Vogel, J. Hughes, G. van Belle and L. Berg (1991). "The Consortium to Establish a Registry for Alzheimer's Disease (CERAD). Part II. Standardization of the neuropathologic assessment of Alzheimer's disease." *Neurology* **41**(4): 479–486.

Montine, T. J., C. H. Phelps, T. G. Beach, E. H. Bigio, N. J. Cairns, D. W. Dickson, C. Duyckaerts, M. P. Frosch, E. Masliah, S. S. Mirra et al. (2012). "National Institute on Aging-Alzheimer's Association guidelines for the neuropathologic assessment of Alzheimer's disease: A practical approach." *Acta Neuropathologica* **123**(1): 1–11.

Morris, J. C., S. Weintraub, H. C. Chui, J. Cummings, C. Decarli, S. Ferris, N. L. Foster, D. Galasko, N. Graff-Radford, E. R. Peskind et al. (2006). "The Uniform Data Set (UDS): Clinical and cognitive variables and descriptive data from Alzheimer Disease Centers." *Alzheimer Disease and Associated Disorders* **20**: 210–216.

Splansky, G. L., D. Corey, Q. Yang, L. D. Atwood, L. A. Cupples, E. J. Benjamin, R. B. D'Agostino Sr., C. S. Fox, M. G. Larson, J. M. Murabito et al. (2007). "The Third Generation Cohort of the National Heart, Lung, and Blood Institute's Framingham Heart Study: Design, recruitment, and initial examination." *American Journal of Epidemiology* **165**(11): 1328–1335.

Thal, D. R., U. Rub, M. Orantes, and H. Braak (2002). "Phases of a beta-deposition in the human brain and its relevance for the development of AD." *Neurology* **58**(12): 1791–1800.

Weintraub, S., D. Salmon, N. Mercaldo, S. Ferris, N. Graff-Radford, H. Chui, J. Cummings, C. DeCarli, N. Foster, D. Galasko et al. (2009). "The Alzheimer's Disease Centers' Uniform Data Set (UDS): The neuropsychologic test battery." *Alzheimer Disease and Associated Disorders* **23**: 91–101.

Chapter 2. Review of Introductory Statistical Methods

Beekly, D. L., E. M. Ramos, W. W. Lee, W. D. Deitrich, M. E. Jacka, J. Wu, J. L. Hubbard, T. D. Koepsell, J. C. Morris and W. A. Kukull (2007). "The National Alzheimer's Coordinating Center (NACC) database: The Uniform Data Set." *Alzheimer Disease and Associated Disorders* **21**(3): 249–258.

Morris, J. C., S. Weintraub, H. C. Chui, J. Cummings, C. Decarli, S. Ferris, N. L. Foster, D. Galasko, N. Graff-Radford, E. R. Peskind et al. (2006). "The Uniform Data Set (UDS): Clinical and cognitive variables and descriptive data from Alzheimer Disease Centers." *Alzheimer Disease and Associated Disorders* **20**: 210–216.

Wasserstein, R. L., and N. A. Lazar (2016). "The ASA's statement on *p*-values: Context, process, and purpose." *American Statistician* **70**(2): 129–133.

Weintraub, S., D. Salmon, N. Mercaldo, S. Ferris, N. Graff-Radford, H. Chui, J. Cummings, C. DeCarli, N. Foster, D. Galasko et al. (2009). "The Alzheimer's Disease

Centers' Uniform Data Set (UDS): The neuropsychologic test battery." *Alzheimer Disease and Associated Disorders* **23**: 91–101.

Chapter 3. Generalized Linear Models

Agresti, A. (1990). *Categorical data analysis*. 3rd ed. New York: John Wiley & Sons.

Box, G. E. P., and D. R. Cox (1964). "An analysis of transformations." *Journal of the Royal Statistical Society Series B* **26**(2): 211–252.

Dobson, A. J., and A. G. Barnett (2008). *An introduction to generalized linear models*. 3rd ed. New York: CRC Press.

Hughes, C., L. Berg, W. Danziger, L. Coben and R. Martin (1982). "A new clinical scale for the staging of dementia." *British Journal of Psychiatry* **140**: 566–572.

Irimata, K. E., B. D. Dugger and J. R. Wilson (2018). "Impact of the presence of select cardiovascular risk factors on cognitive changes among dementia subtypes." *Current Alzheimer Research* **15**(11): 1032–1044.

McCullagh, P., and J. A. Nelder (1989). *Generalized linear models*. 2nd ed. London: Chapman and Hall.

O'Bryant, S., S. Waring, C. Cullum, J. Hall, L. Lacritz, P. Massman, P. Lupo, J. Reisch and R. Doody (2008). "Staging dementia using Clinical Dementia Rating Scale Sum of Boxes scores." *Archives of Neurology* **65**: 1091–1095.

Chapter 4. Hierarchical Regression Models for Continuous Responses

Bergland, A., I. Dalen, A. Larsen, D. Aarsland and H. Soennesyn (2017). "Effect of vascular risk factors on the progression of mild Alzheimer's disease and Lewy body dementia." *Journal of Alzheimer's Disease* **56**: 575–584.

Breslow, N. E., and D. G. Clayton (1993). "Approximate inference in generalized linear mixed models." *Journal of the American Statistical Association* **88**(421): 9–25.

Hu, F. B., J. Goldberg, D. Hedeker, B. R. Flay and M. A. Pentz (1998). "Comparison of population-averaged and subject-specific approaches for analyzing repeated binary outcomes." *American Journal of Epidemiology* **147**(7): 694–703.

Hughes, C., L. Berg, W. Danziger, L. Coben and R. Martin (1982). "A new clinical scale for the staging of dementia." *British Journal of Psychiatry* **140**: 566–572.

Irimata, K. M., and J. R. Wilson (2017). "Identifying intraclass correlation necessitating hierarchical modeling." *Journal of Applied Statistics* **45**(4): 626–641.

Liang, K.-Y., and S. L. Zeger (1986). "Longitudinal data analysis using generalized linear models." *Biometrika* **73**(1): 13–22.

McCulloch, C. E., and S. R. Searle (2000). *Generalized, linear, and mixed models*. New York: Wiley and Sons.

O'Bryant, S., S. Waring, C. Cullum, J. Hall, L. Lacritz, P. Massman, P. Lupo, J. Reisch and R. Doody (2008). "Staging dementia using Clinical Dementia Rating Scale Sum of Boxes scores." *Archives of Neurology* **65**: 1091–1095.

Pan, W. (2001). "Akaike's Information Criterion in generalized estimating equations." *Biometrics* **57**: 120–125.

Pepe, M. S., and G. L. Anderson (1994). "A cautionary note on inference for marginal regression models with longitudinal data and general correlated response data." *Communications in Statistics—Simulation and Computation* 23(4): 939–951.

Stroup, W. (2012). *Generalized linear mixed models: Modern concepts, methods and applications.* Boca Raton, FL: CRC Press.

Verbeke, G., and G. Molenberghs (2000). *Linear mixed models for longitudinal data.* New York: Springer.

Zeger, S. L., and K.-Y. Liang (1986). "Longitudinal data analysis for discrete and continuous outcomes." *Biometrics* 42(1): 121–130.

Chapter 5. Hierarchical Logistic Regression Models

Hardin, J. W., and J. M. Hilbe (2003). *Generalized estimating equations.* Boca Raton, FL: Chapman and Hall / CRC Press.

Hox, J., and I. Kreft (1994). "Multilevel analysis methods." *Sociological Methods and Research* 22(3): 283–299.

Irimata, K. M., and J. R. Wilson (2017). "Identifying intraclass correlations necessitating hierarchical modeling." *Journal of Applied Statistics* 45(4): 626–641.

Liang, K.-Y., and S. L. Zeger (1986). "Longitudinal data analysis using generalized linear models." *Biometrika* 73(1): 13–22.

Zeger, S. L., and K.-Y. Liang (1986). "Longitudinal data analysis for discrete and continuous outcomes." *Biometrics* 42(1): 121–130.

Chapter 6. Bayesian Regression Models

Berger, J. O. (1985). *Statistical decision theory and Bayesian analysis.* New York: Springer-Verlag.

Lunn, D., A. Thomas, N. Best and D. Spiegelhalter (2000). "WinBUGS—A Bayesian modelling framework: Concepts, structure, and extensibility." *Statistics and Computing* 10: 325–337.

Martin, A. D., K. M. Quinn and J. H. Park (2011). "MCMCpack: Markov Chain Monte Carlo in R." *Journal of Statistical Software* 42(9): 1–21.

Chapter 7. Multiple-Membership Models

Armstrong, R. A., P. L. Lantos and N. J. Cairns (2005). "Overlap between neurodegenerative disorders." *Neuropathology* 25(2): 111–124.

Chung, H., and S. Beretvas (2012). "The impact of ignoring multiple membership data structures in multilevel models." *British Journal of Mathematical and Statistical Psychology* 65(2): 185–200.

Dugger, B. N., C. H. Adler, H. A. Shill, J. Caviness, S. Jacobson, E. Driver-Dunckley and T. G. Beach (2014). "Concomitant pathologies among a spectrum of parkinsonian disorders." *Parkinsonism and Related Disorders* 20(5): 525–529.

Hedeker, D. (2014). "Cross-classified and multi-membership multilevel models." MRC Chalk Talk, presented at the Institute for Health Research and Policy, University of Illinois at Chicago, April 15, 2014. https://www.ihrp.uic.edu/content/cross -classified-and-multi-membership-multilevel-models.

Irimata, K. M., and J. R. Wilson (2017). "Identifying intraclass correlations necessitating hierarchical modeling." *Journal of Applied Statistics* 45(4): 626–641.

Kawas, C. H., R. C. Kim, J. A. Sonnen, S. S. Bullain, T. Trieu and M. M. Corrada (2015). "Multiple pathologies are common and related to dementia in the oldest-old: The 90+ Study." *Neurology* 85(6): 535–542.

Rasbash, J., C. M. J. Charlton, W. J. Browne, M. Healy and B. Cameron (2009). *MLwiN*. Bristol: University of Bristol.

Schneider, J. A., Z. Arvanitakis, W. Bang and D. A. Bennett (2007). "Mixed brain pathologies account for most dementia cases in community-dwelling older persons." *Neurology* 69(24): 2197–2204.

Stroup, W. (2012). *Generalized linear mixed models: Modern concepts, methods and applications.* Boca Raton, FL: CRC Press.

Vazquez, E. V., and J. R. Wilson (2019). "Bayesian multiple membership multiple classification logistic regression model of university instructors and majors on student performance." *Unpublished manuscript.*

Zhang, Z., R. M. A. Parker, C. M. J. Charlton, G. Leckie and W. J. Browne (2016). "R2MLwiN: A package to run MLwiN from within R." *Journal of Statistical Software* 72(10): 1–43.

Zhu, M. (2014). *Analyzing multilevel models with the GLIMMIX procedure.* Washington, DC: SAS Global Forum.

Chapter 8. Survival Data Analysis

Breslow, N. (1970). "A generalized Kruskal-Wallis test for comparing K samples subject to unequal patterns of censorship." *Biometrika* 57(3): 579–594.

Cox, D. R. (1972). "Regression models and life-tables." *Journal of the Royal Statistical Society Series B* 34(2): 187–220.

Cox, D. R., and D. Oakes (1984). *Analysis of survival data.* New York: Chapman & Hall.

Gehan, E. A. (1965). "A generalized Wilcoxon test for comparing arbitrarily single-censored samples." *Biometrika* 52: 203–223.

Kaplan, E., and P. Meier (1958). "Nonparametric estimation from incomplete observations." *Journal of the American Statistical Association* 53(282): 457–481.

Lee, E. (1992). *Statistical methods for survival data analysis.* New York: Wiley Interscience.

Mantel, N. (1966). "Evaluation of survival data and two new rank order statistics arising in its consideration." *Cancer Chemotherapy Reports* 50(3): 163–170.

McCullagh, P., and J. A. Nelder (1989). *Generalized linear models.* 2nd ed. London: Chapman and Hall.

Tarone, R., and J. Ware (1977). "On distribution-free tests for equality of survival distributions." *Biometrika* 64: 156–160.

Chapter 9. Modeling Responses with Time-Dependent Covariates

Cai, K. E., and J. R. Wilson (2015). "How to use SAS for GMM logistic regression models for longitudinal data with time-dependent covariates." Presented at the SAS Global Forum, Dallas, April 26–29.

Cai, K. E., and J. R. Wilson (2016). "SAS macro for generalized method of moments estimation for longitudinal data with time-dependent covariates." Presented at the SAS Global Forum, Las Vegas, April 18–21.

Carpenter, A. (2016). *Carpenter's complete guide to the SAS® macro language*. Cary, NC: SAS Institute.

Genz, A. (1992). "Numerical computation of multivariate normal probabilities." *Journal of Computational and Graphical Statistics* 1(2): 141–149.

Genz, A. (1993). "Comparison of methods for the computation of multivariate normal probabilities." *Computing Science and Statistics* 25: 400–405.

Irimata, K. M., and J. R. Wilson (2018). "Using SAS to estimate lagged coefficients with the %partitionedGMM macro." Presented at the SAS Global Forum, Denver, April 8–11.

Irimata, K. M., J. Broatch and J. R. Wilson (2019). "Partitioned GMM logistic regression models for longitudinal data." *Statistics in Medicine* 38(12): 2171–2183.

Lai, T. L., and D. Small (2007). "Marginal regression analysis of longitudinal data with time-dependent covariates: A generalized method-of-moments approach." *Journal of the Royal Statistical Society Series B* 69(1): 79–99.

Lalonde, T. L., J. R. Wilson and J. Yin (2014). "GMM logistic regression models for longitudinal data with time-dependent covariates and extended classifications." *Statistics in Medicine* 33(27): 4756–4769.

Pepe, M. S., and G. L. Anderson (1994). "A cautionary note on inference for marginal regression models with longitudinal data and general correlated response data." *Communications in Statistics—Simulation and Computation* 23(4): 939–951.

Chapter 10. Joint Modeling of Mean and Dispersion

Agresti, A. (1990). *Categorical data analysis*. 3rd ed. New York: John Wiley & Sons.

Aitkin, M. (1987). "Modelling variance heterogeneity in normal regression using GLIM." *Journal of the Royal Statistical Society Series C* 36(3): 332–339.

Carroll, R. J., and D. Ruppert (1982). "Robust estimation in heteroskedastic linear models." *Annals of Statistics* 10: 429–441.

Davidian, M., and R. J. Carroll (1987). "Variance function estimation." *Journal of the American Statistical Association* 82(400): 1079–1091.

Efron, B. (1986). "Double exponential families and their use in generalized linear regression." *Journal of the American Statistical Association* 81: 709–721.

Lee, Y., and J. A. Nelder (2000). "Two ways of modelling overdispersion in non-normal data." *Journal of the Royal Statistical Society Series C* 49(4): 591–598.

Lee, Y., and J. A. Nelder (2006). "Double hierarchical generalized linear models." *Journal of the Royal Statistical Society Series C* 55(2): 139–185.

McCullagh, P., and J. A. Nelder (1989). *Generalized linear models*. 2nd ed. London: Chapman and Hall.

Nelder, J. A., Y. Lee, B. Bergman, A. Hynén, A. F. Huele and J. Engel (1998). "Joint modeling of mean and dispersion." *Technometrics* **40**(2): 168–175.

Neykov, N. M., P. Filzmoser and P. N. Neytchev (2012). "Robust joint modeling of mean and dispersion through trimming." *Computational Statistics and Data Analysis* **56**(1): 34–48.

Pregibon, D. (1984). "Review of generalized linear models (by P. McCullagh and J.A. Nelder)." *Annals of Statistics* **12**: 1589–1596.

Smyth, G. K. (1989). "Generalized linear models with varying dispersion." *Journal of the Royal Statistical Society Series B* **51**(1): 47–60.

Smyth, G. K., and A. P. Verbyla (1999). "Adjusted likelihood methods for modelling dispersion in generalized linear models." *Environmetrics* **10**(6): 695–709.

Chapter 11. Neural Networks and Other Machine Learning Techniques for Big Data

Cheng, B., and D. Titterington (1994). "Neural networks: A review from statistical perspective." *Statistical Science* **9**(1): 49–54.

Eftekhar, B., K. Mohammad, H. Ardebili, M. Ghodsi and E. Ketabchi (2005). "Comparison of artificial neural network and logistic regression models for prediction of mortality in head trauma based on initial clinical data." *BMC Medical Informatics and Decision Making* **5**(1): 3.

Friedman, J., and W. Stuetzle (1981). "Projection pursuit regression." *Journal of the American Statistical Association* **76**: 817–823.

Hastie, T., R. Tibshirani and J. Friedman (2009). *The elements of statistical learning data mining, inference, and prediction*. New York: Springer.

Hosmer, D. W., and S. Lemeshow (1989). *Applied logistic regression*. New York: John Wiley & Sons.

Myers, C. M. (1986). "Analytical thought experiments." *Metaphilosophy* **17**(2–3): 109–118.

Neter, J., and W. Wasserman (1974). *Applied linear statistical models*. New York: McGraw-Hill Irwin.

Paswan, R. P., and S. A. Begum (2013). "Regression and neural networks models for prediction of crop production." *International Journal of Scientific and Engineering Research* **4**(9): 98–108.

Ripley, B. (1994). "Neural networks and related methods for classification." *Journal of the Royal Statistical Society Series B* **56**(3): 409–456.

Sarle, W. S. (1994). "Neural networks and statistical models." Presented at the Annual SAS Users Group International Conference, SAS Institute, Cary, NC, April 10–13.

Schumacher, M., R. Rosner and W. Vach (1996). "Neural networks and logistic regression. Part I." *Computational Statistics and Data Analysis* **21**(6): 661–682.

Setyawati, B., S. Sahirman and R. Creese (2002). "Neural networks for cost estimation." *AACE International Transactions EST13*.

Warner, B., and M. Misra (1996). "Understanding neural networks as statistical tools." *American Statistician* 50(4): 284–293.

Weisberg, S. (1985). *Applied linear regression.* New York: Wiley.

White, H. (1992). *Artificial neural networks: Approximation and learning theory.* Oxford: Blackwell.

Zhao, Y. (2012). *R and data mining—Examples and case studies.* New York: Elsevier.

Chapter 12. Case Study

Beekly, D. L., E. M. Ramos, W. W. Lee, W. D. Deitrich, M. E. Jacka, J. Wu, J. L. Hubbard, T. D. Koepsell, J. C. Morris and W. A. Kukull (2007). "The National Alzheimer's Coordinating Center (NACC) database: The Uniform Data Set." *Alzheimer Disease and Associated Disorders* 21(3): 249–258.

Bergland, A., I. Dalen, A. Larsen, D. Aarsland and H. Soennesyn (2017). "Effect of vascular risk factors on the progression of mild Alzheimer's disease and Lewy body dementia." *Journal of Alzheimer's Disease* 56: 575–584.

Chen, D.-G., D. Fang and J. R. Wilson (2017). "Meta-analysis of two studies with random effects?" *Journal of Minimally Invasive Gynecology* 24(5): 689–690.

Folstein, M., S. Folstein and P. McHugh (1975). "'Mini-mental state': A practical method for grading the cognitive state of patients for the clinician." *Journal of Psychiatric Research* 12: 189–198.

Hughes, C. P., L. Berg, W. L. Danziger, L. A. Coben and R. L. Martin (1982). "A new clinical scale for the staging of dementia." *British Journal of Psychiatry* 140: 566–572.

Irimata, K. E., B. D. Dugger and J. R. Wilson (2018). "Impact of the presence of select cardiovascular risk factors on cognitive changes among dementia subtypes." *Current Alzheimer Research* 15(11): 1032–1044.

Morris, J. C., S. Weintraub, H. C. Chui, J. Cummings, C. Decarli, S. Ferris, N. L. Foster, D. Galasko, N. Graff-Radford, E. R. Peskind et al. (2006). "The Uniform Data Set (UDS): Clinical and cognitive variables and descriptive data from Alzheimer Disease Centers." *Alzheimer Disease and Associated Disorders* 20: 210–216.

Weintraub, S., D. Salmon, N. Mercaldo, S. Ferris, N. Graff-Radford, H. Chui, J. Cummings, C. DeCarli, N. Foster, D. Galasko et al. (2009). "The Alzheimer's Disease Centers' Uniform Data Set (UDS): The neuropsychologic test battery." *Alzheimer Disease and Associated Disorders* 23: 91–101.

Index